Cancer Supportive Care

TRANSLATIONAL MEDICINE SERIES

1. Prostate Cancer: Translational and Emerging Therapies, *edited by Nancy A. Dawson and W. Kevin Kelly*
2. Breast Cancer: Translational Therapeutic Strategies, *edited by Gary H. Lyman and Harold Burstein*
3. Lung Cancer: Translational and Emerging Therapies, *edited by Kishan J. Pandya, Julie R. Brahmer, and Manuel Hidalgo*
4. Multiple Myeloma: Translational and Emerging Therapies, *edited by Kenneth C. Anderson and Irene Ghobrial*
5. Cancer Supportive Care: Advances in Therapeutic Strategies, *edited by Gary H. Lyman and Jeffrey Crawford*
6. Cancer Vaccines: Challenges and Opportunities in Translation, *edited by Adrian Bot and Mihail Obrocea*

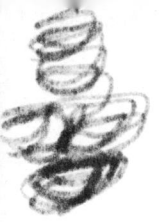

Cancer Supportive Care

Advances in Therapeutic Strategies

Edited by

Gary H. Lyman
*Duke University School of Medicine
Duke Comprehensive Cancer Center
Durham, North Carolina, USA*

Jeffrey Crawford
*Duke University School of Medicine
Duke Comprehensive Cancer Center
Durham, North Carolina, USA*

informa
healthcare

New York   London

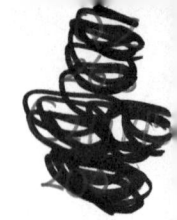

Informa Healthcare USA, Inc.
52 Vanderbilt Avenue
New York, NY 10017

© 2008 by Informa Healthcare USA, Inc.
Informa Healthcare is an Informa business

No claim to original U.S. Government works
Printed in the United States of America on acid-free paper
10 9 8 7 6 5 4 3 2 1

International Standard Book Number-10: 1-4200-5289-6 (Hardcover)
International Standard Book Number-13: 978-1-4200-5289-3 (Hardcover)

This book contains information obtained from authentic and highly regarded sources. Reprinted material is quoted with permission, and sources are indicated. A wide variety of references are listed. Reasonable efforts have been made to publish reliable data and information, but the author and the publisher cannot assume responsibility for the validity of all materials or for the consequence of their use.

No part of this book may be reprinted, reproduced, transmitted, or utilized in any form by any electronic, mechanical, or other means, now known or hereafter invented, including photocopying, microfilming, and recording, or in any information storage or retrieval system, without written permission from the publishers.

For permission to photocopy or use material electronically from this work, please access www.copyright .com (http://www.copyright.com/) or contact the Copyright Clearance Center, Inc. (CCC) 222 Rosewood Drive, Danvers, MA 01923, 978-750-8400. CCC is a not-for-profit organization that provides licenses and registration for a variety of users. For organizations that have been granted a photocopy license by the CCC, a separate system of payment has been arranged.

Trademark Notice: Product or corporate names may be trademarks or registered trademarks, and are used only for identification and explanation without intent to infringe.

Library of Congress Cataloging-in-Publication Data

Cancer supportive care : advances in therapeutic strategies / edited by Gary H. Lyman, Jeffrey Crawford.
    p. ; cm. — (Translational medicine series ; 5)
  Includes bibliographical references and index.
  ISBN-13: 978-1-4200-5289-3 (hardcover : alk. paper)
  ISBN-10: 1-4200-5289-6 (hardcover : alk. paper) 1. Cancer—Palliative treatment. I. Lyman, Gary H., M.D. II. Crawford, Jeffrey, (Jeffrey C.) III. Series.
  [DNLM: 1. Neoplasms—complications. 2. Neoplasms—therapy. 3. Patient Care. 4. Quality of Life. QZ 266 C217145 2008]
  RC271.P33C365 2008
  616.99′406—dc22

                                              2008000658

For Corporate Sales and Reprint Permissions call 212-520-2700 or write to: Sales Department, 52 Vanderbilt Avenue, 16th floor, New York, NY 10017.

Visit the Informa Web site at
www.informa.com

and the Informa Healthcare Web site at
www.informahealthcare.com

Foreword

The management of patients with neoplastic diseases has become a remarkably complex process over the past two decades. New insights into the molecular basis of various forms of cancer have resulted in a proliferation of new diagnostic tools and treatment options. This ever expanding knowledge base presents an ongoing challenge for busy medical oncologists and hematologists to remain abreast of the latest developments. One consequence of this information explosion is an increasing compartmentalization of care where the clinical expertise of practitioners has often become progressively more narrowed in many instances. Despite this trend, there remains a large common base of knowledge that all practitioners caring for patients with cancer must possess if they are to be effective and compassionate caregivers.

An essential element of this common knowledge base is an understanding of the basic principles of the supportive care of the cancer patient. Supportive care undoubtedly conjures up a variety of images to the medical professional, from symptom management to psychological and spiritual support, to end-of-life care. Supportive care certainly encompasses all of these areas but it also is so much more. Supportive care in the most complete sense involves the prevention and management of the adverse effects of cancer and its treatment across the entire continuum of a patient's illness from the time of diagnosis through active treatment to death, including the enhancement of rehabilitation and survivorship. In attempting to optimize the patient experience, therefore, this means harnessing not only the vast array of disease specific information on various antineoplastic treatments, but also bringing to bear all relevant aspects of supportive management as well. This volume represents a timely and invaluable resource for the busy practitioner chronicling the key topics in cancer supportive management. The two editors, each a prominent leader in the supportive care arena, have ably encompassed the full spectrum of supportive care in cancer with comprehensive reviews by authoritative clinical investigators.

Recent therapeutic progress in defining more effective antineoplastic treatments has been heavily dependent on understanding the basic biologic principles of carcinogenesis, growth-signaling, apoptotic pathways, angiogenesis and metatstatic spread. Many of the most significant recent advances in the area of supportive care have also been critically dependent on a better definition of the underlying biologic processes involved in various adverse effects of cancer or antineoplastic treatment. New insights into the pathophysiology of such treatment-induced adverse effects as nausea and vomiting, mucositis and hematopoietic cytopenias have directly led to a number of effective "molecularly targeted" treatment approaches. This volume reviews a number of these new treatment approaches. Traditional supportive care topics such as management of infectious complications, pain, psychological issues and end-of-life care are comprehensively reviewed. In addition, a number of emerging areas which to date remain significant challenges or have received inadequate attention such as fatigue, quality-of-life measurement, cancer survivorship, and the unique needs of the older patient are ably summarized.

Cancer care, as in other areas of medicine, is increasingly being driven by the imperative to be "evidenced-based." Whereas authoritative opinion and tradition may have been sufficient in the past, there is now an expectation to have solid evidence guide treatment. This standard is being increasingly applied in the supportive care arena as well and is equally relevant to agents being introduced to counter adverse effects of antineoplastic treatment as well as those used to treat cancer-related symptoms in a hospice setting. This volume highlights some of the key clinical research developments that have provided us with evidence-based supportive care treatment options.

The unique care requirements of patients with cancer serve to differentiate them in many ways from patients with serious non-neoplastic illnesses. The multidisciplinary care model that has become the standard of care in recent years for patients with cancer perhaps best illustrates this. There is no area in oncology management where the multidisciplinary model has reached a greater level of maturity than in the area of supportive care. Physicians, dentists, nurses, psychologists, social workers and spiritual care providers all play key roles in delivering optimal supportive care. The diverse experience of the authors and the wide spectrum of topics included in this volume provide fitting testimony to the multidisciplinary nature of supportive care in cancer and make this contribution relevant to all who labor to improve the lives of patients with cancer.

For those clinicians whose career caring for patients with cancer extends well back into the prior century, these are both amazing and exciting times as so many significant new advances have been recently realized and the future offers unlimited promise. Going forward it is incumbent that all caregivers retain an appreciation that optimal "patient-centered" care is dependent not simply upon

Foreword

arresting a specific disease process but attending to the full physical, emotional, psychological and spiritual needs of our patients. This volume provides a wealth of information to help the reader work toward this goal.

Paul J. Hesketh, M.D.
Chief, Division of Hematology Oncology
Caritas St. Elizabeth's Medical Center
Professor of Medicine
Tufts University School of Medicine
Boston, Massachusetts, U.S.A.

Preface

The greatest mistake in the treatment of diseases is that there are physicians for the body and physicians for the soul, although the two cannot be separated. ~ Plato

We shall draw from the heart of suffering itself the means of inspiration and survival. ~ Winston Churchill

We are living unquestionably in the most exciting of times for medical care in general and cancer research and treatment in particular. The rate at which scientific advances are occurring and translating into improved medical diagnostics and therapeutics is clearly breathtaking. And anyone familiar with the pipeline of promising new agents as well as novel therapeutic targets arising out of our improved understanding of the basic molecular biology and genetics of cancer stands in awe at what the future almost certainly will provide to future victims of this dread disease. Honest reflection clearly demonstrates that, as important as the development of novel therapeutics has been to our progress against cancer, equally important has been the rapid and continuing progress in our ability to support patients through cancer treatment to better cope with the life changing symptoms of the disease itself.

Cancer Supportive Care: Advances in Therapeutic Strategies brings into a single volume many of the most important advances in supportive care which have enabled exciting improvements in longevity and enhanced the quality of life of patients with cancer each presented by the very leaders that have developed and studied such means of improved patient care. We wish to extend our very sincere thanks to this outstanding representation of thought leaders and investigators who have participated in assembling this impressive repository of information on the latest advances in cancer supportive care.

While many of the recent advances in cancer treatment gaining the attention of both the medical profession as well as the public relate to the introduction of an array of novel agents including small molecules and human monoclonal antibodies targeting and disrupting critical processes in cancer formation, growth, invasion and spread. These new agents have been specifically designed to target critical pathways with the hope of increasing efficacy and reducing the toxicity of more traditional therapies including surgery, radiation therapy and cytotoxic chemotherapy. Studies to date, however, suggest that rather than replacing traditional agents, most of the newer therapies improve patient outcomes by complementing, but not replacing, conventional treatments. Thus many of the toxicities that accompany traditional approaches remain with us and, in some cases, are further aggravated in the effort to improve long-term survival. Whether discussing the classic targeted approach of selective estrogen receptor modulators in hormone receptor positive women with early stage breast cancer or the more recent introduction of anti-HER2 targeted therapy with the humanized monoclonal antibody, trastuzumab, not only did these agents bring with them their own unique set of toxicities but often they have been found to be most effective when administered in combination or sequentially with traditional cytotoxic chemotherapy.

This book has been compiled with the assistance of some of the finest clinical investigators in cancer supportive care in the world today. A fitting introduction to this volume is provided by Paul Hesketh, an authority on cancer supportive care and current president of the Multinational Association of Supportive Care of Cancer (MASCC). Dr. Hesketh provides an insightful look at the breadth of the growing field of cancer supportive care and presents a challenge to all practicing oncologists to embrace the full spectrum of cancer care needs discussed in this volume. The main text begins a comprehensive discussion of the challenge of actually measuring patient symptoms and health-related quality of life by David Cella and colleagues from Northwestern University. For the last two decades, this group has been involved with developing and validating a vast array of patient self assessment tools which have greatly improved our understanding of the various dimensions of quality of life and the impact of cancer and cancer treatment on these measures. Arguably the single most common symptomatic complaint offered by cancer patients, fatigue, is the focus of a chapter by Paul Jacobsen and Heather Jim from the H. Lee Moffitt Cancer Center. This group has developed tools for the assessment of cancer-related fatigue and its many features and relationships with outcomes in patients with cancer and identified potential methods to alleviate patient fatigue symptoms.

The next series of chapters cover the spectrum of treatment-related toxicities largely revolving around the myelosuppressive effects of the majority of systemic cancer therapies producing cytotoxic effects on erythroid, myeloid and megakaryocytic lineages in the bone marrow. The resulting hematologic toxicities of anemia, neutropenia and thrombocytopenia have rightfully been characterized as the most common dose-limiting toxicities of cancer chemotherapy. These "cytopenias" result in serious and potentially life-threatening complications including a wide range of bacterial and fungal infections, and hemorrhagic complications contributing to the symptoms of fatigue mentioned above. The occurrence or anticipation of these complications represent major challenges to the delivery of optimal cancer treatment intensity. In turn, these toxicities have given rise to a wide range of new therapeutic options including newer and more effective antibiotics and an array of recombinant human hematopoietic growth factors. While we are constantly made aware of the need to balance efficacy and safety, the emergence of the erythropoietic stimulating agents discussed by John Glaspy, the myeloid growth factors by Jeffrey Crawford as well as the emerging thrombopoietic agents overviewed by Saroj Vadhan-Raj have had a great impact on the supportive care of patients at risk for these complications enabling the delivery of full dose and dose dense schedules that potentially offer better disease control and long-term survival.

The major contribution that neutropenia and its complications make to morbidity and mortality of cancer chemotherapy is reviewed by David Dale and the related bacterial infections by Kenneth Rolston and Gerald Bodey, and fungal infections by Jean Klastersky. Gary Lyman and Nicole Kuderer put the epidemiology of this problem in the context of assessing patient risk factors for treatment-related complications as we move closer to personalized management of such toxicities. A separate chapter on venous thromboembolism by Alok Khorana and Charles Francis attests to the rising recognition of both the frequency and severity of these complications of cancer and cancer treatment. Toxicities of the gastrointestinal system represent another major set of serious dose limiting complications prompting chapters on mucositis by Doug Peterson and diarrhea and constipation by Joyson Karakunnel. Another increasingly recognized set of complications of cancer and cancer treatment are those of an osseous nature including osteoporosis and the effects of bone metastases. Two chapters highlight this important and rapidly evolving clinical area of supportive care: the first by Alissa Huston on bone metabolism and new novel targeted agents and the second by Allan Lipton on the management of skeletal complications with the bisphosphonates. Two important chapters address a number of special topics including supportive care of the elderly cancer patient by Michelle Shayne and Lodovico Balducci, and late effects and cancer survivorship by Craig Earle and Ann Partridge.

The final chapters of the volume return to the issue of patient quality of life addressed in the initial chapters of the book. Jeanne-Marie Maher and Ann Berger discuss the management of pain, Jimmie Holland and colleagues address the management of depression and anxiety in the cancer patient, while Amy Abernethy and coauthors provide an overview of the multitude of issues related to end-of-life care. In the last chapter, we attempt to lay a framework for the future by discussing the derivation and potential clinical application of risk prediction tools in the supportive care of patients with cancer. The accurate prediction of treatment benefits and toxicities should lay the basis for more individualized, tailored interventions which may alleviate the symptoms of disease and its treatment which often come with their own risks and costs.

The editors share the perspective of the individual authors of this volume that no aspect of cancer care deserves more attention and additional clinical research than the management of the symptoms of the disease and the toxicities associated with cancer treatment. We also share the current excitement and anticipation of all oncologists and cancer researchers that come from the large number of diagnostic and therapeutic breakthroughs of the past decade. At the same time, we recognize the continuing importance of the multitude of supportive care efforts enabling the optimal delivery of modern cancer therapy while improving and sustaining the quality of life of each cancer patient across the entire span of their disease. The primary goal of oncologists and all health care providers must remain the optimal outcome of cancer treatment for each patient in the broadest and most complete sense. While improved cancer treatment with less toxicity and greater efficacy represents the goal of all clinical investigators, more effective and less toxic supportive care measures employed in a more rational, targeted fashion will further enhance these efforts and bring us closer to that ultimate goal of optimal cancer patient care.

Gary H. Lyman
Jeffrey Crawford

Contents

Foreword Paul J. Hesketh ...... *iii*
Preface .... *vii*
Contributors .... *xv*

1. **Measuring Patient Symptoms and Other Aspects of Health-Related Quality of Life** *1*
   Zeeshan Butt, Susan E. Yount, and David Cella

2. **Assessment and Management of Cancer-Related Fatigue** *13*
   Heather S. L. Jim and Paul B. Jacobsen

3. **Anemia and Red Cell Factors** *31*
   John Glaspy

4. **Neutropenia and Its Complications** *59*
   David C. Dale, Jeffrey Crawford, and Gary H. Lyman

5. **Bacterial Infections in Cancer Patients** *73*
   Kenneth V. I. Rolston and Gerald P. Bodey

6. **Management of Fungal Infections in Cancer Patients** *89*
   Mickael Aoun, Jean Klastersky, Kristel Buvé, and Johan Maertens

7. **Myeloid Growth Factors** *115*
   Jeffrey Crawford

8. Thrombocytopenia and Thrombopoetic Growth Factors 135
    Jennifer Wright and Saroj Vadhan-Raj

9. Venous Thromboembolism and Anticoagulation 149
    Maithili V. Rao, Charles W. Francis, and Alok A. Khorana

10. Antiemetic Prophylaxis and Treatment of Chemotherapy-Induced
    Nausea and Vomiting 169
    Karin Jordan, Christoph Sippel, Timo Behlendorf,
    Hans-Heinrich Wolf, and Hans-Joachim Schmoll

11. Mucositis in Patients Receiving High-Dose Cancer Therapy .. 187
    Douglas E. Peterson and Rajesh V. Lalla

12. Diarrhea and Constipation 207
    Joyson Karakunnel and Apurva A. Modi

13. Skeletal Complications: Bone Metabolism and Novel
    Targeted Agents 223
    Alissa Huston

14. The Role of Bisphosphonates to Preserve Bone Health
    in Patients with Breast Cancer 241
    Allan Lipton

15. Supportive Care for Older Cancer Patients 257
    Michelle Shayne and Lodovico Balducci

16. Care of the Cancer Survivor 279
    Craig C. Earle and Ann H. Partridge

17. Pain and Palliation 297
    Jeanne-Marie Maher and Ann Berger

18. Management of Anxiety and Depressive Symptoms 319
    Jimmie C. Holland, Talia R. Weiss, and Maria Rueda-Lara

19. **End-of-Life Care** *337*
    Amy P. Abernethy, Joshua S. Barclay, Jane L. Wheeler,
    and David C. Currow

20. **Risk Prediction of Chemotherapy-Associated Toxicity
    in Patients Receiving Cancer Chemotherapy** *359*
    Gary H. Lyman and Nicole M. Kuderer

Index *377*

Contributors

Amy P. Abernethy Division of Medical Oncology, Department of Medicine, Duke University Medical Center (DUMC), Durham, North Carolina, U.S.A. and Department of Palliative and Supportive Services, Flinders University, Bedford Park, South Australia, Australia

Mickael Aoun Institut Jules Bordet, Université Libre de Bruxelles, Brussels, Belgium

Lodovico Balducci H. Lee Moffitt Cancer Center, University of South Florida, Tampa, Florida, U.S.A.

Joshua S. Barclay Division of General Internal Medicine, Department of Medicine, Duke University Medical Center (DUMC), Durham, North Carolina, U.S.A.

Timo Behlendorf Department of Internal Medicine IV, Oncology/Hematology, Martin-Luther-University Halle-Wittenberg, Halle (Saale), Germany

Ann Berger Bethesda, Maryland, U.S.A.

Gerald P. Bodey Department of Infectious Diseases, Infection Control and Employee Health, Division of Internal Medicine, The University of Texas M.D. Anderson Cancer Center, Houston, Texas, U.S.A.

Zeeshan Butt Center on Outcomes, Research, and Education (CORE), Evanston Northwestern Healthcare, Evanston, and Department of Psychiatry and Behavioral Sciences, Northwestern University, Feinberg School of Medicine, Chicago, Illinois, U.S.A.

Kristel Buvé Department of Hematology, University Hospital Gasthuisberg, Acute Leukemia and Transplantation Unit, Leuven, Belgium

David Cella Center on Outcomes, Research, and Education (CORE), Evanston Northwestern Healthcare, Evanston; Department of Psychiatry and Behavioral Sciences, and Institute for Healthcare Studies, Northwestern University, Feinberg School of Medicine, Chicago, Illinois, U.S.A.

Jeffrey Crawford Department of Medicine, Duke University School of Medicine and the Duke Comprehensive Cancer Center, Durham, North Carolina, U.S.A.

David C. Currow Department of Palliative and Supportive Services, Flinders University, Bedford Park, South Australia, and Cancer Australia, Canberra, Australia

David C. Dale Department of Medicine, University of Washington, Seattle, Washington, U.S.A.

Craig C. Earle Dana Farber Cancer Institute, Center for Outcomes/Policy Research, Harvard Medical School, Boston, Massachusetts, U.S.A.

Charles W. Francis James P. Wilmot Cancer Center and the Department of Medicine, University of Rochester, Rochester, New York, U.S.A.

John Glaspy Division of Hematology-Oncology, Department of Medicine, UCLA School of Medicine, Los Angeles, California, U.S.A.

Jimmie C. Holland Department of Psychiatry and Behavioral Sciences, Memorial Sloan-Kettering Cancer Center, New York, New York, U.S.A.

Alissa Huston James P. Wilmot Cancer Center, University of Rochester, Rochester, New York, U.S.A.

Paul B. Jacobsen Health Outcomes & Behavior Program, H. Lee Moffitt Cancer Center, Tampa, Florida, U.S.A.

Heather S. L. Jim Health Outcomes & Behavior Program, H. Lee Moffitt Cancer Center, Tampa, Florida, U.S.A.

Karin Jordan Department of Internal Medicine IV, Oncology/Hematology, Martin-Luther-University Halle-Wittenberg, Halle (Saale), Germany

Joyson Karakunnel National Institutes of Health, Bethesda, Maryland, U.S.A.

Alok A. Khorana James P. Wilmot Cancer Center and the Department of Medicine, University of Rochester, Rochester, New York, U.S.A.

Jean Klastersky Institut Jules Bordet, Université Libre de Bruxelles, Brussels, Belgium

Nicole M. Kuderer   Department of Medicine, Duke University School of Medicine and the Duke Comprehensive Cancer Center, Durham, North Carolina, U.S.A.

Rajesh V. Lalla   Section of Oral Medicine, Department of Oral Health and Diagnostic Sciences and Head & Neck/Oral Oncology Program, Neag Comprehensive Cancer Center, University of Connecticut Health Center, Farmington, Connecticut, U.S.A.

Allan Lipton   Penn State Cancer Center, Milton S. Hershey Medical Center, Hershey, Pennsylvania, U.S.A.

Gary H. Lyman   Department of Medicine, Duke University School of Medicine and the Duke Comprehensive Cancer Center, Durham, North Carolina, U.S.A.

Johan Maertens   Department of Hematology, University Hospital Gasthuisberg, Acute Leukemia and Transplantation Unit, Leuven, Belgium

Jeanne-Marie Maher   Home Health and Hospice Care, Nashua, New Hampshire, U.S.A.

Apurva A. Modi   National Institutes of Health, Bethesda, Maryland, U.S.A.

Ann H. Partridge   Dana Farber Cancer Institute, Center for Outcomes/Policy Research, Harvard Medical School, Boston, Massachusetts, U.S.A.

Douglas E. Peterson   Section of Oral Medicine, Department of Oral Health and Diagnostic Sciences and Head & Neck/Oral Oncology Program, Neag Comprehensive Cancer Center, University of Connecticut Health Center, Farmington, Connecticut, U.S.A.

Maithili V. Rao   James P. Wilmot Cancer Center and the Department of Medicine, University of Rochester, Rochester, New York, U.S.A.

Kenneth V. I. Rolston   Department of Infectious Diseases, Infection Control and Employee Health, Division of Internal Medicine, The University of Texas M.D. Anderson Cancer Center, Houston, Texas, U.S.A.

Maria Rueda-Lara   Department of Psychiatry and Behavioral Sciences, Memorial Sloan-Kettering Cancer Center, New York, New York, U.S.A.

Hans-Joachim Schmoll   Department of Internal Medicine IV, Oncology/Hematology, Martin-Luther-University Halle-Wittenberg, Halle (Saale), Germany

Michelle Shayne   James P. Wilmot Cancer Center, University of Rochester, Rochester, New York, U.S.A.

Christoph Sippel   Department of Internal Medicine IV, Oncology/Hematology, Martin-Luther-University Halle-Wittenberg, Halle (Saale), Germany

Saroj Vadhan-Raj   The University of Texas M.D. Anderson Cancer Center, Houston, Texas, U.S.A.

Talia R. Weiss   Department of Psychiatry and Behavioral Sciences, Memorial Sloan-Kettering Cancer Center, New York, New York, U.S.A.

Jane L. Wheeler   Division of Medical Oncology, Department of Medicine, Duke University Medical Center (DUMC), Durham, North Carolina, U.S.A.

Hans-Heinrich Wolf   Department of Internal Medicine IV, Oncology/Hematology, Martin-Luther-University Halle-Wittenberg, Halle (Saale), Germany

Jennifer Wright   Baylor College of Medicine, Houston, Texas, U.S.A.

Susan E. Yount   Center on Outcomes, Research, and Education (CORE), Evanston Northwestern Healthcare, Evanston, and Institute for Healthcare Studies, Northwestern University, Feinberg School of Medicine, Chicago, Illinois, U.S.A.

1

Measuring Patient Symptoms and Other Aspects of Health-Related Quality of Life

Zeeshan Butt

Center on Outcomes, Research, and Education (CORE), Evanston Northwestern Healthcare, Evanston, and Department of Psychiatry and Behavioral Sciences, Northwestern University, Feinberg School of Medicine, Chicago, Illinois, U.S.A.

Susan E. Yount

Center on Outcomes, Research, and Education (CORE), Evanston Northwestern Healthcare, Evanston, and Institute for Healthcare Studies, Northwestern University, Feinberg School of Medicine, Chicago, Illinois, U.S.A.

David Cella

Center on Outcomes, Research, and Education (CORE), Evanston Northwestern Healthcare, Evanston; Department of Psychiatry and Behavioral Sciences, and Institute for Healthcare Studies, Northwestern University, Feinberg School of Medicine, Chicago, Illinois, U.S.A.

INTRODUCTION

With increased rates of survival for cancer, there is an increasing focus on the health-related quality of life (HRQL) of patients. An individual who has undergone treatment for cancer may experience improved HRQL across several domains, or a more mixed, symptomatic recovery. Because of the numerous physical, mental, and social changes that cancer survivors may experience years following their treatment, ongoing HRQL assessment should be considered. Formal, systematic assessment of patients can serve as a useful gauge of treatment success, assist in the identification of long-term complications that should continue to be monitored by medical personnel, or identify potential teaching and learning moments where health promotion interventions could be implemented (1,2).

As outlined by the World Health Organization, health is "not merely the absence of disease or infirmity" (3). We define HRQL building off of the WHO model of health as a multidimensional concept that refers to an individual's usual or expected physical, emotional, and social well-being. Figure 1 depicts a conceptual model of HRQL, with measurable concepts subsumed under each broad dimension. Although organized as discrete domains, physical, emotional, and social well-being are likely interrelated. Similarly, HRQL refers to the subjective experience and well-being of a patient as impacted by a medical condition or its treatment (4). To study HRQL in the medical context, it is customary to narrow the field of study to those areas of life quality that can be related (directly or indirectly) to one's health. However, given the multidimensional nature of HRQL it may be useful to assess targeted life quality domains as well as domains less directly affected by the medical condition or its treatment. At its broadest, HRQL encompasses not only disease symptoms

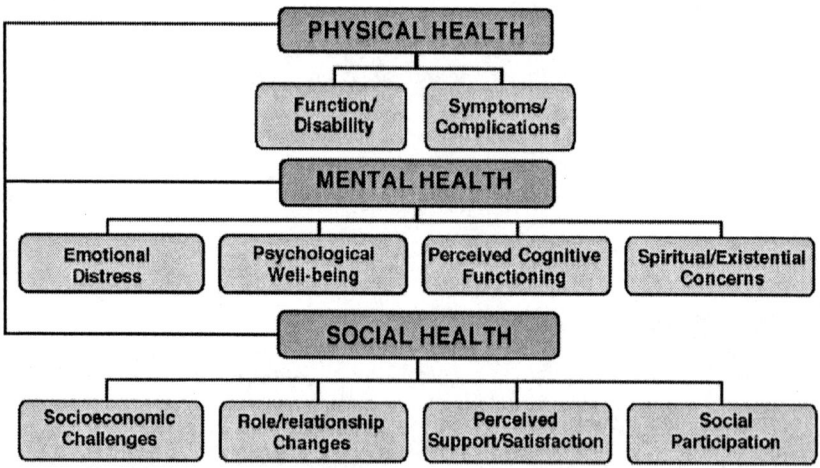

Figure 1 Conceptual model of health-related quality of life. *Source*: Adapted from Victorson, Cella, Wagner, Kramer, and Smith (2007). Measuring quality of life in cancer survivors. In: Handbook of Cancer Survivorship (Ed. M. Feuerstein), Springer, New York, NY (p. 81, Fig 1) with kind permission of Springer Science and Business Media.

and functional consequences, but also more subjective domains such as life satisfaction, happiness, and the value that one places on life at any given time. Notably, such patient-reported outcome (PRO) instruments that assess this range of concepts are increasingly becoming emphasized in clinical trials and other areas of medicine (5,6).

ISSUES IN PATIENT-REPORTED OUTCOME ASSESSMENT

FDA Draft Guidance

In February 2006, the U.S. Food and Drug Administration (FDA) (7) issued draft guidance for the pharmaceutical industry that describes how the FDA evaluates PRO instruments used as effectiveness endpoints in clinical trials. In this document, the FDA described their perspective on how industry sponsors can develop and use study results measured by PRO instruments to support claims in approved product labeling. As defined by the FDA, a PRO is a measurement of any aspect of a patient's health status that comes directly from the patient (i.e., without the interpretation of the patient's responses by a physician or anyone else). In clinical trials, a PRO may be used to measure the impact of an intervention on one or multiple aspects of patients' health status. This could range from a specific symptom response (e.g., pain relief) to more general concepts such as HRQL. The guidance also advises that PRO measures that assess a simple concept (e.g., a specific symptom) may not be viewed by the FDA as adequate to substantiate a more complex claim, such as HRQL benefit. The guidance includes recommendations on the conceptual bases and criteria on which PRO measures should be developed, assessed for reliability and validity, and modified. However, it is important to note that the main focus of the FDA guidance is on the evidentiary support for claims of PRO benefit, not general HRQL research (8).

NCCN/FACIT Experience

No single instrument currently in use meets all HRQL assessment needs in the context of cancer. The challenge in developing an HRQL instrument for a specific population is to write items that are relevant, targeted, and responsive to change. Cella and colleagues have developed a measurement system (i.e., Functional Assessment of Chronic Illness Therapy—FACIT) (9,10) with HRQL scales for a number of populations, including cancer, multiple sclerosis, HIV/AIDS, Parkinson's disease, and rheumatoid arthritis. Scale development within the FACIT system proceeds through a series of iterative steps for all measures: (1) item generation based on patient/clinician input and literature review, (2) item review and reduction, (3) scale construction, (4) initial psychometric evaluation, and (5) additional evaluation.

Using items drawn from the FACIT system and methods consistent with the recent FDA guidance, our group has recently developed symptom indexes for patients with advanced lymphoma and bladder, brain, breast, colorectal, head/neck, hepatobiliar/pancreatic, kidney, lung, ovarian, and prostate cancer (www.facit.org). Input on the most important symptoms was obtained from 550 patients recruited from National Comprehensive Cancer Network (NCCN) member institutions and four nonprofit social service organizations. Physician experts in each of the eleven diseases were also surveyed to differentiate symptoms that are predominantly disease based from those that are predominantly treatment induced. Results are currently being evaluated alongside previously published indexes for 9 of these 11 advanced cancers that were created on the basis of expert provider surveys, also at NCCN institutions (11). The end product will include symptom indexes specific to each advanced cancer site. Beyond the clinical value of such indices, they may also contribute significantly to satisfying regulatory requirements for a standardized tool to evaluate drug efficacy with respect to relevant symptoms. Further, by aligning the perspectives of physicians and nurses, as well as patients diagnosed with these various advanced cancers, the most current set of symptom indexes will represent a comprehensive list of the symptoms prioritized by the most integral stakeholders involved in patient care.

GENERIC AND TARGETED HRQL ASSESSMENT

The use of both generic and targeted HRQL instruments is a frequently implemented strategy in health care research (12–14), in an effort to maximize the utility of the assessment. Generic HRQL instruments tend to ask questions general enough for broad applicability, including for use among individuals in good health. On the other hand, targeted measures may focus on specific symptoms (e.g., pain, mood) that are common in many health conditions or concerns and symptoms specific to a disease or to its treatment.

Both generic and targeted HRQL measures can be useful, as they discriminate people and groups of people at different levels of focus. With the difference in focus comes a different profile of strengths and limitations. General health status measures quantify overall health and functioning, are applicable across multiple populations, can provide cross-disease and cross-intervention comparisons, are sensitive to comorbid conditions, and because of their broad scope may identify unexpected findings. In contrast, targeted instruments offer fine-grained assessment of narrower domains and symptoms. Advantages to targeted instruments include the focus on relevant areas, sensitivity to change in clinical status over time, and perceived relevance and practicality by clinicians and patients. In a sense, generic and targeted measures are at two ends of the spectrum of HRQL assessment. Both types of instruments likely have a role in the comprehensive assessment of HRQL (13,15).

While there are a number of reliable and valid HRQL instruments currently in use in cancer research, none can be considered the gold standard outcome to be used in all situations. Ideally, scale selection should be guided by the specific population under study, reason for the assessment, the outcomes of interest, and characteristics of the instruments themselves (e.g., psychometrics, item length).

INNOVATIVE MEASUREMENT APPROACHES FOR HRQL ASSESSMENT

Quality-of-life outcomes in cancer can be improved by refining the measurement of common symptoms and other health status variables. While there may be room for the development of new HRQL instruments specific for cancer, it may also be useful to consider improving HRQL assessment via the adoption of several unique statistical/methodological perspectives. Below, we consider three of these innovative approaches: the use of minimally important difference scores; the development of item banks and their applications, such as customized short forms and computerized adaptive testing (CAT); and real-time symptom monitoring.

Minimally Important Differences

In many cases, scores obtained on patient-reported measures of HRQL can be referenced against a normative sample to provide *relative* meaning to such scores. However, changes in HRQL scores can be difficult to interpret without a similar reference. Determining meaningful change in HRQL scores is a necessary step for interpreting change in HRQL over time, both within and across experimental treatment arms. Furthermore, quantification of meaningful change in HRQL scores can be useful for statistical power analyses in preparation for new clinical trials. Jaeschke, Singer, and Guyatt have described the minimal clinically important difference (MCID) on a HRQL score as "the smallest difference in score in the domain of interest which patients perceive as beneficial and which would mandate, in the absence of troublesome side effects and excessive cost, a change in the patient's management" (16). Ideally, clinically significant change in HRQL scores should be assessed from the perspective of both patients and clinicians. Responsive instruments are capable of detecting changes and will correlate positively with other measures of change (e.g., markers of disease progression). Meaningful change in HRQL scores is also referred to as the minimally important difference (MID) (17), as well, and is the term we prefer (18–20).

There are a number of ways to determine the clinical significance of changes in patient-reported HRQL outcome scores (21). For example, anchor-based methods for determining MIDs map HRQL difference scores onto differences in clinical results via cross-sectional and/or longitudinal comparisons. Distribution-based methods establish MIDs based on the statistical score distributions of HRQL scores, including use of the standard deviation or standard error of measurement calculated in a given study (22). The MID for a HRQL instrument is most accurately represented as a range of values and perhaps best calculated based on the convergence of more than one approach (18–20).

Item Response Theory and Its Applications

Item response theory (IRT) is an alternate approach to traditional test construction with relatively long roots (23–26). Notably, IRT estimates group-independent item parameters (e.g., difficulty, discrimination), expresses test-independent estimates of a concept (e.g., HRQL), and provides an estimate of precision for all levels of the symptom or other aspect of HRQL (27,28). Said another way, in IRT, item parameters are invariant with regard to the sample of respondents. Unlike traditional test theory, which describes scores against group-specific norms, IRT models the probability of a particular item response to the respondent's underlying symptom level. An IRT approach can be useful for examining the item-level properties of an instrument as well as the information provided by items (or groups of items) across the full range of the concept.

An item bank is comprised of carefully calibrated questions that develop, define, and quantify a common theme and thus provide an operational definition of a symptom or other aspect of HRQL. In a traditional testing situation, examinees are given fixed-length tests that may contain questions that are inappropriate for the sample being tested (i.e., they endorse none or all of the symptoms). IRT models the probability that a person, at a particular level of an underlying trait (e.g., fatigue), will endorse any given response option to any particular item in an item bank. Unlike the classical approach of adding up responses to all questions to produce a score, IRT models estimate the position of the respondent based upon the pattern of responses to the questions administered from the item bank. This enables one to control test length and even content of the questions administered from the bank. Since IRT methods make it possible to estimate HRQL using any set of items in an item bank, the approach also lends itself to the application of CAT.

Given a calibrated bank of discriminating items of varying difficulty levels, it is possible to develop a computerized algorithm that systematically administers items to an examinee to hone in on their HRQL score. At each item administration, the algorithm estimates examinee trait level and an associated standard error. Once the standard error drops below an acceptable level, CAT is terminated, producing a patient's score range (29,30). While CAT assessments are only starting to emerge in real-world healthcare applications, they are an exciting proposition. CAT-administered assessments are, on average, half as long as paper-and-pencil measures with equal or better precision (31–33). CAT applications may allow for briefer assessments, more efficient assessments, and assessment of more symptoms and domains of interest.

Without a doubt, an instrument's sensitivity to detect change at an individual level is an important consideration for both researchers and clinicians. IRT scores can also assist researchers to measure change over time. Reise, Haviland, and colleagues (34,35) have described that equal changes on an IRT-defined symptom or HRQL domain can result in unequal changes on an instrument's raw score, depending on where on the scale the change takes place.

In certain areas, such as in the measurement of HRQL (29), IRT strategies for measuring change may help alleviate some of the scaling problems of raw scores, allowing for a better understanding of individual (as opposed to group) change over time.

HRQL outcomes for cancer can be improved by refining the measurement of common symptoms and other health status variables. Our ability to evaluate innovative medical advances from the patient's perspective will be improved to the extent that researchers and clinicians can attach meaning to HRQL scores (or change in scores). There are a number of HRQL instruments from which to chose; additional research will be useful toward further advances in this area. Of particular interest, in 2004, the U.S. National Institutes of Health (NIH) funded a cooperative group to develop and validate item banks to measure self-reported health status. This group, the Patient-Reported Outcomes Measurement Information System (PROMIS) (36,37), has made available several IRT-based tools to measure PROs in clinical research (see also www.nihpromis.org).

Real-Time Symptom Monitoring

People with advanced cancer often experience multiple, debilitating symptoms related to their disease and treatment. Outpatient chemotherapy is usually administered over several months, with office visits scheduled two to four weeks apart. As a result, many symptoms emerge when patients are home, between scheduled clinic appointments. This creates challenges for the effective and timely monitoring and management of these symptoms. Unrecognized symptoms over time can cause emergency room visits and hospitalizations for management, interrupted therapy, reduced doses of chemotherapy, and reduced HRQL (38–41).

Effective symptom management begins with accurate symptom assessment (40). Numerous organizations, including the NCCN, have recommended "routine" monitoring of symptoms, psychosocial problems, and/or distress to ensure overall good quality of patient care. Despite the potential benefits of active, systematic assessment with patient-driven measures (42,43), this is seldom performed in clinical practice (39,40).

There are a number of patient, physician, and system barriers to adequate symptom management. Two of the most widely reported barriers are inadequate symptom assessment (38) and limited patient–provider communication regarding symptoms (44). While there is growing evidence suggesting that routine, formal assessment of patient-reported symptoms and health status may improve communication between patients and physicians, satisfaction with care, and HRQL, there remain some unanswered questions.

For example, additional research is needed to determine the impact of routine screening on symptom detection, treatment, and outcome over time. Rosenbloom and colleagues (45) recently reported results of their three-armed trial of HRQL assessment among 213 patients with metastatic breast, lung, or colorectal cancer. Notably, they found no differences in HRQL or treatment satisfaction across patients receiving usual care, HRQL assessment, or assessment with discussion of results. Symptom monitoring and management may be improved via patient education efforts regarding these and other cancer-related symptoms. Routine screening with the appropriate follow-up may be useful for symptom control, objective functional status, and quality of life.

Through the application of information technology resources, routine, systematic patient-reported symptom and HRQL assessments could be conducted on patients in "real time," while they are at home or in the clinic, with minimal burden on staff and patients. Such assessments may provide the detailed and specific knowledge necessary to allow for early and accurate identification and reporting of symptoms to the clinical team, which may alter symptom burden and allow for more effective management.

Several recent studies have demonstrated the feasibility, acceptability, and clinical utility of collecting and integrating symptom and HRQL information into routine outpatient visits (40). Critical elements for feasible, routine, clinic-based symptom assessment include: (a) the ability to assess multiple symptoms (46); (b) the use of brief measures that place minimal burden on patients (47); (c) data collection, analysis, interpretation, and delivery of patient responses to clinicians in real time at the point of care (48,49); (d) presentation of individual symptom profiles rather than total symptom scores (50); and (e) inclusion of cut points for decision thresholds (51).

Routine, real-time assessment of HRQL in cancer may prove most beneficial when assessment results are coupled with specific clinical suggestions for symptom treatment or management. At present such practice is rare, in part because HRQL instruments have diverse scaling properties and may not be clearly interpretable by clinicians. For these reasons, results from HRQL assessments need to be presented in an efficient user-friendly format that includes reference or normative data (52) and guides intervention (50). Such a practice may allow clinicians to monitor individual patients and detect small but important changes in HRQL. Specific care recommendations can then be based on the level, or change in level, of a given symptom.

Our group has recently begun using novel approaches for real-time, telecommunication-based assessment of HRQL for patients with advanced cancer. Briefly, on a weekly basis for 12 weeks, enrolled patients with advanced lung cancer receiving chemotherapy telephone a computerized survey system to complete a brief lung cancer-specific symptom index. In addition, patients complete periodic measures of HRQL and treatment satisfaction. A research nurse monitors patients' weekly responses and within 24 hours, contacts any patient who endorses any symptom severity as "very much" or "quite a bit" or reports a two-point worsening from the previous week. At that point, the nurse verifies the accuracy of the report and either provides education or counseling (e.g., energy conservation for fatigue, reminders on medication adherence) to the patient and/or calls the patient's physician for further consultation on symptom management (e.g., medication change, diagnostic tests, office visit). Summary

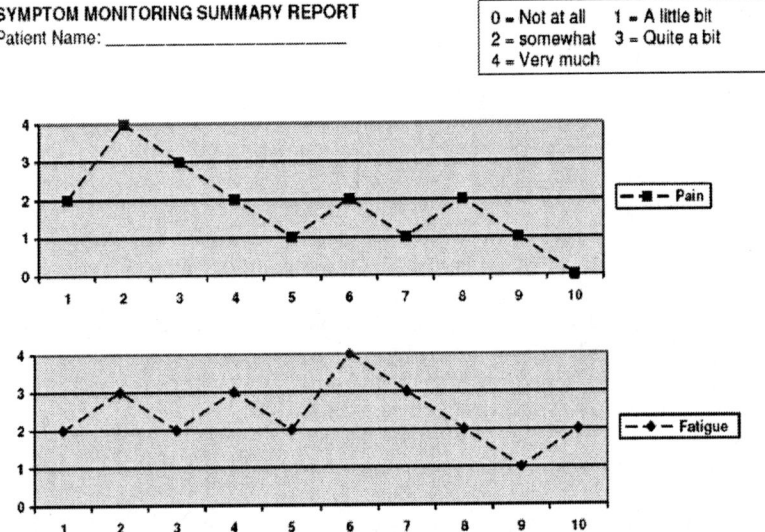

Figure 2 Sample symptom monitoring report.

reports with graphic displays of cumulative symptom and HRQL information are generated, reviewed, and discussed with patients at each physician visit (Fig. 2). Results from a pilot trial support the use of computer and telephone technology as a means of collecting HRQL data as well as the utility and understandability of graphic reports as part of routine physician visits (53). Full trials using this approach are currently underway within our group for advanced lung and breast cancer.

SUMMARY

We define quality of life as a multidimensional concept encompassing an individual's usual or expected physical, emotional, and social well-being. From that perspective, assessment of a cancer patients' HRQL necessarily involves measurement of cancer-related symptoms. Since symptom presentation often changes over the course of cancer treatment, ongoing HRQL assessment should be considered as part of routine clinical care. This is especially important now that PRO measures are increasingly being used to index cancer treatment efficacy. In addition, there has been increasing interest in the degree to which instrument content should be general vs. more targeted in scope. Ongoing developments in HRQL assessment include the establishment of clinical significance thresholds, applications of modern psychometric theory, and real-time symptom monitoring. These innovative assessment approaches hold promise to improve our ability to reliably, validly, and meaningfully assess the patient experience in cancer.

REFERENCES

1. Cella D, Webster K. Linking outcomes management to quality-of-life measurement. Oncology (Williston Park) 1997; 11(11A):232–235.
2. Cella D, Nowinski CJ. Measuring quality of life in chronic illness: the functional assessment of chronic illness therapy measurement system. Arch Phys Med Rehabil 2002; 83(12 suppl 2):S10–S17.
3. World Health Organization. Constitution of the World Health Organization. Geneva: WHO, 1946.
4. Cella DF. Methods and problems in measuring quality of life. Support Care Cancer 1995; 3(1):11–22.
5. Atherton PJ, Sloan JA. Rising importance of patient-reported outcomes. Lancet Oncol 2006; 7(11):883,884.
6. Leidy NK, Beusterien K, Sullivan E, et al. Integrating the patient's perspective into device evaluation trials. Value Health 2006; 9(6):394–401.
7. Food and Drug Administration. Guidance for industry: patient-reported outcome measures, use in medical product development to support labelling claims (Draft Guidance), 2006.
8. Revicki DA. FDA draft guidance and health-outcomes research. Lancet 2007; 369 (9561):540–542.
9. Lent L, Hahn E, Eremenco S, Webster K, et al. Using cross-cultural input to adapt the Functional Assessment of Chronic Illness Therapy (FACIT) scales. Acta Oncol 1999; 38(6):695–702.
10. Webster K, Cella D, Yost K. The Functional Assessment of Chronic Illness Therapy (FACIT) measurement system: properties, applications, and interpretation. Health Qual Life Outcomes 2003; 1(1):79.
11. Cella D, Paul D, Yount S, et al. What are the most important symptom targets when treating advanced cancer? A survey of providers in the National Comprehensive Cancer Network (NCCN). Cancer Invest 2003; 21(4):526–535.
12. Wu AW, Fink NE, Marsh-Manzi JV, et al. Changes in quality of life during hemodialysis and peritoneal dialysis treatment: generic and disease specific measures. J Am Soc Nephrol 2004; 15(3):743–753.
13. Ware Jr., JE, Kemp JP, Buchner DA, et al. The responsiveness of disease-specific and generic health measures to changes in the severity of asthma among adults. Qual Life Res 1998; 7(3):235–244.
14. Patrick DL, Deyo RA. Generic and disease-specific measures in assessing health status and quality of life. Med Care 1989; 27(3 suppl):S217–S232.
15. Guyatt GH, Feeny DH, Patrick DL. Measuring health-related quality of life. Ann Intern Med 1993; 118(8):622–629.
16. Jaeschke R, Singer J, Guyatt GH. Measurement of health status. Ascertaining the minimal clinically important difference. Control Clin Trials 1989; 10(4):407–415.
17. Wyrwich KW. Minimal important difference thresholds and the standard error of measurement: is there a connection? J Biopharm Stat 2004; 14(1):97–110.
18. Eton DT, Cella D, Yost KJ, et al. A combination of distribution- and anchor-based approaches determined minimally important differences (MIDs) for four endpoints in a breast cancer scale. J Clin Epidemiol 2004; 57(9):898–910.
19. Yost KJ, Cella D, Chawla A, et al. Minimally important differences were estimated for the Functional Assessment of Cancer Therapy-Colorectal (FACT-C) instrument

using a combination of distribution- and anchor-based approaches. J Clin Epidemiol 2005; 58(12):1241–1251.
20. Yost KJ, Eton DT. Combining distribution- and anchor-based approaches to determine minimally important differences: the FACIT experience. Eval Health Prof 2005; 28(2):172–191.
21. Schunemann HJ, Akl EA, Guyatt GH. Interpreting the results of patient reported outcome measures in clinical trials: the clinician's perspective. Health Qual Life Outcomes 2006; 4:62.
22. Hays RD, Farivar SS, Liu H. Approaches and recommendations for estimating minimally important differences for health-related quality of life measures. COPD 2005; 2(1):63–67.
23. Anastasi A, Urbina S. Psychological Testing. 7th ed. Upper Saddle River, NJ: Prentice Hall, 1997.
24. Lord FM. Application of item response theory to practical testing problems. Hillsdale, NJ: Erlbaum, 1980.
25. Richardson MW. The relationship between difficulty and the differential validity of a test. Psychometrika 1936; 1:33–49.
26. Streiner DL, Norman GR. Health measurement scales: a practical guide to their development and use. 2nd ed. Oxford: Oxford University Press, 1995.
27. Hambleton RK, Swaminathan H, Rogers HJ. Fundamentals of item response theory. Newbury Park, CA: Sage, 1991.
28. Steinberg L, Thissen D. Item response theory in personality research. In: Shrout PE, ed. Personality Research, Methods, and Theory: A Festschrift Honoring Donald W. Fiske. Hillsdale, NJ: Lawrence Erlbaum Associates, Inc., 1995:161–181.
29. Cella D, Chang CH. A discussion of item response theory and its applications in health status assessment. Medical Care 2000; 38:II66–II72.
30. Hays RD, Morales LS, Reise SP. Item response theory and health outcomes measurement in the 21st century. Medical Care 2000; 38(9 suppl):II28–II42.
31. Embretson SE, Reise SP. Item response theory for psychologists. Mahwah, NJ: Erlbaum, 2000.
32. Embretson SE. The continued search for nonarbitrary metrics in psychology. American Psychologist 2006; 61:50–55.
33. Weiss DJ. Computerized adaptive testing for effective and efficient measurement in counseling and education. Meas Eval Counsel Dev 2004; 37:70–84.
34. Reise SP, Haviland MG. Item response theory and the measurement of clinical change. J Pers Assess 2005; 84(3):228–238.
35. Reise SP, Ainsworth AT, Haviland MG. Item response theory: fundamentals, applications, and promise in psychological research. Curr Dir Psychol Sci 2005; 14:95–101.
36. Cella D, Yount S, Rothrock N, et al. The Patient-Reported Outcomes Measurement Information System (PROMIS): progress of an NIH roadmap cooperative group during its first two years. Med Care 2007; 45(5 suppl 1):S3–S11.
37. Garcia SF, Cella D, Clauser S, et al. Standardizing patient-reported outcomes assessment in cancer clinical trials: a PROMIS initiative. J Clin Oncol 2007; 25(32): 5106–5112.
38. Von Roenn JH, Cleeland CS, Gonin R, et al. Physician attitudes and practice in cancer pain management. A survey from the Eastern Cooperative Oncology Group. Ann Intern Med 1993; 119(2):121–126.

39. Cleeland CS. Cancer-related symptoms. Semin Radiat Oncol 2000; 10(3):175–190.
40. Naughton M, Homsi J. Symptom assessment in cancer patients. Curr Oncol Rep 2002; 4(3):256–263.
41. Meyers CA, Seabrooke LF, Albitar M, Estey EH. Association of cancer-related symptoms with physiological parameters. J Pain Symptom Manage 2002; 24(4): 359–361.
42. Schuit KW, Sleijfer DT, Meijler WJ, et al. Symptoms and functional status of patients with disseminated cancer visiting outpatient departments. J Pain Symptom Manage 1998; 16(5):290–297.
43. Butt Z, Wagner LI, Beaumont JL, et al. Use of a single item screening tool to detect clinically significant fatigue, pain, distress, and anorexia in ambulatory cancer practice. J Pain Symptom Manage 2008; 35(1):20–30.
44. Butt Z, Wagner LI, Beaumont JL, et al. Longitudinal screening and management of fatigue, pain, and emotional distress associated with cancer therapy. Support Care Cancer 2008 Feb; 16(2):151–159. Epub 2007 July 3.
45. Rosenbloom SK, Victorson DE, Hahn EA, et al. Assessment is not enough: a randomized controlled trial of the effects of HRQL assessment on quality of life and satisfaction in oncology clinical practice. Psychooncology 2007; 16(12):1069–1079.
46. Donnelly S, Walsh D, Rybicki L. The symptoms of advanced cancer: identification of clinical and research priorities by assessment of prevalence and severity. J Palliat Care 1995; 11(1):27–32.
47. Cleeland CS, Mendoza TR, Wang XS, et al. Assessing symptom distress in cancer patients: the M.D. Anderson Symptom Inventory. Cancer 2000; 89(7):1634–1646.
48. Buxton J, White M, Osoba D. Patients' experiences using a computerized program with a touch-sensitive video monitor for the assessment of health-related quality of life. Qual Life Res 1998; 7(6):513–519.
49. Davis K, Cella D. Assessing quality of life in oncology clinical practice: a review of barriers and critical success factors. J Clin Outcomes Manage 2002; 9:327–332.
50. Velikova G, Booth L, Smith AB, et al. Measuring quality of life in routine oncology practice improves communication and patient well-being: a randomized controlled trial. J Clin Oncol 2004; 22(4):714–724.
51. Fortner B, Okon T, Schwartzberg L, et al. The Cancer Care Monitor: psychometric content evaluation and pilot testing of a computer administered system for symptom screening and quality of life in adult cancer patients. J Pain Symptom Manage 2003; 26(6):1077–1092.
52. Liang MH. Longitudinal construct validity: establishment of clinical meaning in patient evaluative instruments. Med Care 2000; 38(9 suppl):II84–II90.
53. Davis K, Yount S, Del Ciello K, et al. An innovative symptom monitoring tool for people with advanced lung cancer: a pilot demonstration. J Support Oncol 2007; 5(8):381–387.

2

Assessment and Management of Cancer-Related Fatigue

Heather S. L. Jim and Paul B. Jacobsen
Health Outcomes & Behavior Program, H. Lee Moffitt Cancer Center, Tampa, Florida, U.S.A.

INTRODUCTION

Fatigue is a common experience for cancer patients which can have devastating effects on quality of life. Considerable recent progress has been made in defining, assessing, and diagnosing cancer-related fatigue. This progress has enabled clinicians and researchers to better understand which patients are at greater risk for fatigue, as well as identify potential etiological factors in the development and maintenance of cancer-related fatigue. Although cancer-related fatigue is still not well understood, several behavioral and pharmacological interventions show promise in its management. This chapter begins with a definition of cancer-related fatigue, and then reviews current research regarding its prevalence, assessment, and management.

DEFINITION OF CANCER-RELATED FATIGUE

The National Comprehensive Cancer Network's (NCCN) Cancer-Related Fatigue Management Guidelines define fatigue as "a distressing persistent, subjective sense of tiredness or exhaustion related to cancer or cancer treatment that is not proportional to recent activity and interferes with usual functioning" (1). Research suggests that the fatigue experienced by cancer patients is both quantitatively and qualitatively different from that of healthy individuals. As Poulson (2) notes, "The deadening fatigue which invades the very bones of cancer patients is totally unlike even the most profound fatigue of an otherwise well person." Normal fatigue is usually described as physical exhaustion or sleepiness that is alleviated by rest (3). In contrast, cancer-related fatigue endures; energy is not replenished even after long periods of sleep or rest (4). In addition, cancer-related fatigue is distressing; patients often describe fatigue as one of the most difficult and disruptive aspects of the cancer experience (5,6). Finally, cancer-related fatigue is pervasive; it saps the energy to function effectively in cognitive, physical, and psychological domains. Patients often report problems with short-term memory and concentration, generalized weakness, reduced ability to carry out normal activities, decreased motivation, and heightened frustration and depression (3,7,8). Thus, reduction of cancer-related fatigue has the potential to greatly improve quality of life across multiple domains.

PREVALENCE OF CANCER-RELATED FATIGUE

Cancer-related fatigue is extremely common. Depending on the patient sample and methodology, an estimated 70% to 100% of cancer patients experience fatigue (1). Neither demographic (e.g., age, race, ethnicity, marital status, education) nor medical variables (e.g., disease stage) appear to be strongly correlated with fatigue severity (9). Instead, the type of treatment appears to be the most important contributor. Chemotherapy is reliably associated with increases in fatigue (10), which can persist months or years after treatment completion (11). Bone marrow transplant (BMT) patients are also at risk for increased and persistent fatigue (12). With radiotherapy, fatigue levels tend to peak during treatment, then decrease (13) to rates comparable to healthy controls (14). Fatigue also tends to be high in palliative care settings (15). For example, in a study comparing the fatigue scores of palliative care inpatients to those of age- and sex-matched healthy controls, 75% of patients scored in excess of the 95th percentile of controls (16).

COGNITIVE-BEHAVIORAL MODEL OF CANCER-RELATED FATIGUE

Factors that precipitate and perpetuate cancer-related fatigue can be conceptualized via a cognitive-behavioral framework (Fig. 1). This model indicates that fatigue is likely due to a myriad of contributing factors rather than any single cause. One contributing factor is the presence of preexisting conditions, such as congestive heart failure and pulmonary dysfunction, which may exacerbate cancer-related fatigue (17). The tumor itself (i.e., tumor burden) may contribute to fatigue through abnormalities of energy metabolism (18), muscle functioning (18), and hormonal changes (18,19). Symptoms of the tumor, such as nausea, pain, and shortness of breath, may require significant compensatory energy expenditures that also result in fatigue (17). Treatment is theorized to contribute to fatigue through biological mechanisms such as anemia (20), hypothyroidism (1), and

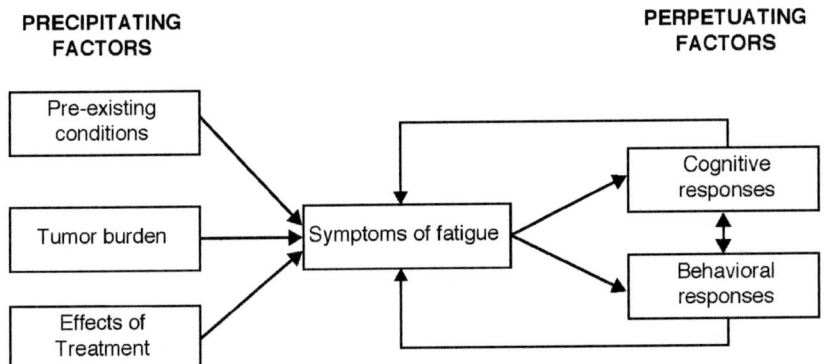

Figure 1 Cognitive-behavioral model of cancer-related fatigue.

increased cytokine production (18,19,21), as well as secondary effects such as nausea, vomiting, pain, dehydration, and malnutrition (22). Once treatment is completed, persistent immune changes and late effects may contribute to fatigue among long-term survivors (21). Taken together, these factors individually and jointly may precipitate the subjective experience of fatigue, cognitive and behavioral manifestations of fatigue, and disability. In addition, the cognitions and behaviors that patients employ to cope with fatigue may perpetuate the problem. Patients who catastrophize, or make negative statements about themselves and the future, tend to report greater fatigue than patients who do not (9,11). Patients who cope with fatigue through behavioral inactivity also tend to report greater fatigue (10,23), perhaps due to muscle wasting. Disruptions in sleeping patterns, including both insomnia and hypersomnia, may also contribute to fatigue (23). In sum, the factors that precipitate and perpetuate fatigue are multifaceted and present multiple targets for assessment and intervention.

ASSESSMENT OF FATIGUE

Reliable and valid measures of fatigue are essential to evaluating the efficacy of new interventions and to determining whether intervention is clinically warranted in individual patients. However, fatigue is a complex, subjective phenomenon that makes assessment difficult. This difficulty led Muscio to suggest in 1921 that "the term [fatigue] be absolutely banished from scientific discussion, and consequently that attempts to obtain a fatigue test be abandoned" (24). Considerable progress has been made in defining and assessing fatigue since Muscio wrote, but no gold standard measure has yet emerged. Existing measures vary widely in terms of the definition of fatigue, development process, known psychometric properties, and intended population. Despite their heterogeneity, instruments can be broadly categorized as single-dimensional or multidimensional measures (Table 1).

Table 1 Commonly Used Measures of Cancer-Related Fatigue

Measure	Description	Domain(s) assessed	Development/ validity sample(s)	Concurrent and discriminant validity	Reliability
Single-dimensional scales					
Profile of Mood States (POMS) fatigue and vigor subscales (27)	7 fatigue items, 8 vigor items rated on five-point Likert scales	Fatigue severity, vigor	148 cancer patients	*Fatigue subscale* PANAS positive affect: −0.10 PANAS negative affect: 0.40	Cronbach's alpha (fatigue subscale): 0.95 2 day test-retest: 0.74
Functional Assessment of Cancer Therapy— Fatigue (FACT-F) (26)	13 items rated on five-point Likert scales	Fatigue severity	50 cancer patients during treatment	POMS fatigue: −0.74 Piper fatigue: −0.75 Marlowe Crowne: 0.04	Cronbach's alpha (full scale): 0.93–0.95 1 week test-retest (full scale): 0.90
Symptom Distress Scale (SDS) (32)	1 fatigue item rated on five-point Likert scale	Fatigue severity	52 patients with advanced medical conditions	SDS mood: 0.60 SDS insomnia: 0.55 SDS pain: 0.37	Not available for fatigue item
Rotterdam Symptom Checklist (RSCL) (33)	1 fatigue item rated on point Likert scale	Fatigue severity	95 female cancer patients, 56 ovarian cancer patients, 20 healthy controls	Not available for fatigue item	Not available for fatigue item

Scale	Description	Measures	Sample	Validity	Reliability
Linear Analog Scale Assessment (LASA) (35)	1 fatigue item rated on 11-point Likert scale	Fatigue severity	103 cancer patients	Functional living index cancer: 0.39 Perceived adjustment to chronic illness: 0.33 Psychological adjustment to cancer: 0.53	Not available for fatigue item
Visual Analog Scale (VAS) (7)	1 item, 100 mm line	Fatigue severity	38 cancer patients	Fatigue assessment questionnaire: 0.73 HADS anxiety: 0.47 HADS depression: 0.62	Not available for fatigue item
Multidimensional scales					
Brief Fatigue Inventory (BFI) (36)	9 items rated on 11-point Likert scales	Fatigue severity, interference	305 cancer patients, 290 community-dwelling adults	FACT-F: −0.88 POMS fatigue: 0.84 Hemoglobin: −0.36	Cronbach's alpha (full scale): 0.96
Fatigue Symptom Inventory (FSI) (37,38)	14 items rated on 11-point Likert scales	Fatigue severity, duration, effect on daily functioning	107 breast cancer patients on treatment, 113 breast cancer patients posttreatment, 50 healthy women, 342 cancer patients	*Individual items* POMS-fatigue: 0.51–0.80 SF-36 vitality: −0.52 to −0.77 Marlowe Crowne: −0.02 to −0.23 *Interference subscale* CES-D: 0.47 Satisfaction with life domains—cancer: −0.53	Cronbach's alpha (full scale): 0.92–0.95 2–3 week test-retest (individual items): 0.10–0.75

(Continued)

Table 1 Commonly Used Measures of Cancer-Related Fatigue (*Continued*)

Measure	Description	Domain(s) assessed	Development/ validity sample(s)	Concurrent and discriminant validity	Reliability
Piper Fatigue Scale (PFS) (40,41)	27 items: 5 qualitative, 22 items rated on 11-point Likert scales	Behavioral/severity, affective meaning, sensory, cognitive/mood	50 breast and lung cancer patients, 382 breast cancer patients	POMS total mood disturbance: 0.50 POMS fatigue: 0.42 Fatigue symptom checklist: 0.47	Cronbach's alpha (subscales): 0.92–0.97
Multidimensional Fatigue Scale (MFSI) (42,43)	30 items rated on five-point Likert scales	General fatigue, physical fatigue, emotional fatigue, mental fatigue, vigor	146 breast cancer patients in treatment, 92 breast cancer patients posttreatment, 54 healthy women	*Subscales* State Trait Anxiety Inventory: 0.51–0.80 CES-D: 0.61–0.80 Marlowe Crowne: −0.14 to −0.26	Cronbach's alpha (subscales): 0.87–0.96 2–3 week test-retest (individual items): 0.51–0.70

Instruments Assessing Fatigue as a Single Dimension

Single-dimensional measures define fatigue as a unitary construct, yielding information regarding presence and severity. They tend to be shorter than multidimensional measures, making them useful when time is limited or participant burden is high. In clinical settings, single-dimensional measures are most frequently selected when the goal of assessment is screening; fatigue severity is used to determine when intervention is warranted. In research settings, single-dimensional measures are often favored when fatigue is one of many constructs assessed. Single-dimensional measures fall into two categories: (1) subscales of longer instruments, and (2) single-item measures.

Single-dimensional measures may be subscales of longer instruments designed to assess mood and quality of life. Use of these measures enables researchers to assess fatigue and other outcomes simultaneously. Two examples are the Profile of Mood States (POMS) (25) and the Functional Assessment of Cancer Therapy (FACT) (26). The POMS fatigue and vigor subscales have been used to assess cancer-related fatigue (27–29). The POMS requires patients to rate a list of adjectives on 5-point Likert scales; the vigor subscale consists of eight items and the fatigue subscale consists of seven. Although the POMS was originally designed as a measure of mood in psychiatric outpatients (25), the fatigue subscale displays acceptable reliability and validity for assessment of cancer-related fatigue (27). However, the vigor and fatigue subscales should not be viewed as opposite ends of a continuum, as they are only moderately correlated with one another in cancer patients (28). Unlike the POMS, the fatigue subscale of the FACT (FACT-F) was developed specifically to assess cancer-related fatigue (26). The FACT-F can be used independently (26) or can be administered with the FACT-General scale (FACT-G) (30), which assesses general health-related quality of life. The FACT-F was developed via interviews with cancer patients and clinicians regarding the experience of fatigue (26). Patients rate thirteen fatigue-related concerns on 5-point Likert scales; item responses are summed to produce a single fatigue score. The FACT-F displayed good psychometric properties in two validation studies (26,31). A score of 34 has been proposed as a cutoff for clinically significant fatigue (31).

Alternately, single items allow for very brief assessment of cancer-related fatigue. For instance, fatigue may be assessed using a single item from a larger symptom checklist, such as the Symptom Distress Scale (SDS) (32) or the Rotterdam Symptom Checklist (RSCL) (33). Single-item measures can also be used independently, such as the Rhoten Fatigue Scale (RFS) (34), Linear Analog Scale Assessment (LASA) (35), and the Visual Analog Scale (VAS) (7). Single-item measures are quick, easy to administer, have high face validity, and are useful for screening. However, psychometric properties for single items are not well established.

Instruments Assessing Multiple Dimensions of Fatigue

Although single-dimensional measures are convenient to administer, multidimensional measures enable a more comprehensive assessment of fatigue. In terms of content, they generally fall into two categories: (1) measures that assess duration, severity, and interference of fatigue; and (2) measures that assess domains of fatigue symptoms. As such, multidimensional measures are useful when a more nuanced picture of fatigue is needed. However, they tend to be longer than single-dimensional measures and may be burdensome for patients who are very fatigued or ill.

Examples of multidimensional measures that have been developed to examine fatigue duration, severity, and interference include the Brief Fatigue Inventory (BFI) (36) and the Fatigue Symptom Inventory (FSI) (37,38). The BFI was developed for use with cancer patients as a shorter alternative to other multidimensional measures of fatigue. It consists of nine items and yields information regarding the severity and interference of fatigue. Patients are asked to rate the severity of the worst, average, and current fatigue as well as the extent that fatigue interferes with daily activities in the previous 24 hours. The BFI displays good psychometric properties in cancer samples (36,39) and offers a cutoff score for severe fatigue (36). The FSI was developed to assess the severity and duration of cancer-related fatigue as well as its effect on daily functioning. Patients are asked to rate fatigue in the past week on fourteen Likert-scale items. The FSI displays good reliability and validity in cancer patients (37,38). An advantage of the BFI and FSI is that they do not assume the presence of fatigue, and thus are appropriate for all patients.

Measures developed to assess domains of fatigue symptoms include the Piper Fatigue Scale (PFS) (40,41) and the Multidimensional Fatigue Symptom Inventory (MFSI) (42,43). The PFS measures behavioral/severity, affective meaning, sensory, and cognitive/mood aspects of fatigue (41). The revised version consists of twenty-seven items: five items are qualitative and twenty-two require patients to rate fatigue on 11-point, adjective-anchored Likert scales. Although validity data are published only for the original version, the revised PFS demonstrates good internal consistency in breast and lung cancer patients (41). The PFS has been frequently used in studies of cancer-related fatigue (44–46). It assumes that patients are experiencing fatigue, and thus may not be appropriate for use in all cancer patients. In contrast, the MFSI does not assume the presence of fatigue. It was designed to measure general, physical, emotional, and mental fatigue as well as vigor in cancer patients. Patients are asked to rate the extent to which they experienced 30 symptoms of fatigue during the past week on 5-point Likert scales (42,43). The measure yields five subscale scores and a total score. The MFSI displays good internal consistency and is well-validated in cancer samples (42,43).

MANAGEMENT OF CANCER-RELATED FATIGUE

The consensus-based NCCN Cancer-Related Fatigue Management Guidelines recommend that patients reporting fatigue in the moderate or severe range receive further evaluation and treatment (1). Management of fatigue should occur in two stages: 1) health care professionals should identify and treat contributing factors to fatigue; and 2) residual fatigue should be treated (1). The NCCN has identified seven contributing factors to fatigue: pain, emotional distress, sleep disturbance, anemia, nutrition, activity level, and comorbidities. The complexity of the mechanisms underlying fatigue is reflected in these guidelines, as well as in current management strategies. Interventions target a broad array of possible causes and as a result, multiple interventions may be required to reduce fatigue.

Patient Education and Energy Conservation

Patient education is an important aspect of fatigue management. The focus of patient education is to dispel misconceptions about cancer-related fatigue and to teach behavioral strategies to conserve energy. Energy conservation strategies include delegation, priority setting, pacing, following a daily schedule, and planning energy-intensive activities during times of peak energy. Patients are encouraged to use daily diaries to discern patterns of fatigue and plan activities accordingly (1). Originally developed for use with other chronic conditions such as chronic fatigue syndrome and rheumatoid arthritis (47,48), three clinical trials with cancer patients have shown beneficial effects on fatigue, sleep quality, and mood (49–51).

Exercise Training

Exercise training is one of the best-studied interventions for cancer-related fatigue. It is based on the rationale that patients typically increase sleep and rest behaviors and engage in less activity in response to cancer-related fatigue (5,52). These strategies are largely ineffective (52) and may even contribute to greater fatigue and decreased energy through decreased physical capacity (53). Exercise can reduce or reverse loss of physical capacity (54), which theoretically reduces fatigue by decreasing the effort needed to engage in daily activities. Both supervised (55) and home-based exercise (56) interventions have been examined. Walking (57,58) or cycle ergometers (59), alone or in combination with resistance training (60,61), have been examined most often. Meta-analyses (62–65) suggest that exercise interventions result in improvements on a variety of outcomes, including cardiorespiratory fitness, symptoms/side effects, vigor/vitality, fatigue, and physical functioning. Individual studies have reported additional benefits including better sleep quality (57), improved lean body weight (54), decreased nausea (59), and reduced depression and anxiety (58). Mild- to moderate-intensity exercise is generally well tolerated among cancer patients (64,65), with adherence rates above 70% (58,61,65). While exercise training can help improve physical capacity and quality of life in cancer patients, it should be noted that not all patients are appropriate candidates for exercise. The presence of bone metastases, immunosuppression, neutropenia, thrombocytopenia, and anemia are potential contraindications to exercise (1). Physical therapy may be indicated for individuals who are particularly deconditioned or have significant comorbidities (1).

Psychosocial Intervention

Like exercise training, the effects of psychosocial interventions on cancer-related fatigue have been extensively studied. Both structured and individually-tailored interventions have been examined. Structured interventions typically educate patients on cognitive and behavioral strategies to reduce stress, enhance adaptive coping skills, and/or increase emotional support. They may be self-administered or administered by a clinician. Clinician-administered education and emotional support have been found to limit fatigue in breast cancer patients (46), and coping skills training has been found to reduce fatigue and nausea in patients undergoing BMT (66). Self-administered interventions appear to be a viable alternative to resource-intensive professionally administered interventions. In one clinical trial of chemotherapy patients (67), a self-administered stress management intervention was compared to a professionally-administered stress management intervention and usual care. Patients who received the self-administered intervention but not the professionally-administered intervention reported better outcomes (i.e., physical functioning, vitality, and mental health) than patients who received usual care. These results suggest that outcomes are not compromised by a cost-effective, self-administered format.

Individually-tailored psychosocial interventions typically ask patients to rate the degree to which they are experiencing a list of problems at the beginning of each intervention contact. If the rating meets a threshold criterion, a manualized treatment for that problem is administered. Tailored interventions also show promise in the management of fatigue. For example, Gielissen and colleagues (68) found that tailored, individual cognitive-behavioral therapy resulted in significant improvements in fatigue, functional impairment, and psychological distress in cancer survivors as compared to wait-list controls. Other clinical trials (69,70) have reported beneficial effects of tailored cognitive behavioral therapy on symptoms during chemotherapy, although in one study benefits were not statistically significant (70). Similar to other fatigue management strategies, the mechanisms of action for psychosocial treatments remain unclear.

Treatment of Disrupted Sleep

Sleep disruptions are a natural target for interventions to reduce fatigue. Patients who are fatigued often spend more time resting, but their sleep is commonly disrupted with frequent awakenings (71). Nonpharmacological treatment of insomnia (72–74) targets multiple sleep-related behaviors. Patients are advised to go to bed when sleepy, to go to bed at the same time each night, to rise at the same time each day, to avoid long naps, and to limit time in bed. In addition, it is suggested that patients avoid caffeine late in the day, develop relaxing rituals before bedtime, and establish a dark, quiet, comfortable environment that is conducive to sleep (1). Data suggest that this type of treatment may be efficacious in improving sleep quality, decreasing use of sleep medication, improving mood, reducing fatigue, and enhancing quality of life (73,74).

Pharmacologic Treatment

Pharmacological treatments for fatigue generally take two forms: 1) erythropoiesis-stimulating agents (ESAs) for treatment of anemia; and 2) use of psychostimulants. While ESAs have traditionally been used only for severe anemia (i.e., hemoglobin <10 g/dL) (75), their use has become increasingly common in patients with mild to moderate anemia (76). Increased hemoglobin levels in cancer patients during treatment are associated with decreases in fatigue and improvements in quality of life (75). However, the Food and Drug Administration recently issued a warning regarding potential adverse effects of ESAs in cancer patients who are not receiving them for treatment of chemotherapy-related anemia (77). Accordingly, future use of ESAs in the management of fatigue is uncertain.

Psychostimulants have been less frequently used to manage fatigue, due in part to concerns over side effects (78). Methylphenidate has been used to treat opioid-induced somnolence (79) and improve mood (80) and cognitive functioning (80) in cancer patients. Evidence is conflicting regarding the effects of psychostimulants on cancer-related fatigue. In an open-label study (81), methylphenidate was associated with a 30% reduction in mean fatigue in patients with advanced cancer. However, a double-blind, randomized clinical trial (82) of methylphenidate did not result in significant differences in fatigue between groups. Consequently, NCCN Guidelines for the Treatment of Cancer-Related Fatigue (1) note that evidence for psychostimulants is currently insufficient to recommend their use.

Complementary Therapies

Although research examining the effects of complementary therapies on fatigue is still in its infancy, data suggest that massage, acupuncture, and yoga may be beneficial. For example, massage appears to be associated with transient reductions in fatigue. In an observational study (83) comparing symptoms before and after massage sessions, treatment resulted in a 43% reduction in fatigue. Benefits were temporary in inpatients, returning to baseline scores in two to five hours (83). Benefits were stronger and more persistent in outpatients, remaining lower than baseline during the 48-hour follow-up period (83). In addition, a clinical trial (84) in patients receiving autologous BMT found that patients who received massage reported greater reductions in fatigue over time than patients in standard care. Acupuncture is also associated with reductions in fatigue. A single-group design (85) was conducted with patients who had completed adjuvant treatment but continued to report severe fatigue. Patients received acupuncture twice a week for four weeks or once a week for six weeks. At two-week follow-up, there was a 31% mean reduction in fatigue. Finally, yoga has been found to improve quality of life across a number of domains. Data from two clinical trials (86,87) suggest significant improvements in sleep quality, mood, and quality of life relative to controls.

SUMMARY

The prevalence of cancer-related fatigue and its debilitating effects on quality of life argue for intensive efforts to accurately assess and aggressively manage it. Significant advances have been made in defining and identifying cancer-related fatigue. To this end, both single-dimensional and multidimensional measures of fatigue have been developed. Clinicians and researchers interested in brief screening for fatigue may wish to choose a single-dimensional measure, such as the LASA or FACT-F. If a more extensive or nuanced picture of fatigue is desired, measures such as the FSI, BFI, MFSI, and PFS have been shown to be both reliable and valid in cancer samples. Factors precipitating and perpetuating cancer-related fatigue are complex and further research is needed to determine the relative influences of disease, treatment, cognitive, behavioral, and other factors. A better understanding of fatigue may help to drive the development of new interventions. To date, exercise training and cognitive-behavioral treatments have shown the greatest efficacy in managing fatigue and deconditioning. Other treatments, such as psychostimulants, patient education and energy conservation, and complementary therapies may also prove beneficial with further research. In sum, just as the causes and symptoms of cancer-related fatigue are multifaceted, so too are effective assessment and treatment strategies.

REFERENCES

1. NCCN. Clinical Practice Guidelines in Oncology: Cancer-Related Fatigue. 2007 (Accessed March 22, 2007, at http://www.nccn.org/professionals/physician_gls/PDF/fatigue.pdf).
2. Poulson MJ. Not just tired. J Clin Oncol 2001; 19(21):4180–4181.
3. Glaus A, Crow R, Hammond S. A qualitative study to explore the concept of fatigue/tiredness in cancer patients and in healthy individuals. Eur J Cancer Care 1996; 5 (2 suppl):8–23.
4. Cella D, Davis K, Breitbart W, et al. Cancer-related fatigue: prevalence of proposed diagnostic criteria in a United States sample of cancer survivors. J Clin Oncol 2001; 19(14):3385–3391.

5. Rhodes VA, Watson PM, Hanson BM. Patients' descriptions of the influence of tiredness and weakness on self-care abilities. Cancer Nurs 1988; 11(3):186–194.
6. Baker F, Denniston M, Smith T, et al. Adult cancer survivors: how are they faring? Cancer 2005; 104(11 suppl):2565–2576.
7. Geinitz H, Zimmermann FB, Thamm R, et al. Fatigue in patients with adjuvant radiation therapy for breast cancer: long-term follow-up. J Cancer Res Clin Oncol 2004; 130(6):327–333.
8. Jacobsen PB, Donovan KA, Weitzner MA. Distinguishing fatigue and depression in patients with cancer. Sem Clin Neuropsychiatry 2003; 8(4):229–240.
9. Jacobsen PB, Andrykowski MA, Thors CL. Relationship of catastrophizing to fatigue among women receiving treatment for breast cancer. J Consult Clin Psychol 2004; 72(2):355–361.
10. Jacobsen PB, Hann DM, Azzarello LM, et al. Fatigue in women receiving adjuvant chemotherapy for breast cancer: characteristics, course, and correlates. J Pain Symptom Manage 1999; 18(4):233–242.
11. Broeckel JA, Jacobsen PB, Horton J, et al. Characteristics and correlates of fatigue after adjuvant chemotherapy for breast cancer. J Clin Oncol 1998; 16(5):1689–1696.
12. Hann DM, Jacobsen PB, Martin SC, et al. Fatigue in women treated with bone marrow transplantation for breast cancer: a comparison with women with no history of cancer. Support Care Cancer 1997; 5(1):44–52.
13. Greenberg DB, Sawicka J, Eisenthal S, et al. Fatigue syndrome due to localized radiation. J Pain Symptom Manage 1992; 7(1):38–45.
14. Hann DM, Jacobsen P, Martin S, et al. Fatigue and quality of life following radiotherapy for breast cancer: a comparative study. J Clin Psychol Med Settings 1998; 5(1):19–33.
15. Stone P, Richards M, A'Hern R, et al. A study to investigate the prevalence, severity and correlates of fatigue among patients with cancer in comparison with a control group of volunteers without cancer. Ann Oncol 2000; 11(5):561–567.
16. Stone P, Hardy J, Broadley K, et al. Fatigue in advanced cancer: a prospective controlled cross-sectional study. Br J Cancer 1999; 79(9–10):1479–1486.
17. Cella D, Peterman A, Passik S, et al. Progress toward guidelines for the management of fatigue. Oncology 1998; 12(11A):369–377.
18. Stasi R, Abriani L, Beccaglia P, et al. Cancer-related fatigue: evolving concepts in evaluation and treatment. Cancer 2003; 98(9):1786–1801.
19. Gutstein HB. The biologic basis of fatigue. Cancer 2001; 92(6 suppl):1678–1683.
20. Groopman JE, Itri LM. Chemotherapy-induced anemia in adults: incidence and treatment. J Natl Cancer Inst 1999; 91(19):1616–1634.
21. Bower JE, Ganz PA, Aziz N, et al. Fatigue and proinflammatory cytokine activity in breast cancer survivors. Psychosom Med 2002; 64(4):604–611.
22. Cella D. Factors influencing quality of life in cancer patients: anemia and fatigue. Sem Oncol 1998; 25(3 suppl 7):43–46.
23. Roscoe JA, Morrow GR, Hickok JT, et al. Temporal interrelationships among fatigue, circadian rhythm and depression in breast cancer patients undergoing chemotherapy treatment. Support Care Cancer 2002; 10(4):329–336.
24. Alberts M, Vercoulen JHMM, Bleijenberg G. Assessment of fatigue: the practical utility of the subjective feeling of fatigue in research and clinical practice. In: Vingerhoets A, ed. Assessment in Behavioral Medicine. New York: Taylor & Francis, 2001:301–328.

25. McNair PM, Lorr M, Droppleman LF. POMS Manual, 2 ed.San Diego: Educational and Industrial Testing Service, 1981.
26. Yellen SB, Cella DF, Webster K, et al. Measuring fatigue and other anemia-related symptoms with the Functional Assessment of Cancer Therapy (FACT) measurement system. J Pain Symptom Manage 1997; 13(2):63–74.
27. Meek PM, Nail LM, Barsevick A, et al. Psychometric testing of fatigue instruments for use with cancer patients. Nurs Res 2000; 49(4):181–190.
28. Schwartz AL, Nail LM, Chen S, et al. Fatigue patterns observed in patients receiving chemotherapy and radiotherapy. Cancer Invest 2000; 18(1):11–19.
29. Brown P, Clark MM, Atherton P, et al. Will improvement in quality of life (QOL) impact fatigue in patients receiving radiation therapy for advanced cancer? Am J Clin Oncol 2006; 29(1):52–58.
30. Cella DF, Tulsky DS, Gray G, et al. The Functional Assessment of Cancer Therapy scale: development and validation of the general measure. J Clin Oncol 1993; 11(3): 570–579.
31. Van Belle S, Paridaens R, Evers G, et al. Comparison of proposed diagnostic criteria with FACT-F and VAS for cancer-related fatigue: proposal for use as a screening tool. Support Care Cancer 2005; 13(4):246–254.
32. McCorkle R, Young K. Development of a symptom distress scale. Cancer Nurs 1978; 1(5):373–378.
33. de Haes JC, van Knippenberg FC, Neijt JP. Measuring psychological and physical distress in cancer patients: structure and application of the Rotterdam Symptom Checklist. Br J Cancer 1990; 62(6):1034–1038.
34. Rhoten D. Fatigue and the postsurgical patient. In: Norris C, ed. Concept Clarification in Nursing. Rockville, MD: Aspen, 1982:277–300.
35. Butow P, Coates A, Dunn S, et al. On the receiving end. IV: Validation of quality of life indicators. Ann Oncol 1991; 2(8):597–603.
36. Mendoza TR, Wang XS, Cleeland CS, et al. The rapid assessment of fatigue severity in cancer patients: use of the Brief Fatigue Inventory. Cancer 1999; 85(5): 1186–1196.
37. Hann DM, Jacobsen PB, Azzarello LM, et al. Measurement of fatigue in cancer patients: development and validation of the Fatigue Symptom Inventory. Qual Life Res 1998; 7(4):301–310.
38. Hann DM, Denniston MM, Baker F. Measurement of fatigue in cancer patients: further validation of the Fatigue Symptom Inventory. Qual Life Res 2000; 9(7): 847–854.
39. Hwang SS, Chang VT, Cogswell J, et al. Clinical relevance of fatigue levels in cancer patients at a Veterans Administration Medical Center. Cancer 2002; 94(9): 2481–2489.
40. Piper BF, Lindsey AM, Dodd MJ, et al. The development of an instrument to measure the subjective dimension of fatigue. In: Funk SG, Tournquist EM, Champagne MT, Copp LA, Weise RA, eds. Key aspects of comfort: Management of pain, fatigue, and nausea. New York: Springer, 1989:199–208.
41. Piper BF, Dibble SL, Dodd MJ, et al. The revised Piper Fatigue Scale: psychometric evaluation in women with breast cancer. Oncol Nurs Forum 1998; 25(4):677–684.
42. Stein KD, Jacobsen PB, Blanchard CM, et al. Further validation of the multidimensional fatigue symptom inventory-short form. J Pain Symptom Manage 2004; 27(1):14–23.

43. Stein KD, Martin SC, Hann DM, et al. A multidimensional measure of fatigue for use with cancer patients. Cancer Pract 1998; 6(3):143–152.
44. Berger AM, Farr LA, Kuhn BR, et al. Values of sleep/wake, activity/rest, circadian rhythms, and fatigue prior to adjuvant breast cancer chemotherapy. J Pain Symptom Manage 2007; 33(4):398–409.
45. de Jong N, Candel MJ, Schouten HC, et al. Course of the fatigue dimension "activity level" and the interference of fatigue with daily living activities for patients with breast cancer receiving adjuvant chemotherapy. Cancer Nurs 2006; 29(5): E1–E13.
46. Yates P, Aranda S, Hargraves M, et al. Randomized controlled trial of an educational intervention for managing fatigue in women receiving adjuvant chemotherapy for early-stage breast cancer. J Clin Oncol 2005; 23(25):6027–6036.
47. Friedberg F, Krupp LB. A comparison of cognitive behavioral treatment for chronic fatigue syndrome and primary depression. Clin Infect Dis 1994; 18(suppl 1):S105–S110.
48. Furst GP, Gerber LH, Smith CC, et al. A program for improving energy conservation behaviors in adults with rheumatoid arthritis. Am J Occup Ther 1987; 41(2):102–111.
49. Barsevick AM, Dudley W, Beck S, et al. A randomized clinical trial of energy conservation for patients with cancer-related fatigue. Cancer 2004; 100(6):1302–1310.
50. Kim Y, Roscoe JA, Morrow GR. The effects of information and negative affect on severity of side effects from radiation therapy for prostate cancer. Support Care Cancer 2002; 10(5):416–421.
51. Ream E, Richardson A, Alexander-Dann C. Supportive intervention for fatigue in patients undergoing chemotherapy: a randomized controlled trial. J Pain Symptom Manage 2006; 31(2):148–161.
52. Richardson A, Ream EK. Self-care behaviours initiated by chemotherapy patients in response to fatigue. Int J Nurs Stud 1997; 34(1):35–43.
53. Ahlberg K, Ekman T, Gaston-Johansson F, et al. Assessment and management of cancer-related fatigue in adults. Lancet 2003; 362(9384):640–650.
54. Courneya KS, Friedenreich CM, Sela RA, et al. The group psychotherapy and home-based physical exercise (group-hope) trial in cancer survivors: physical fitness and quality of life outcomes. Psychooncology 2003; 12(4):357–374.
55. Dimeo FC, Stieglitz RD, Novelli-Fischer U, et al. Effects of physical activity on the fatigue and psychologic status of cancer patients during chemotherapy. Cancer 1999; 85(10):2273–2277.
56. Pinto BM, Frierson GM, Rabin C, et al. Home-based physical activity intervention for breast cancer patients. J Clin Oncol 2005; 23(15):3577–3587.
57. Mock V, Burke MB, Sheehan P, et al. A nursing rehabilitation program for women with breast cancer receiving adjuvant chemotherapy. Oncol Nurs Forum 1994; 21(5): 899–907; discussion 8.
58. Segal R, Evans W, Johnson D, et al. Structured exercise improves physical functioning in women with stages I and II breast cancer: results of a randomized controlled trial. J Clin Oncol 2001; 19(3):657–665.
59. Winningham ML, MacVicar MG. The effect of aerobic exercise on patient reports of nausea. Oncol Nurs Forum 1988; 15(4):447–450.
60. Coleman EA, Hall-Barrow J, Coon S, et al. Facilitating exercise adherence for patients with multiple myeloma. Clin J Oncol Nurs 2003; 7(5):529–534, 540.

61. Nieman DC, Cook VD, Henson DA, et al. Moderate exercise training and natural killer cell cytotoxic activity in breast cancer patients. Int J Sports Med 1995; 16(5): 334–337.
62. McNeely ML, Campbell KL, Rowe BH, et al. Effects of exercise on breast cancer patients and survivors: a systematic review and meta-analysis. CMAJ 2006; 175(1): 34–41.
63. Conn VS, Hafdahl AR, Porock DC, et al. A meta-analysis of exercise interventions among people treated for cancer. Support Care Cancer 2006; 14(7):699–712.
64. Stevinson C, Lawlor DA, Fox KR. Exercise interventions for cancer patients: systematic review of controlled trials. Cancer Causes Control 2004; 15(10):1035–1056.
65. Schmitz KH, Holtzman J, Courneya KS, et al. Controlled physical activity trials in cancer survivors: a systematic review and meta-analysis. Cancer Epidemiol Biomarkers Prev 2005; 14(7):1588–1595.
66. Gaston-Johansson F, Fall-Dickson JM, Nanda J, et al. The effectiveness of the comprehensive coping strategy program on clinical outcomes in breast cancer autologous bone marrow transplantation. Cancer Nurs 2000; 23(4):277–285.
67. Jacobsen PB, Meade CD, Stein KD, et al. Efficacy and costs of two forms of stress management training for cancer patients undergoing chemotherapy. J Clin Oncol 2002; 20(12):2851–2862.
68. Gielissen MF, Verhagen S, Witjes F, et al. Effects of cognitive behavior therapy in severely fatigued disease-free cancer patients compared with patients waiting for cognitive behavior therapy: a randomized controlled trial. J Clin Oncol 2006; 24(30): 4882–4887.
69. Given C, Given B, Rahbar M, et al. Effect of a cognitive behavioral intervention on reducing symptom severity during chemotherapy. J Clin Oncol 2004; 22(3):507–516.
70. Given B, Given CW, McCorkle R, et al. Pain and fatigue management: results of a nursing randomized clinical trial. Oncol Nurs Forum 2002; 29(6):949–956.
71. Berger AM, Farr L. The influence of daytime inactivity and nighttime restlessness on cancer-related fatigue. Oncol Nurs Forum 1999; 26(10):1663–1671.
72. Savard J, Morin CM. Insomnia in the context of cancer: a review of a neglected problem. J Clin Oncol 2001; 19(3):895–908.
73. Savard J, Simard S, Ivers H, et al. Randomized study on the efficacy of cognitive-behavioral therapy for insomnia secondary to breast cancer, part II: Immunologic effects. J Clin Oncol 2005; 23(25):6097–6106.
74. Quesnel C, Savard J, Simard S, et al. Efficacy of cognitive-behavioral therapy for insomnia in women treated for nonmetastatic breast cancer. J Consult Clin Psychol 2003; 71(1):189–200.
75. Crawford J, Cella D, Cleeland CS, et al. Relationship between changes in hemoglobin level and quality of life during chemotherapy in anemic cancer patients receiving epoetin alfa therapy. Cancer 2002; 95(4):888–895.
76. Straus DJ, Testa MA, Sarokhan BJ, et al. Quality-of-life and health benefits of early treatment of mild anemia: a randomized trial of epoetin alfa in patients receiving chemotherapy for hematologic malignancies. Cancer 2006; 107(8):1909–1917.
77. Information for Healthcare Professionals Erythropoiesis Stimulating Agents (ESA) [Aranesp (darbepoetin), Epogen (epoetin alfa), and Procrit (epoetin alfa)], Feburary 16, 2007 (Accessed May 9, 2007, at http://www.fda.gov/cder/drug/InfoSheets/HCP/RHE2007HCP.htm)

78. Alert for Healthcare Professionals Pemoline Tablets and Chewable Tablets (marketed as Cylert), October 24, 2005 (Accessed May 9, 2007, at http://www.fda.gov/cder/drug/InfoSheets/HCP/pemolineHCP.htm)
79. Bruera E, Chadwick S, Brenneis C, et al. Methylphenidate associated with narcotics for the treatment of cancer pain. Cancer Treat Rep 1987; 71(1):67–70.
80. Meyers CA, Weitzner MA, Valentine AD, et al. Methylphenidate therapy improves cognition, mood, and function in brain tumor patients. J Clin Oncol 1998; 16(7): 2522–2527.
81. Sugawara Y, Akechi T, Shima Y, et al. Efficacy of methylphenidate for fatigue in advanced cancer patients: a preliminary study. Palliat Med 2002; 16(3):261–263.
82. Bruera E, Valero V, Driver L, et al. Patient-controlled methylphenidate for cancer fatigue: a double-blind, randomized, placebo-controlled trial. J Clin Oncol 2006; 24(13):2073–2078.
83. Cassileth BR, Vickers AJ. Massage therapy for symptom control: outcome study at a major cancer center. J Pain Symptom Manage 2004; 28(3):244–249.
84. Ahles TA, Tope DM, Pinkson B, et al. Massage therapy for patients undergoing autologous bone marrow transplantation. J Pain Symptom Manage 1999; 18(3): 157–163.
85. Vickers AJ, Straus DJ, Fearon B, et al. Acupuncture for postchemotherapy fatigue: a phase II study. J Clin Oncol 2004; 22(9):1731–1735.
86. Cohen L, Warneke C, Fouladi RT, et al. Psychological adjustment and sleep quality in a randomized trial of the effects of a Tibetan yoga intervention in patients with lymphoma. Cancer 2004; 100(10):2253–2260.
87. Culos-Reed SN, Carlson LE, Daroux LM, et al. A pilot study of yoga for breast cancer survivors: physical and psychological benefits. Psychooncology 2006; 15(10): 891–897.

3

Anemia and Red Cell Factors

John Glaspy
*Division of Hematology-Oncology,
Department of Medicine, UCLA School of
Medicine, Los Angeles, California, U.S.A.*

INTRODUCTION

Anemia is the most common hematological abnormality observed in cancer patients. Its consequences include a reduction in oxygen delivery to the tissues, a decline in functional status and quality of life, and an increase in the frequency of red blood cell transfusions. The primary regulator of erythropoiesis in humans, erythropoietin, was one of the first human proteins cloned and developed for clinical application. Recombinant erythropoietin (rEPO) transformed the management of anemia in several settings, including that occurring during cancer chemotherapy. Determining the optimal management of anemia in this setting has proven to be more challenging than was initially assumed and the field continues to evolve rapidly as additional data relevant to the pathophysiology of anemia and the benefits and safety or treatment are developed.

BACKGROUND: THE PREVALENCE AND PATHOPHYSIOLOGY OF ANEMIA IN ONCOLOGY

Anemia is observed frequently in cancer patients (1), and is multifactorial, with contributing factors including general malnutrition or specific nutritional deficiencies of iron, folate, or vitamin B_{12}, bleeding, hemolysis, myelosuppressive chemotherapy (2), radiation to bone marrow, and, most importantly, the anemia of chronic disease (ACD). B-cell malignancies and malignancies with extensive involvement of the marrow disrupt the interactions of erythroid progenitors with the marrow microenvironment that support and regulate hematopoiesis. Not infrequently, modest renal insufficiency related to comorbid illnesses or paraproteins is a factor in the anemia. In the important special case of myelodysplasia, the hematopoietic stem cells themselves are reduced in number and ineffective as progenitors.

The most important recent advance in our understanding of the biology of anemia in patients with cancer has been the elucidation of the molecular biology of chronic inflammatory illness as it relates to iron kinetics. Initially, it was recognized that a decreased endogenous erythropoietin response to anemia is frequent in patients with chronic illnesses such as cancer (3). Subsequently, it has been shown that inflammation is associated with increased production of the iron-regulatory peptide, hepcidin, by the liver (4–7). Hepcidin binds to and inactivates ferroportin, the transporter required for transfer of iron across cell membranes, thereby impairing both absorption of dietary iron and access to storage iron pools in the reticuloendothelial system (8,9). This biology indicates that the central cause of the anemia observed in patients with chronic illnesses such as cancer is the combined effects of relative erythropoietin deficiency and erythropoiesis that is iron restricted despite the presence of adequate, though inadequately accessible, body iron stores. Placed in the larger context of the multiple contributing factors, our current understanding of the biology of anemia in cancer patients is shown schematically in Figure 1, together with potential strategies for intervention.

MANAGEMENT OF ANEMIA DURING CANCER CHEMOTHERAPY

It is not well appreciated that anemia in cancer patients is frequently due to reversible factors such as iron loss in surgery, bleeding, or unsuspected nutritional deficiencies. In one recent study, 5% of anemic cancer chemotherapy patients being evaluated for eligibility for a clinical trial were found upon screening to have decreased serum vitamin B_{12} concentrations (10). Historically, the only available treatments for anemic cancer patients without these easily reversible causes were red cell transfusions and, ultimately, successful eradication of the underlying malignancy. Transfusions have risks, and the available blood supply is limited. Appropriately, prior to the introduction of erythropoiesis stimulating agents (ESAs), anemia treatment was reserved for patients with severe anemia (hemoglobin levels 8 g/dL or lower) or ominous cardiovascular symptoms, such as chest pain or dyspnea at rest.

The Erythropoietic Agents

The primary regulator of red cell production in mammals is the glycoprotein erythropoietin. The cloning, introduction into clinical use of rEPO represented a watershed in anemia management, initially in nephrology and later in oncology.

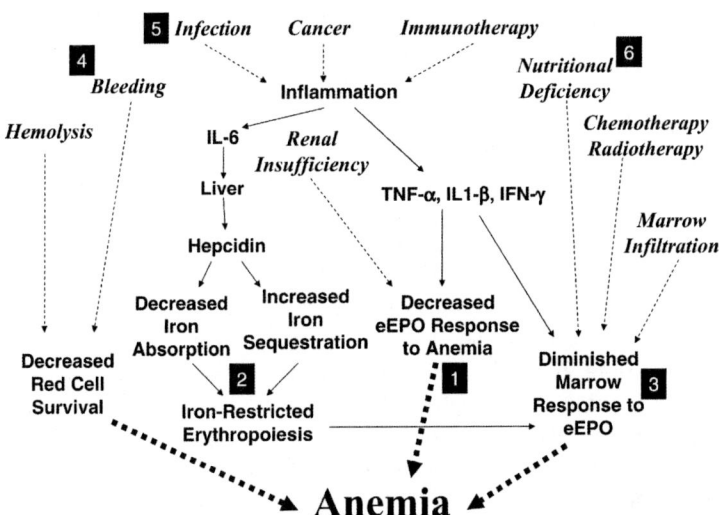

Figure 1 The biology of anemia in patients receiving cancer chemotherapy and potential interventions. Type I cytokines promote a decrease in the endogenous EPO response to anemia and directly suppress the marrow. Type II inflammatory cytokines induce hepcidin production by the liver, which decreases both gastrointestinal absorption of iron and accessibility of storage iron. Potential sites for interventions are shown in numbered black boxes: (1) erythropoietic agents or stabilizers of hypoxia-inducible factor (HIF), (2) parenteral iron, (3) possibly HIF stabilizers, (4) address bleeding, (5) treat infections, (6) improve nutritional status. *Abbreviations*: eEPO, endogenous erythropoietin; TNF-α, tumor necrosis factor alpha; IL1-β, interleukin-1 beta; IFN-α, interferon gamma; IL-6, interleukin-6. *Source*: Adapted from Glaspy, in Abeloff, et. al. Clinical Oncology.

Two preparations are available in the United States, epoetin alfa and the hyper-gycosylated rEPO, darbepoetin alfa (11), which has a longer half life. Additional agents are available outside the United States or are under development (12). In randomized, placebo-controlled trials carried out in anemic cancer patients receiving chemotherpy, both epoetin alfa (13–17) and darbepoetin alfa (18,19) were shown to increase hemoglobin levels and reduce red cell transfusion rates. Both ESAs are approved by the Food and Drug Administration for this indication.

Fatigue is a common complaint of cancer patients. Two large patient surveys have demonstrated that fatigue is often the dominant symptom in cancer patients, limiting functional status and decreasing quality of life (20,21). This fatigue is clearly multifactorial, with contributions from local and systemic effects of the tumor, treatment toxicities, depression, malnutrition, and sleep disturbances. For years, it remained an open question whether the anemia that was frequent in cancer patients was contributing to this fatigue, and to what degree.

Once there was an alternative to transfusions for increasing hemoglobin levels in cancer patients with anemia that was not due to an easily reversible cause, it became feasible to explore the effects of moderate degrees of anemia on cancer patients and their reported fatigue levels. Previous data had suggested that anemia, even when of mild or moderate magnitude, can impair functional status and productivity in healthy adults (22). When rEPO was used to treat anemia in patients with chronic renal failure, it was found that quality of life improved when hemoglobin levels increased, even at hemoglobin levels above traditional transfusion threshold (23–26). Similar findings were subsequently reported in anemic cancer chemotherapy patients treated with ESAs (13,17,27–41). Not surprisingly, comparisons of results from studies of ESAs for anemia treatment in dialysis patients to those in cancer patients demonstrated that the benefits of treatment in terms of improved quality of life and energy level were similar in the two settings (42). To explore the relationship of each specific 1 g increase in hemoglobin to energy level and patient-reported quality of life, data from two large community-based observational trials of epoetin alfa for chemotherapy-induced anemia (30,43) were subjected to an analysis using an incremental gain model (44). The results demonstrated that larger incremental improvements in patient-reported outcomes were observed with hemoglobin increases from 11 to 12 g/dL than with any other 1 g increase. It is tempting to dichotomize the two benefits, transfusion reduction and symptom relief, of ESAs for anemic cancer chemotherapy patients. In fact, the two are not separable. A significant proportion of the red cell transfusions given to cancer patients in the United States are given in response to symptoms rather than for a specific hemoglobin trigger level. Transfusions and patient-reported outcomes are two aspects of the same endpoint, with transfusions being a conveniently quantifiable reflection of a physician's and patient's assessment of the magnitude of anemia symptoms, and it is not surprising that effective anemia intervention affects both.

Both of the available ESAs are currently utilized for the treatment of anemia in patients with cancer receiving chemotherapy. Randomized trials to date have failed to demonstrate that either agent is superior in terms of transfusion prevention or fatigue reduction when utilized at starting doses of epoetin alfa of 40,000 U/wk and darbepoetin alfa of 200 µg every two weeks (45,46). Darbepoetin alfa is effective for the treatment of chemotherapy-associated anemia when given every three weeks at doses of either 300 µg (47) or 500 µg (48); dosing by this schedule on the same day as chemotherapy is as effective as asynchronous dosing (49). Studies utilizing initial weekly dosing of epoetin alfa followed by every three weeks at a dose of 120,000 U have demonstrated that this schedule is also feasible (50). There is little evidence that higher doses of either ESP result in improved responses for cancer patients. Although the problems of nonresponse and hyporesponse remain significant challenges in chemotherapy patients, the common practice, supported by FDA labeling, of increasing dose in this setting has never been studied in randomized trials and its benefit, if any, is unknown.

Anemia and Red Cell Factors

At least three other rEPO preparations are in use in other parts of the world and several erythropoietic agents, including pegylated peptides, small-molecule erythropoietin receptor (EPO-R) agonists, and hypoxia inducible factor (HIF) stabilizers are under development (12). At present, in the United States, epoetin alfa and darbepoetin alfa are the two erythropoietic agents available to treat anemia during cancer chemotherapy.

When to Intervene

Weeks are usually required for ESAs to increase hemoglobin levels and there is a role for red cell transfusion for acute intervention in severe anemia with ominous symptoms. Hence, when a patient's hemoglobin has already fallen by 2 to 3 g/dL and further chemotherapy is planned, the risk that patient will require transfusion if ESA therapy is not initiated is very high. When intervention is withheld until the hemoglobin level is less than 10 g/dL, some ultimately responsive patients will require transfusions for management of severe anemia or symptoms before they respond to treatment (Fig. 2). Several trials have approached the question of early versus late intervention, and taken in aggregated the results strongly suggest that later intervention is associated with a significant increase in transfusion risk (51). Additionally, later intervention results in more fatigue. Recent guidelines by the National Comprehensive Cancer Network (52) and the European Organization for

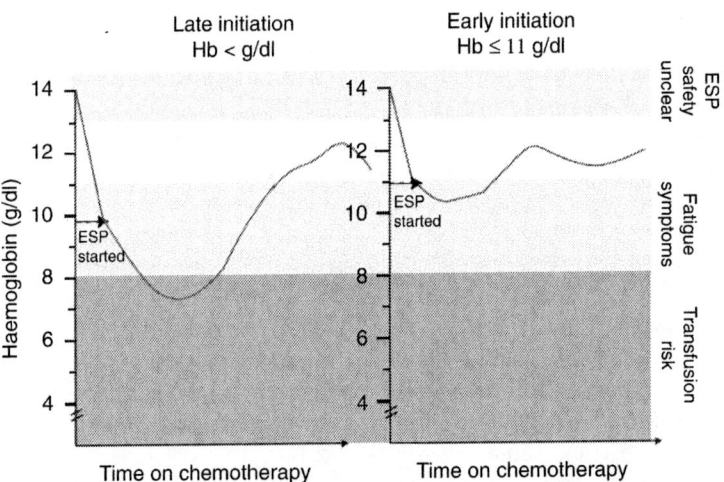

Figure 2 The theoretical paradigm supporting earlier intervention with erythropoiesis stimulating proteins in anemic cancer patients scheduled to receive additional chemotherapy. When intervention is withheld until the hemoglobin is less than 10 g/dL, the risk of a red cell transfusion before a response occurs will be higher, and patients will be more symptomatic for long, reducing the cost effectiveness of the agents. *Source*: Adapted from Ref. 12.

Research and Treatment of Cancer (EORTC) (53) supported the initiation of treatment when hemoglobin levels fall to 11 g/dL, especially when symptoms are present and continued chemotherapy is planned. However, recent concerns regarding the safety of ESAs in cancer patients (see below) have resulted in restrictive reimbursement policies that will make early intervention less feasible, at least until further analyses of safety data are available.

Once ESP treatment is initiated, it should be continued, with dose or frequency adjusted to maintain a hemoglobin level of ≤ 12 g/dL. The safety of targeting higher hemoglobin levels has not been demonstrated (see below). This titrated treatment should be continued until the chemotherapy is completed and hemoglobin levels remain in the target range without ESA support.

Entering the Iron Age

One of the most vexing challenges for ESA therapy in oncology has been the relative resistance of anemia in this setting to ESA treatment, a significant proportion (approximately 35% of patients) do not respond when treated, and those who do respond require doses approximately threefold higher than the effective doses in the dialysis setting. The recent advances in our understanding of the biology of the anemia of chronic illness (Fig. 1) has provided a potential explanation and a promising future. When patients are treated with ESAs, evidence of iron-restricted erythropoiesis often develops, even in the presence of apparently adequate body iron stores (54). This phenomenon, caused by an inability to mobilize storage iron in sufficient quantities to support the accelerated erythropoiesis associated with treatment, has been termed functional iron deficiency (FID) to distinguish it from absolute iron deficiency, which refers to diminished body stores. The limited quantity of oral iron that can be absorbed on a daily basis and the poor compliance with oral iron makes parenteral iron an attractive option for reversing FID during ESA treatment. In the setting of chronic renal failure and dialysis, treatment with parenteral iron is now commonly used with ESAs and appears to decrease the ESA dose required (55). Early preparations of iron dextran were associated with infrequent but potentially life-threatening anaphylactic reactions and made parenteral iron relatively unattractive and infrequently administered. The introduction of low-molecular-weight dextran preparations and the iron salts, ferric gluconate, and ferric succrate are relatively safe (56–59). Current parenteral iron preparations and practical aspects of their use are summarized in Table 1.

We now know that chronic illness is associated with diminished absorption of oral iron and decreased accessibility of body iron stores. When patients in whom this biology is relevant are treated with ESAs, the increased iron demand of the erythron results in a significant degree of FID. This may explain at least part of the relative resistance to ESAs observed in patients with inflammatory illnesses such as cancer. A few studies have now addressed the effect of parenteral iron on response to ESAs in anemic cancer patients during chemotherapy. In one randomized study, iron

Table 1 Currently Available Parenteral Iron Preparations and Practical Aspects of Their Use

	Low-molecular-weight iron dextran	Iron saccharate	Ferric gluconate	High-molecular-weight iron dextran
Test dose required	Yes	No	No	Yes
Vial volume (mL)	2	5	5	1–2
Iron per vial (mg/mL)	50	20	12.5	50
Black box warning	Yes	No	No	Yes
Total dose infusion	Yes	No	No	Yes
Premedication	TDI only	No	No	TDI only
Preservative	None	None	Benzyl alcohol	None
Molecular weight measured by manufacturer (Da)	165,000	34,000–60,000	289,000–440,000	265,000

Abbreviation: TDI, total dose infusion.

dextran, given either as a weekly fixed dose of 100 mg of elemental iron or as a single total dose infusion of the calculated iron deficit, was associated with a significantly better response to epoetin alfa than that observed with either oral iron or no iron (60). Similar results have now been reported in trials utilizing ferric gluconate (10) and darbepoetin alfa. These data strongly suggest that parenteral iron will play a substantially greater role in the future in the management of anemia in cancer patients and patients with other inflammatory illnesses (61,62).

For iron support during ESA treatment in oncology to be rational, methods for the reliable detection of iron-restricted erythropoiesis will need to be developed. The anemia of chronic illness is associated with reductions in serum iron and iron binding capacity and chronic illness itself frequently causes increases in serum ferritin levels, rendering transferrin saturation and ferritin determinations less reliable indicators of adequate iron delivery to the marrow or of body iron stores (63). Serum levels of soluble transferrin receptors are normal in patients with the ACD and increased in patients with iron deficiency anemia and might be useful in distinguishing the two conditions, at least prior to any therapy (64). Unfortunately, this laboratory test is not widely available and levels are increased by ESA treatment and fluctuate during the chemotherapy cycle, making this test much less useful for monitoring iron supply to the marrow in cancer patients during ESP therapy. Similar limitations exist for the transferrin receptor to ferritin ratio (65–67). Two promising parameters that can be determined using flow cytometric techniques available in some hemogram autoanalyzers are the percentage of hypochromic red cells (68–70) and the reticulocyte hemoglobin content (69,71–75). The relationship of these parameters with iron delivery to the marrow is not affected by the cytokine milieu of chronic disease, ESP therapy, or chemotherapy, and both have been shown to be useful in guiding iron therapy in patients with renal failure receiving ESP therapy. When the proportion of red cells with a hemoglobin concentration of less than 28 g/dL exceeds 5% it is concluded that there has been iron deficient erythropoiesis during the preceding two weeks. When the reticulocyte hemoglobin content is less than 29 pg, iron-deficient erythropoiesis occurs during the preceding two days. These two tests should become more widely available for monitoring iron delivery during ESA treatment of chemotherapy-induced anemia. Until they are available, it is rational to consider parenteral iron therapy whenever the transferrin saturation is less than 25% to 30% or when the response to ESA therapy is inadequate.

Treatment of Anemia in Cancer Patients Not Receiving Chemotherapy

Because cancer patients not receiving chemotherapy do not have the myelosuppressive effects of ongoing marrow toxic treatment, it would be logical to assume that they would be more likely to benefit from ESA treatment for anemia than patients receiving chemotherapy. The results of earlier randomized clinical trials in this setting demonstrated that ESA therapy is associated with an increase in hemoglobin concentration and appears to be well tolerated, although no randomized trial had sufficiently documented a statistically significant reduction in red blood cell transfusion rates (76,77). Recently, the results of a well-powered, randomized, placebo-controlled trial of darbepoetin alfa for anemic cancer patients not receiving chemotherapy that enrolled 985 patients were reported (78). Darbepoetin therapy was associated with increases in hemoglobin concentration, but did not achieve its endpoint of documenting a statistically significant reduction in transfusion risk. More importantly, a decreased survival was observed in the darbepoetin group (hazard ratio = 1.29). Although the survival disparity was not observed in all patient subsets in this heterogeneous population and there were baseline disparities in prognostic factors favoring survival in the placebo group, the safety of ESAs for anemia in cancer patients not receiving chemotherapy has not been established and these agents should not be routinely used to treat anemia in this setting until safety has been established.

Myelodysplastic Syndrome

For the anemia that occurs in these patients, both rEPO (79–87) and darbepoetin alfa (88–91) have been shown to increase hemoglobin levels or reduce transfusion requirements in 30% to 60% of patients with low or intermediate-1 stage disease. There is some evidence that simultaneous administration of a myeloid growth factor may enhance erythropoietic response (92–99), although the cost effectiveness of this approach has been questioned (100). It is reasonable to treat a patient with either transfusion-dependent or symptomatic anemia, who has an

IPSS low or intermediate-1 myelodysplastic syndrome (MDS) with and ESA with or without a myeloid growth factor and to continue this therapy if it is effective in improving clinical status and not associated with increasing thrombocytopenia or the percentage of circulating blasts.

THE SAFETY OF ESAs IN CANCER PATIENTS

Erythropoietic agents are generally well tolerated, although there are three issues regarding their safety of which the oncologist must be aware in informing patients and making sound, rational decisions.

Anti-Erythropoietin Antibodies and Pure Red Cell Aplasia

Following the introduction of a new formulation of epoetin alfa in Europe and Canada, an increase in the incidence of pure red cell aplasia (PRCA) was noted in chronic renal failure patients receiving ESA therapy (101). The PRCA was caused by anti-erythropoietin autoantibodies that were induced by an otherwise undetectable alteration in the tertiary structure of the recombinant molecule and were cross-reactive with endogenous erythropoietin. With changes in the production, storage, and handling of this preparation, the incidence of PRCA decreased again, and is no longer an issue (102). PRCA was not reported in patients with cancer receiving ESP therapy, probably because of the short duration of treatment in this setting and the immunosuppressed status of oncology patients. This episode did establish the absolute importance of careful handling and storage of rEPO preparations and the need for extensive pharmacovigilance programs, especially when new preparations are introduced, even when biochemical data suggest that the new preparation is identical to previous preparations.

Venous Thromboembolism

When ESAs were developed for the treatment of the anemia occurring in patients with chronic renal insufficiency, an increase in the incidence of hypertension and thromboses was reported. There was some evidence that these complications were more likely to occur when hemoglobin levels increased rapidly and it was assumed that the physiology involved a rapid expansion in red cell mass in patients lacking the ability to respond with a compensatory reduction in plasma volume. If this were the only mechanism of thrombosis associated with ESA therapy, it would not be expected to occur in patients with reasonably intact renal function.

Since the time of Trousseau, it has been recognized that cancer is a hypercoaguable condition. The pathophysiology of this increase in thrombosis rates is complex and multifactorial (103,104), with contributing factors including production of tissue factor (a transmembrane protein that binds Factor VII and generates thrombin) (105,106) and cancer procoagulant (a vitamin K dependent protease that activates Factor X) (107,108) by tumor cells, the thrombogenic effects of chemotherapy, hormonal agents and antiangiogenic drugs used in treatment, indwelling vascular devices, venous compression by tumors, and immobility (109,110). Because the risk of thrombosis varies widely across tumor types, tumor stages, and tumor treatments, it is especially difficult to accurately assess risk in a given patient and to detect an increase in risk induced by a particular agent. Indeed, in individual randomized clinical trials, ESAs did not initially appear to significantly increase thrombosis risk.

However, in meta-analyses of randomized, placebo-controlled trials of ESAs administered to patients with cancer during chemotherapy an increased risk of thromboses, predominantly venous, has been observed (relative risk 1.4–1.7, absolute increase from 2–3% to 5–6%, Fig. 3) (111–113). This appears to be a class effect, with similar results obtained in rEPO and darbepoetin alfa; this observed class effect is similar in patients with cancer, whether or not they are receiving chemotherapy (113). A review of the trials utilized to generate this meta-analysis suggests that the increment in risk is not spread evenly over all trials and clinical settings; the increase in risk conferred by ESAs is most consistently observed in patients with cancers of the uterine cervix and in patients receiving combined radiotherapy and chemotherapy treatment (114,115). Nevertheless, an increase in risk of thrombosis rates has been observed, and this potential must be considered in therapeutic decision making by patients and their physicians.

It is widely assumed that thromboses during ESA therapy in cancer patients are due to alterations in blood rheology induced by increasing red cell mass; in fact, there is little evidence to support this in the oncology setting. If rapid expansion of red cell mass in cancer patients were a major factor driving thrombotic risk, a significant incidence of thrombosis would be observed immediately following red blood cell transfusion. Although the risks of red cell transfusion have been extensively studied and well documented, a significant increase in venous thrombosis has not been demonstrated. Moreover, there is no clear relationship observed between hemoglobin response following initiation of ESA therapy and thrombosis; thrombosis occurs in nonresponders as well as responders. In a detailed analysis of data from more than 2000 patients, no significant relationship between initial ESA dose or rate of hemoglobin rise and observed thrombosis could be identified (116). These authors concluded that if a predictor of thrombosis based upon hemoglobin rise must be chosen, the best predictor would be a rise of 2 g/dL in 28 days; a rise of 1 g/dL in 14 days had no predictive value. Because very few patients treated with ESAs in the oncology setting develop "overshoot" polycythemia, avoiding supranormal hemoglobin levels, a very prudent goal, would not be expected to reduce thrombosis risk.

In contrast, there is persuasive evidence that vascular endothelial cells express functional EPO-R's. Clinically, an increase in diastolic blood pressure is sometimes noted when subjects are treated with ESAs; this is frequently manifest before an increase in hemoglobin has occurred, suggesting a direct effect of the

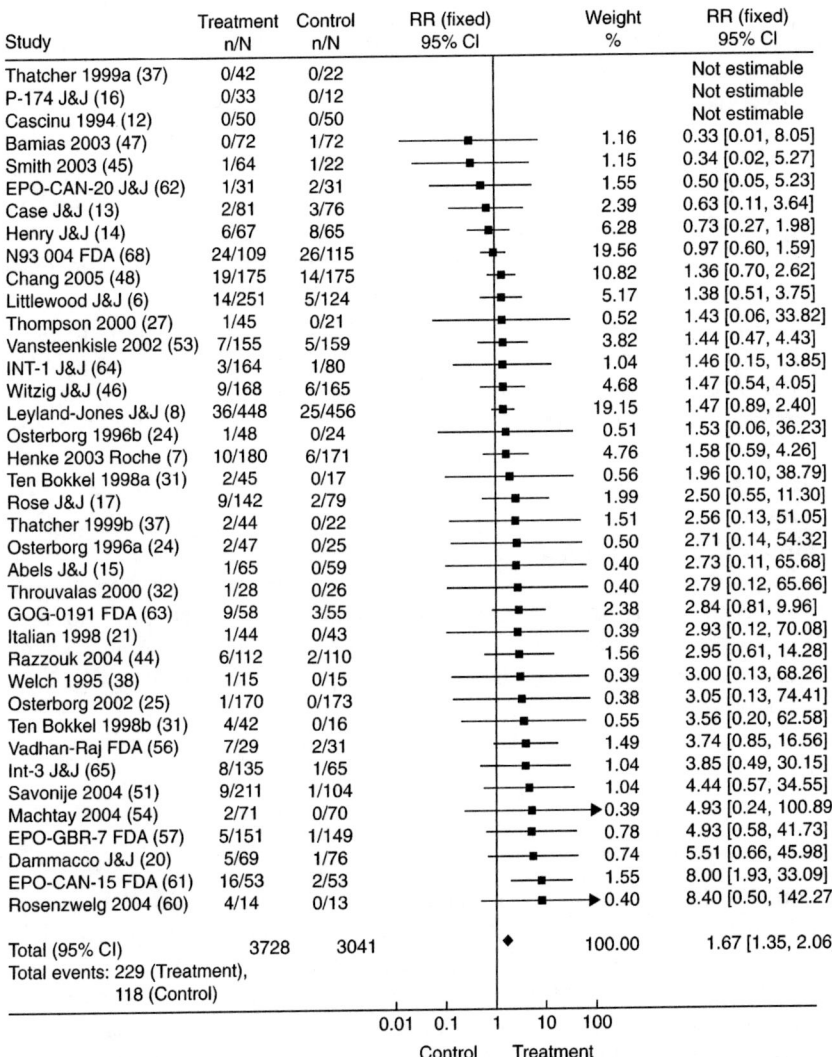

Figure 3 Results of a meta-analysis of reported thromboembolism rates in randomized trials of ESAs during cancer chemotherapy. *Source*: Adapted from Ref. 171.

hormone on vasculature. Human endothelial cells express EPO-R messenger RNA (117), and activation of these receptors by erythropoietin results in a characteristic molecular response in these cells (118). In vitro, erythropoietin induces nitric oxide production by endothelial cells (119,120); in vivo, it promotes vasculogenesis (121) and appears to be involved in endothelial cell recruitment and mobilization (122,123). In an important clinical trial in healthy volunteer subjects treated with rEPO, increases in serum E-selectin levels were observed, demonstrating endothelial activation and with evidence of increased platelet reactivity (124). A direct effect of ESAs in vascular endothelium increasing the propensity for interactions with platelets and the initiation of hemostasis is clearly a viable mechanism for ESA-induced thrombosis.

There is some in vitro evidence that red blood cells may play a role in enhancing the recruitment of platelets by activated platelets during thrombus formation, with a direct relationship between hematocrit and the ultimate extent of platelet activation (125). There is some evidence that erythropoietin may synergize with thrombopoietin in the activating effects of that ligand on mature platelets (126). Finally, it has been suggested that ESA therapy may in some way increase inflammation, which would be expected to increase thrombotic potential (127). None of these alternative explanations have convincing evidence that they are important in the increase in thrombosis rates observed with ESA therapy in cancer patients. To date, vascular activation is the explanation with the most convincing supportive evidence. If this is the major mechanism, it suggests that antiplatelet agents may be effective in abrogating the effects of ESAs on coagulation.

The role of prophylactic anticoagulation in patients with cancer has always been and remains controversial. Given this background, it is not surprising that there is no agreed-upon approach to the prevention of thrombosis associated with ESA therapy during chemotherapy. It is not surprising that low-dose warfarin does not lower risk (128). Clearly, more data are needed, and our current understanding of the biology indicates that trials of antiplatelet agents are of particular interest.

Tumor Progression and Survival

For sound reasons, it was initially expected that treatment of anemia in cancer patients would be associated with improved tumor outcomes and survival. Anemia is associated with cellular hypoxia, and this is especially true for tumor cells (129–135). Tumor cell hypoxia has been associated with genomic instability and increased tumor cell mutation rates, promotion of more apoptosis-resistant and invasive phenotypes (132,136–152), and increased resistance to both radiation (138,153–158) and chemotherapy (159–161). Anemia is an independent negative prognostic factor across a wide range of malignancies (162); while this is an association rather than a demonstrated cause-effect relationship, the observation indicates the potential importance of rational anemia management to optimal cancer care and outcomes. One critical issue that remains to be addressed is the "optimal" hemoglobin level for cancer patients. The vasculature of tumors is more tortuous than that in normal tissue and the relationship between hemoglobin level, blood viscosity, and oxygen delivery to malignant tissue is unique. Tumor tissue oxygenation drops off rapidly as hemoglobin levels fall below 12 g/dL (132,163,164) and may actually decline as hemoglobin levels rise above 13 g/dL (133–135,165). If tumor cell hypoxia is an important factor in tumor progression and resistance to treatment, it may be deleterious to patients to allow hemoglobin levels to fall below 11 to 12 g/dL or to increase them to levels much greater than 13 g/dL. This hypothesis has been and will remain very difficult to test in clinical trials, but the answer is obviously essential to rational oncology care aimed at optimizing outcomes.

In two randomized trials of ESAs utilized to prevent, rather than treat, anemia in patients with breast cancer receiving chemotherapy (166) or with head and neck cancer undergoing radiation therapy (167) an increase in the rate of tumor progression or a decreased survival was observed in the ESA-treated patients. In both of these trials, hemoglobin levels were increased to levels greater than 13 g/dL and increased tumor progression and/or decreased survival could have resulted, paradoxically, from the induction of hypoxia in tumor tissues. Nevertheless, the results are of concern and highlight the need for further large, well-designed trials assessing the impact of ESAs on tumor outcomes. It is reassuring that two subsequent trials of ESAs during chemotherapy in breast cancer designed with survival as an outcome, one in metastatic disease and one in early-stage adjuvant treatment have been completed, and reportedly no negative impact of ESAs on survival was observed.

More recently, the results of two additional clinical trials in which ESA therapy was associated with a decrease in observed survival in the ESA-treated arm were reported. In a large randomized, placebo-controlled trial of darbepoetin alfa in patients with cancer not receiving chemotherapy, a reduction in overall survival was observed in the ESA-treated arm (78). This trial differed from previous trials of ESAs for the anemia of cancer in that patients with cancer in remission were not eligible and all enrolled patients had active cancer that was not being treated, either because no further treatment was available or because no treatment was necessary. The trial was not designed with survival as a primary endpoint and all stratification factors were chosen to equalize transfusion risk, not survival, in the two arms. Indeed, there were imbalances in baseline prognostic factors favoring survival in the placebo group that at least partially explained the observed differences in survival. Most deaths were attributed by the investigators to tumor progression, although no formal investigations of causes of death were undertaken. The findings in this trial remain unexplained. It is of concern that, unlike the previous two trials with a negative signal in terms or cancer outcomes, hemoglobin levels in excess of 13 g/dL were not attained, and hence the findings cannot be explained by excessive hemoglobin levels. The second report was of a very small randomized trial in patients with non–small cell lung cancer (NSCLC), who had advanced disease and were receiving either salvage chemotherapy or palliative care and who were randomized to receive epoetin alfa or placebo (168). A decreased survival was observed in the ESA-treated arm, although both the small size of the study and the existence of a much larger randomized trial in patients with NSCLC with no observed negative impact or survival (18) make these findings much less concerning. At the same time, the results of two randomized trials of ESAs in patients undergoing chemotherapy for small cell lung cancer were released, and demonstrated noninferiority of ESA treatment in terms of response to chemotherapy (169) and no difference in overall survival.

It is important to note that in the majority of randomized trials of ESAs in patients with cancer no difference in survival is observed, and that a decrease in survival or increase in tumor progression has never been observed in a clinical trial in which ESAs were being used as they are in typical oncology practice: to treat, rather than to prevent, anemia in patients with cancer undergoing chemotherapy, with a target hemoglobin level of ≤ 12 g/dL. Moreover, meta-analyses of randomized, controlled trials of ESP treatment during cancer chemotherapy have not shown an increase in tumor progression or a decrease in overall survival in anemic patients treated with ESPs (Fig. 4) (170–173). For the present, there is no evidence of decreased survival or enhanced tumor progression when anemic cancer chemotherapy patients receive ESPs. Until there is a much better demonstration of the safety of ESAs used to prevent anemia or to normalize hemoglobin levels in these chemotherapy patients, or to treat anemia in cancer patients not receiving chemotherapy, these practices cannot be supported.

If ESA therapy is associated with tumor progression and/or diminished survival, the mechanism for this effect is unknown. Some recent papers have reported the detection of EPO-R protein in human cancer cells (174–177). In these studies, immunohistochemistry with polyclonal rabbit antisera has been used to detect EPO-R in tumor specimens. However, careful analysis of these antisera has demonstrated that they also bind tumor-associated proteins, other than EPO-R, including heat shock protein 70-2, and therefore lack the required specificity to demonstrate tumor EPO-R (178). Moreover, unlike the case with endothelial cell EPO-R, data have not been published that provide evidence that any EPO-R on tumor cells are functional or that activation of these receptors meaningfully alters tumor cell biology. The issue of the potential of ESPs to directly induce proliferation or apoptosis resistance in human cancers is obviously a very important one, and deserves more attention in future work rigorously addressing both the specificity of techniques utilized in EPO-R detection and the functionality of any true EPO-R found. To date, in vitro work with human cancer cell lines and in vivo studies using human tumor xenografts have not demonstrated any effect of ESPs on cancer cell proliferation or tumor progression (179,180).

Another area worthy of further attention concerns the thrombogenic potential of ESAs. There is accumulating evidence that coagulation may play a role in tumor progression (105,108,181). Interestingly, there is some indication that anticoagulation may improve survival in cancer patients (182–184). It is conceivable that the thrombosis-promoting activity of ESAs mediates an effect on tumor progression and/or survival in some cancer patients. If this were to be the case, any strategy developed to decrease thrombosis risk in ESA-treated patients would likely ameliorate any negative effects on tumor outcomes.

Anemia and Red Cell Factors

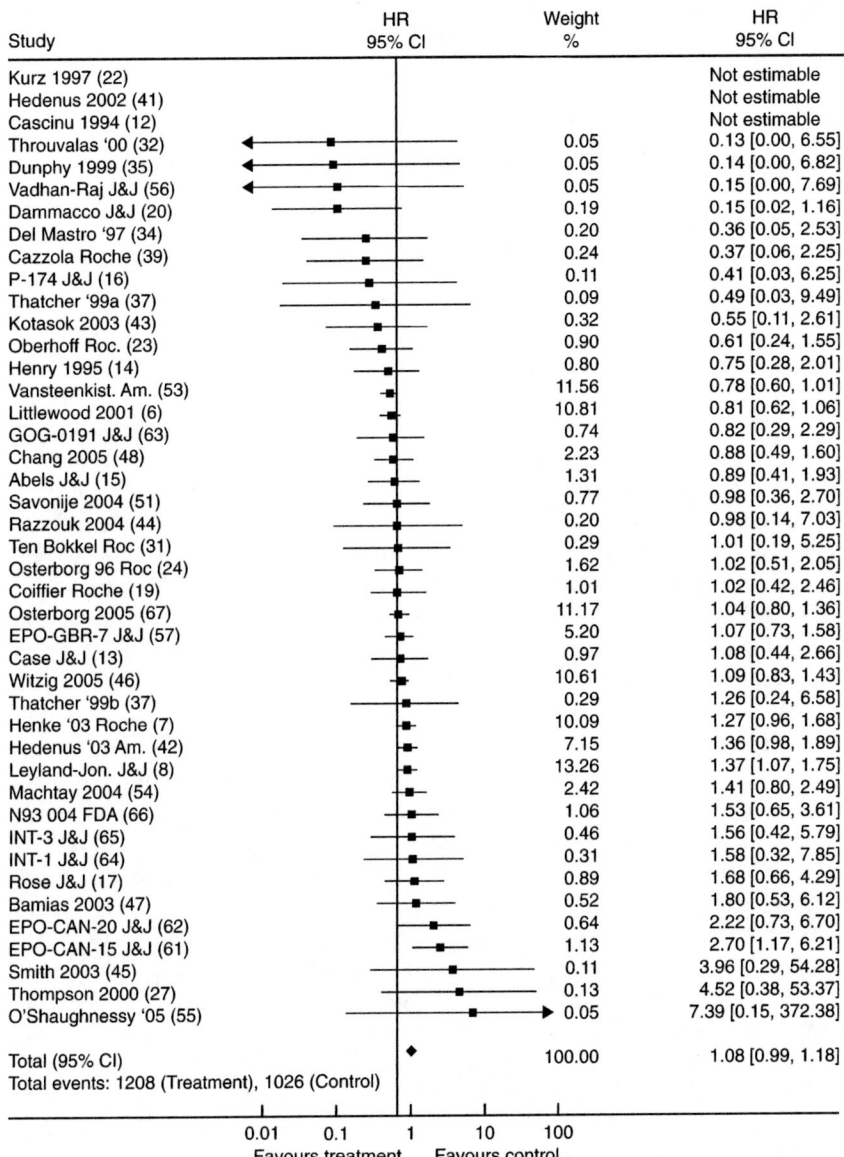

Figure 4 Results of a meta-analysis of reported mortality rates in randomized trials of ESAs during cancer chemotherapy. *Source*: Adapted from Ref. 171.

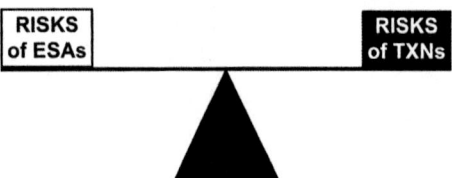

Figure 5 Balancing the risks of ESAs and transfusions (TXNs)

CONCLUSION

Therapy with ESAs for anemia due to cancer chemotherapy has clear benefits for patients in reducing the incidence of red cell transfusions and the symptoms of anemia that frequently cause those transfusions to be given. Red cell transfusions have very well documented risks and a reduction exposure to those risks is a recognized benefit. Advances in our understanding of the biology of anemia and resistance to ESA therapy during cancer chemotherapy promise to provide strategies for increasing the benefits and decreasing the costs of ESA treatment in this setting, with the most promising immediate strategy being parenteral iron administration. Although ESAs are generally well tolerated, we have learned that, like all medical interventions, they have risks, with the best documented risk being an increase in the incidence of venous thrombosis. Our understanding of the physiology underlying this thrombotic tendency is incomplete, but current data point toward antiplatelet agents, which might offset the thrombogenic effects of endothelial activation, as a possible preventative approach. There have also been three important trials in which either enhanced tumor progression or decreased survival was observed in ESA-treated patients. However, there has been no consistent safety signal from any cancer primary site as a direct effect of ESAs on tumors. The effects, if any, of ESAs on tumor progression and survival are poorly understood, apparently inconsistent across studies, and are clearly the most important safety issue facing this field. Obviously, further studies are needed, including careful studies of ESAs used in the fashion that most benefits patients, for the treatment of chemotherapy-induced anemia initiated early enough to maximally reduce transfusion risks, with dosing strategies aimed at maintaining hemoglobin levels in the range between 11 and 12 g/dL, and approaches that, to date, have not been associated with a negative effect upon tumor outcomes. There are real, known risks of transfusions and good clinical trial design and patient treatment decisions should be aimed at balancing these risks against the known thrombosis risk and the totality of the available tumor progression/survival data in a fashion that achieves optimal outcomes for cancer patients (Fig. 5).

REFERENCES

1. Ludwig H, Van Belle S, Barrett-Lee P, et al. The European Cancer Anaemia Survey (ECAS): a large, multinational, prospective survey defining the prevalence, incidence, and treatment of anaemia in cancer patients. Eur J Cancer 2004; 40:2293–2306.
2. Groopman JE, Itri LM. Chemotherapy-induced anemia in adults: incidence and treatment. J Natl Cancer Inst 1999; 91:1616–1634.
3. Miller CB, Jones RJ, Piantadosi S, Abeloff MD, Spivak JL. Decreased erythropoietin response in patients with the anemia of cancer. N Engl J Med 1990; 322:1689–1692.
4. Nicolas G, Chauvet C, Viatte L, et al. The gene encoding the iron regulatory peptide hepcidin is regulated by anemia, hypoxia, and inflammation. J Clin Invest 2002; 110:1037–1044.
5. Ganz T. Hepcidin, a key regulator of iron metabolism and mediator of anemia of inflammation. Blood 2003; 102:783–788.
6. Andrews NC. Anemia of inflammation: the cytokine-hepcidin link. J Clin Invest 2004; 113:1251–1253.
7. Nemeth E, Valore EV, Territo M, Schiller G, Lichtenstein A, Ganz T. Hepcidin, a putative mediator of anemia of inflammation, is a type II acute-phase protein. Blood 2003; 101:2461–2463.
8. Nemeth E, Tuttle MS, Powelson J, et al. Hepcidin regulates cellular iron efflux by binding to ferroportin and inducing its internalization. Science 2004; 306:2090–2093.
9. Fleming RE, Bacon BR. Orchestration of iron homeostasis. N Engl J Med 2005; 352:1741–1744.
10. Henry D, Dahl N, Auerbach D, Tchekmedyian S, Laufman L. Intravenous ferric gluconate (FG) for increasing response to epoetin (EPO) in patients with anemia of cancer chemotherapy: results of a multi-center, randomized trial. Blood 2004; 104: abstract 3696.
11. Egrie JC, Browne JK. Development and characterization of novel erythropoiesis stimulating protein (NESP). Br J Cancer 2001; 1:3–10.
12. Glaspy JA. The development of erythropoietic agents in oncology. Expert Opin Emerg Drugs 2005; 10:553–567.
13. Case DC, Bukowski RM, Carey RW, et al. Recombinant human erythropoietin therapy for anemic cancer patients on combination chemotherapy. J Natl Cancer Inst 1993; 85:801–806.
14. Henry DH, Abels RI. Recombinant human erythropoietin in the treatment of cancer and chemotherapy-induced anemia: results of double-blind and open-label follow-up studies. Semin Oncol 1994; 21:21–28.
15. Wilkinson PM, Antonopoulos M, Lahousen M, et al. Epoetin alfa in platinum-treated ovarian cancer patients: results of a multinational, multicentre, randomised trial. Br J Cancer 2006; 94:947–954.
16. Razzouk BI, Hord JD, Hockenberry M, et al. Double-blind, placebo-controlled study of quality of life, hematologic end points, and safety of weekly epoetin alfa in children with cancer receiving myelosuppressive chemotherapy. J Clin Oncol 2006; 24:3583–3589.
17. Littlewood TJ, Bajetta E, Nortier JW, et al. Effects of epoetin alfa on hematologic parameters and quality of life in cancer patients receiving nonplatinum

chemotherapy: results of a randomized, double-blind, placebo-controlled trial. J Clin Oncol 2001; 19:2865–2874.
18. Vansteenkiste J, Pirker R, Massuti B, et al. Double-blind, placebo-controlled, randomized phase III trial of darbepoetin alfa in lung cancer patients receiving chemotherapy. J Natl Cancer Inst 2002; 94:1211–1220.
19. Hedenus M, Adriansson M, San Miguel J, et al. Efficacy and safety of darbepoetin alfa in anaemic patients with lymphoproliferative malignancies: a randomized, double-blind, placebo-controlled study. Br J Haematol 2003; 122:394–403.
20. Vogelzang NJ, Breitbart W, Cella D, et al. Patient, caregiver, and oncologist perceptions of cancer-related fatigue: results of a tripart assessment survey. The Fatigue Coalition. Semin Hematol 1997; 34:4–12.
21. Curt GA, Breitbart W, Cella D, et al. Impact of cancer-related fatigue on the lives of patients: new findings from the Fatigue Coalition. Oncologist 2000; 5:353–360.
22. Basta SS, Soekirman, Karyadi D, et al. Iron deficiency anemia and the productivity of adult males in Indonesia. Am J Clin Nutr 1979; 32:916–925.
23. Evans RW, Rader B, Manninen DL. The quality of life of hemodialysis recipients treated with recombinant human erythropoietin. Cooperative Multicenter EPO Clinical Trial Group. JAMA 1990; 263:825–830.
24. Levin NW, Lazarus JM, Nissenson AR. National Cooperative rHu Erythropoietin Study in patients with chronic renal failure: an interim report. The National Cooperative rHu Erythropoietin Study Group. Am J Kidney Dis 1993; 22:3–12.
25. Parsons DS, Harris DC. A review of quality of life in chronic renal failure. Pharmacoeconomics 1997; 12:140–160.
26. Nissenson AR. Optimal hematocrit in patients on dialysis therapy. Am J Kidney Dis 1998; 32:S142–S146.
27. Leitgeb C, Pecherstorfer M, Fritz E, Ludwig H. Quality of life in chronic anemia of cancer during treatment with recombinant human erythropoietin. Cancer 1994; 73:2535–2542.
28. Ludwig H, Sundal E, Pecherstorfer M, et al. Recombinant human erythropoietin for the correction of cancer associated anemia with and without concomitant cytotoxic chemotherapy. Cancer 1995; 76:2319–2329.
29. Pawlicki M, Jassem J, Bosze P, et al. A multicenter study of recombinant human erythropoietin (epoetin alpha) in the management of anemia in cancer patients receiving chemotherapy. Anticancer Drugs 1997; 8:949–957.
30. Glaspy J, Bukowski R, Steinberg D, et al. Impact of therapy with epoetin alfa on clinical outcomes in patients with nonmyeloid malignancies during cancer chemotherapy in community oncology practice. Procrit Study Group. J Clin Oncol 1997; 15:1218–1234.
31. Glimelius B, Linne T, Hoffman K, et al. Epoetin beta in the treatment of anemia in patients with advanced gastrointestinal cancer. J Clin Oncol 1998; 16:434–440.
32. Cella D, Bron D. The effect of Epoetin alfa on quality of life in anemic cancer patients. Cancer Pract 1999; 7:177–182.
33. Quirt I, Robeson C, Lau CY, et al. Epoetin alfa therapy increases hemoglobin levels and improves quality of life in patients with cancer-related anemia who are not receiving chemotherapy and patients with anemia who are receiving chemotherapy. J Clin Oncol 2001; 19:4126–4134.
34. Cella D. The effects of anemia and anemia treatment on the quality of life of people with cancer. Oncology 2002; 16:125–132.

35. Daneryd P. Epoetin alfa for protection of metabolic and exercise capacity in cancer patients. Semin Oncol 2002; 29:69–74.
36. Osterborg A, Brandberg Y, Molostova V, et al. Randomized, double-blind, placebo-controlled trial of recombinant human erythropoietin, epoetin Beta, in hematologic malignancies. J Clin Oncol 2002; 20:2486–2494.
37. Cella D, Dobrez D, Glaspy J. Control of cancer-related anemia with erythropoietic agents: a review of evidence for improved quality of life and clinical outcomes. Ann Oncol 2003; 14:511–519.
38. Cella D, Zagari MJ, Vandoros C, et al. Epoetin alfa treatment results in clinically significant improvements in quality of life in anemic cancer patients when referenced to the general population. J Clin Oncol 2003; 21:366–373.
39. Cella D, Kallich J, McDermott A, et al. The longitudinal relationship of hemoglobin, fatigue and quality of life in anemic cancer patients: results from five randomized clinical trials. Ann Oncol 2004; 15:979–986.
40. Jones M, Schenkel B, Just J, et al. Epoetin alfa improves quality of life in patients with cancer: results of metaanalysis. Cancer 2004; 101:1720–1732.
41. Chang J, Couture F, Young S, et al. Weekly epoetin alfa maintains hemoglobin, improves quality of life, and reduces transfusion in breast cancer patients receiving chemotherapy. J Clin Oncol 2005; 23:2597–2605.
42. Ross SD, Fahrbach K, Frame D, et al. The effect of anemia treatment on selected health-related quality-of-life domains: a systematic review. Clin Ther 2003; 25:1786–1805.
43. Demetri GD, Kris M, Wade J, et al. Quality-of-life benefit in chemotherapy patients treated with epoetin alfa is independent of disease response or tumor type: results from a prospective community oncology study. Procrit Study Group. J Clin Oncol 1998; 16:3412–3425.
44. Crawford J, Cella D, Cleeland CS, et al. Relationship between changes in hemoglobin level and quality of life during chemotherapy in anemic cancer patients receiving epoetin alfa therapy. Cancer 2002; 95:888–895.
45. Witzig TE, Silberstein PT, Loprinzi CL, et al. Phase III, randomized, double-blind study of epoetin alfa compared with placebo in anemic patients receiving chemotherapy. J Clin Oncol 2005; 23:2606–2617.
46. Glaspy J, Vadhan-Raj S, Patel R, et al. Randomized comparison of every-2-week darbepoetin alfa and weekly epoetin alfa for the treatment of chemotherapy-induced anemia: the 20030125 Study Group Trial. J Clin Oncol 2006; 24:2290–2297.
47. Boccia R, Malik IA, Raja V, et al. Darbepoetin alfa administered every three weeks is effective for the treatment of chemotherapy-induced anemia. Oncologist 2006; 11:409–417.
48. Canon JL, Vansteenkiste J, Bodoky G, et al. Randomized, double-blind, active-controlled trial of every-3-week darbepoetin alfa for the treatment of chemotherapy-induced anemia. J Natl Cancer Inst 2006; 98:273–284.
49. Glaspy J, Henry D, Patel R, et al. Effects of chemotherapy on endogenous erythropoietin levels and the pharmacokinetics and erythropoietic response of darbepoetin alfa: a randomised clinical trial of synchronous versus asynchronous dosing of darbepoetin alfa. Eur J Cancer 2005; 41:1140–1149.
50. Steensma DP, Molina R, Sloan JA, et al. Phase III study of two different dosing schedules of erythropoietin in anemic patients with cancer. J Clin Oncol 2006; 24:1079–1089.

51. Lyman GH, Glaspy J. Are there clinical benefits with early erythropoietic intervention for chemotherapy-induced anemia? A systematic review. Cancer 2006; 106: 223–233.
52. Rodgers Gea. National Comprehensive Cancer Network—Clinical Practice Guidelines in Oncology, 2008 (www.nccn.org).
53. Bokemeyer C, Aapro MS, Courdi A, et al. EORTC guidelines for the use of erythropoietic proteins in anaemic patients with cancer. Eur J Cancer 2004; 40: 2201–2216.
54. Glaspy J, Cavill I. Role of iron in optimizing responses of anemic cancer patients to erythropoietin. Oncology 1999; 13:461–473.
55. Eschbach JW. Iron requirements in erythropoietin therapy. Best Pract Res Clin Haematol 2005; 18:347–361.
56. Sheashaa H, El-Husseini A, Sabry A, et al. Parenteral iron therapy in treatment of anemia in end-stage renal disease patients: a comparative study between iron saccharate and gluconate. Nephron Clin Pract 2005; 99:c97–c101.
57. Chertow GM, Mason PD, Vaage-Nilsen O, et al. On the relative safety of parenteral iron formulations. Nephrol Dial Transplant 2004; 19:1571–1575.
58. Chertow GM, Mason PD, Vaage-Nilsen O, et al. Update on adverse drug events associated with parenteral iron. Nephrol Dial Transplant 2006; 21:378–382.
59. Auerbach M, Ballard H, Glaspy J. Clinical update: Intravenous iron for anaemia. The Lancet 2007; 369:1502–1504.
60. Auerbach M, Ballard H, Trout JR, et al. Intravenous iron optimizes the response to recombinant human erythropoietin in cancer patients with chemotherapy-related anemia: a multicenter, open-label, randomized trial. J Clin Oncol 2004; 22:1301–1307.
61. Henry DH. The role of intravenous iron in cancer-related anemia. Oncology 2006; 20:21–24.
62. Ludwig H. Iron metabolism and iron supplementation in anemia of cancer. Semin Hematol 2006; 43:S13–S17.
63. Weiss G, Goodnough LT. Anemia of chronic disease. N Engl J Med 2005; 352: 1011–1023.
64. Ferguson BJ, Skikne BS, Simpson KM, et al. Serum transferrin receptor distinguishes the anemia of chronic disease from iron deficiency anemia. J Lab Clin Med 1992; 119:385–390.
65. Cook JD, Flowers CH, Skikne BS. The quantitative assessment of body iron. Blood 2003; 101:3359–3364.
66. Thomas C, Thomas L. Biochemical markers and hematologic indices in the diagnosis of functional iron deficiency. Clin Chem 2002; 48:1066–1076.
67. Thomas C, Thomas L. Anemia of chronic disease: pathophysiology and laboratory diagnosis. Lab Hematol 2005; 11:14–23.
68. Macdougall IC, Cavill I, Hulme B, et al. Detection of functional iron deficiency during erythropoietin treatment: a new approach. BMJ 1992; 304:225–226.
69. Tessitore N, Solero GP, Lippi G, et al. The role of iron status markers in predicting response to intravenous iron in haemodialysis patients on maintenance erythropoietin. Nephrol Dial Transplant 2001; 16:1416–1423.
70. Richardson D, Bartlett C, Jolly H, et al. Intravenous iron for CAPD populations: proactive or reactive strategies? Nephrol Dial Transplant 2001; 16:115–119.

71. Brugnara C, Laufer MR, Friedman AJ, et al. Reticulocyte hemoglobin content (CHr): early indicator of iron deficiency and response to therapy [letter]. Blood 1994; 83:3100–3101.
72. Fishbane S, Galgano C, Langley RC, et al. Reticulocyte hemoglobin content in the evaluation of iron status of hemodialysis patients. Kidney Int 1997; 52:217–222.
73. Cullen P, Soffker J, Hopfl M, et al. Hypochromic red cells and reticulocyte haemglobin content as markers of iron-deficient erythropoiesis in patients undergoing chronic haemodialysis. Nephrol Dial Transplant 1999; 14:659–665.
74. Mast AE, Blinder MA, Lu Q, et al. Clinical utility of the reticulocyte hemoglobin content in the diagnosis of iron deficiency. Blood 2002; 99:1489–1491.
75. Tsuchiya K, Okano H, Teramura M, et al. Content of reticulocyte hemoglobin is a reliable tool for determining iron deficiency in dialysis patients. Clin Nephrol 2003; 59:115–123.
76. Abels RI. Use of recombinant human erythropoietin in the treatment of anemia in patients who have cancer. Semin Oncol 1992; 19:29–35.
77. Smith RE, Tchekmedyian NS, Chan D, et al. A dose- and schedule-finding study of darbepoetin alpha for the treatment of chronic anaemia of cancer. Br J Cancer 2003; 88:1851–1858.
78. Glaspy J, Smith R, Aapro MS, et al. Results from a phase III, randomized, double-blind, placebo-conrolled study of darbepoetin alfa for the treatment of anemia in patients not receiving chemotherapy or radiotherapy. Proceedings, the Annual Meeting of the Americal Association for Cancer Research 2007; Late Breaking Abstract LB-3.
79. Stebler C, Tichelli A, Dazzi H, et al. High-dose recombinant human erythropoietin for treatment of anemia in myelodysplastic syndromes and paroxysmal nocturnal hemoglobinuria: a pilot study. Exp Hematol 1990; 18:1204–1208.
80. Bowen D, Culligan D, Jacobs A. The treatment of anaemia in the myelodysplastic syndromes with recombinant human erythropoietin. Br J Haematol 1991; 77:419–423.
81. Bessho M, Jinnai I, Matsuda A, et al. Improvement of anemia by recombinant erythropoietin in patients with myelodysplastic syndromes and aplastic anemia. Int J Cell Cloning 1990; 8:445–458.
82. Hellstrom E, Birgegard G, Lockner D, et al. Treatment of myelodysplastic syndromes with recombinant human erythropoietin. Eur J Haematol 1991; 47:355–360.
83. Stein RS, Abels RI, Krantz SB. Pharmacologic doses of recombinant human erythropoietin in the treatment of myelodysplastic syndromes. Blood 1991; 78: 1658–1663.
84. Cazzola M, Ponchio L, Beguin Y, et al. Subcutaneous erythropoietin for treatment of refractory anemia in hematologic disorders. Results of a phase I/II clinical trial [see comments]. Blood 1992; 79:29–37.
85. Rafanelli D, Grossi A, Longo G, et al. Recombinant human erythropoietin for treatment of myelodysplastic syndromes. Leukemia 1992; 6:323–327.
86. Goy A, Belanger C, Casadevall N, et al. High doses of intravenous recombinant erythropoietin for the treatment of anaemia in myelodysplastic syndrome. Br J Haematol 1993; 84:232–237.
87. Stone RM, Bernstein SH, Demetri G, et al. Therapy with recombinant human erythropoietin in patients with myelodysplastic syndromes. Leuk Res 1994; 18:769–776.
88. Musto P, Lanza F, Balleari E, et al. Darbepoetin alpha for the treatment of anaemia in low-intermediate risk myelodysplastic syndromes. Br J Haematol 2005; 128:204–209.

89. Stasi R, Abruzzese E, Lanzetta G, et al. Darbepoetin alfa for the treatment of anemic patients with low- and intermediate-1-risk myelodysplastic syndromes. Ann Oncol 2005; 16:1921–1927.
90. Patton JF, Sullivan T, Mun Y, et al. A retrospective cohort study to assess the impact of therapeutic substitution of darbepoetin alfa for epoetin alfa in anemic patients with myelodysplastic syndrome. J Support Oncol 2005; 3:419–426.
91. Mannone L, Gardin C, Quarre MC, et al. High-dose darbepoetin alpha in the treatment of anaemia of lower risk myelodysplastic syndrome results of a phase II study. Br J Haematol 2006; 133:513–519.
92. Negrin RS, Stein R, Vardiman J, et al. Treatment of the anemia of myelodysplastic syndromes using recombinant human granulocyte colony-stimulating factor in combination with erythropoietin [see comments]. Blood 1993; 82:737–743.
93. Negrin RS, Stein R, Doherty K, et al. Maintenance treatment of the anemia of myelodysplastic syndromes with recombinant human granulocyte colony-stimulating factor and erythropoietin: evidence for in vivo synergy. Blood 1996; 87: 4076–4081.
94. Hansen PB, Johnsen HE, Hippe E, Hellstrom-Lindberg E, Ralfkiaer E. Recombinant human granulocyte-macrophage colony-stimulating factor plus recombinant human erythropoietin may improve anemia in selected patients with myelodysplastic syndromes. Am J Hematol 1993; 44:229–236.
95. Hellstrom-Lindberg E, Ahlgren T, Beguin Y, et al. Treatment of anemia in myelodysplastic syndromes with granulocyte colony-stimulating factor plus erythropoietin: results from a randomized phase II study and long-term follow-up of 71 patients. Blood 1998; 92:68–75.
96. Stasi R, Pagano A, Terzoli E, et al. Recombinant human granulocyte-macrophage colony-stimulating factor plus erythropoietin for the treatment of cytopenias in patients with myelodysplastic syndromes. Br J Haematol 1999; 105:141–148.
97. Mantovani L, Lentini G, Hentschel B, et al. Treatment of anaemia in myelodysplastic syndromes with prolonged administration of recombinant human granulocyte colony-stimulating factor and erythropoietin. Br J Haematol 2000; 109:367–375.
98. Thompson JA, Gilliland DG, Prchal JT, et al. Effect of recombinant human erythropoietin combined with granulocyte/macrophage colony-stimulating factor in the treatment of patients with myelodysplastic syndrome. GM/EPO MDS Study Group. Blood 2000; 95:1175–1179.
99. Jadersten M, Montgomery SM, Dybedal I, et al. Long-term outcome of treatment of anemia in MDS with erythropoietin and G-CSF. Blood 2005; 106:803–811.
100. Casadevall N, Durieux P, Dubois S, et al. Health, economic, and quality-of-life effects of erythropoietin and granulocyte colony-stimulating factor for the treatment of myelodysplastic syndromes: a randomized, controlled trial. Blood 2004; 104: 321–327.
101. Casadevall N, Nataf J, Viron B, et al. Pure red-cell aplasia and antierythropoietin antibodies in patients treated with recombinant erythropoietin. N Engl J Med 2002; 346:469–475.
102. Bennett CL, Luminari S, Nissenson AR, et al. Pure red-cell aplasia and epoetin therapy. N Engl J Med 2004; 351:1403–1408.
103. Adess M, Eisner R, Nand S, et al. Thromboembolism in cancer patients: pathogenesis and treatment. Clin Appl Thromb Hemost 2006; 12:254–266.

104. Zwicker JI, Furie BC, Furie B. Cancer-associated thrombosis. Crit Rev Oncol Hematol 2007; 62:126–136.
105. Rak J, Milsom C, May L, et al. Tissue factor in cancer and angiogenesis: the molecular link between genetic tumor progression, tumor neovascularization, and cancer coagulopathy. Semin Thromb Hemost 2006; 32:54–70.
106. Tesselaar ME, Romijn FP, Van Der Linden IK, et al. Microparticle-associated tissue factor activity: a link between cancer and thrombosis? J Thromb Haemost 2007; 5: 520–527.
107. Gale AJ, Gordon SG. Update on tumor cell procoagulant factors. Acta Haematol 2001; 106:25–32.
108. Franchini M, Montagnana M, Targher G, et al. Pathogenesis, clinical and laboratory aspects of thrombosis in cancer. J Thromb Thrombolysis 2007; 24:29–38.
109. Lee AY. Epidemiology and management of venous thromboembolism in patients with cancer. Thromb Res 2003; 110:167–172.
110. Lee AY, Levine MN, Butler G, et al. Incidence, risk factors, and outcomes of catheter-related thrombosis in adult patients with cancer. J Clin Oncol 2006; 24: 1404–1408.
111. Bohlius J, Langensiepen S, Schwarzer G, et al. Erythropoietin for patients with malignant disease. Cochrane Database Syst Rev 2004; 3:CD003407.
112. Bohlius J, Wilson J, Seidenfeld J, et al. Erythropoietin or darbepoetin for patients with cancer. Cochrane Database Syst Rev 2006; 3:CD003407.
113. Ross SD, Allen IE, Henry DH, et al. Clinical benefits and risks associated with epoetin and darbepoetin in patients with chemotherapy-induced anemia: a systematic review of the literature. Clin Ther 2006; 28:801–831.
114. Wun T, Law L, Harvey D, et al. Increased incidence of symptomatic venous thrombosis in patients with cervical carcinoma treated with concurrent chemotherapy, radiation, and erythropoietin. Cancer 2003; 98:1514–1520.
115. Lavey RS, Liu PY, Greer BE, et al. Recombinant human erythropoietin as an adjunct to radiation therapy and cisplatin for stage IIB-IVA carcinoma of the cervix: a Southwest Oncology Group study. Gynecol Oncol 2004; 95:145–151.
116. Hedenus M, Canon J, Kotasek D, et al. Effects of dose adjustment rules on safety during erythropoietic therapy: a retrospective analysis of darbepoetin alfa administered either every 3 weeks or weekly. Proceedings, the American Society of Hematology Annual Meeting 2005; Abstract 3376.
117. Anagnostou A, Liu Z, Steiner M, et al. Erythropoietin receptor mRNA expression in human endothelial cells. Proc Natl Acad Sci U S A 1994; 91:3974–3978.
118. Fodinger M, Fritsche-Polanz R, Buchmayer H, et al. Erythropoietin-inducible immediate-early genes in human vascular endothelial cells. J Investig Med 2000; 48:137–149.
119. Banerjee D, Rodriguez M, Nag M, et al. Exposure of endothelial cells to recombinant human erythropoietin induces nitric oxide synthase activity. Kidney Int 2000; 57:1895–1904.
120. Beleslin-Cokic BB, Cokic VP, Yu X, et al. Erythropoietin and hypoxia stimulate erythropoietin receptor and nitric oxide production by endothelial cells. Blood 2004; 104:2073–2080.
121. Ashley RA, Dubuque SH, Dvorak B, et al. Erythropoietin stimulates vasculogenesis in neonatal rat mesenteric microvascular endothelial cells. Pediatr Res 2002; 51:472–478.

122. Satoh K, Kagaya Y, Nakano M, et al. Important role of endogenous erythropoietin system in recruitment of endothelial progenitor cells in hypoxia-induced pulmonary hypertension in mice. Circulation 2006; 113:1442–1450.
123. Urao N, Okigaki M, Yamada H, et al. Erythropoietin-mobilized endothelial progenitors enhance reendothelialization via Akt-endothelial nitric oxide synthase activation and prevent neointimal hyperplasia. Circ Res 2006; 98:1405–1413.
124. Stohlawetz PJ, Dzirlo L, Hergovich N, et al. Effects of erythropoietin on platelet reactivity and thrombopoiesis in humans. Blood 2000; 95:2983–2989.
125. Valles J, Santos MT, Aznar J, et al. Platelet-erythrocyte interactions enhance alpha (IIb)beta(3) integrin receptor activation and P-selectin expression during platelet recruitment: down-regulation by aspirin ex vivo. Blood 2002; 99:3978–3984.
126. Wun T, Paglieroni T, Hammond WP, et al. Thrombopoietin is synergistic with other hematopoietic growth factors and physiologic platelet agonists for platelet activation in vitro. Am J Hematol 1997; 54:225–232.
127. Tobu M, Iqbal O, Fareed D, et al. Erythropoietin-induced thrombosis as a result of increased inflammation and thrombin activatable fibrinolytic inhibitor. Clin Appl Thromb Hemost 2004; 10:225–232.
128. Lin A, Ryu J, Harvey D, et al. Low-dose warfarin does not decrease the rate of thrombosis in patients with cervix and vulvo-vaginal cancer treated with chemotherapy, radiation, and erythropoeitin. Gynecol Oncol 2006; 102:98–102.
129. Stone HB, Brown JM, Phillips TL, et al. Oxygen in human tumors: correlations between methods of measurement and response to therapy. Summary of a workshop held November 19–20, 1992, at the National Cancer Institute, Bethesda, Maryland. Radiat Res 1993; 136:422–434.
130. Kelleher DK, Mattheinsen U, Thews O, et al. Blood flow, oxygenation, and bioenergetic status of tumors after erythropoietin treatment in normal and anemic rats. Cancer Res 1996; 56:4728–4734.
131. Fyles AW, Milosevic M, Pintilie M, et al. Cervix cancer oxygenation measured following external radiation therapy. Int J Radiat Oncol Biol Phys 1998; 42:751–753.
132. Hockel M, Vaupel P. Tumor hypoxia: definitions and current clinical, biologic, and molecular aspects. J Natl Cancer Inst 2001; 93:266–276.
133. Vaupel P, Thews O, Mayer A, et al. Oxygenation status of gynecologic tumors: what is the optimal hemoglobin level? Strahlenther Onkol 2002; 178:727–731.
134. Vaupel P, Mayer A, Briest S, et al. Oxygenation gain factor: a novel parameter characterizing the association between hemoglobin level and the oxygenation status of breast cancers. Cancer Res 2003; 63:7634–7637.
135. Vaupel P, Mayer A, Briest S, et al. Hypoxia in breast cancer: role of blood flow, oxygen diffusion distances, and anemia in the development of oxygen depletion. Adv Exp Med Biol 2005; 566:333–342.
136. Graeber TG, Osmanian C, Jacks T, et al. Hypoxia-mediated selection of cells with diminished apoptotic potential in solid tumours [see comments]. Nature 1996; 379:88–91.
137. Semenza GL. Hypoxia, clonal selection, and the role of HIF-1 in tumor progression. Crit Rev Biochem Mol Biol 2000; 35:71–103.
138. Krishnamachary B, Berg-Dixon S, Kelly B, et al. Regulation of colon carcinoma cell invasion by hypoxia-inducible factor 1. Cancer Res 2003; 63:1138–1143.

139. Semenza GL. Involvement of hypoxia-inducible factor 1 in human cancer. Intern Med 2002; 41:79–83.
140. Stoeltzing O, McCarty MF, Wey JS, et al. Role of hypoxia-inducible factor 1alpha in gastric cancer cell growth, angiogenesis, and vessel maturation. J Natl Cancer Inst 2004; 96:946–956.
141. Bos R, Zhong H, Hanrahan CF, et al. Levels of hypoxia-inducible factor-1 alpha during breast carcinogenesis. J Natl Cancer Inst 2001; 93:309–314.
142. Buchler P, Reber HA, Buchler M, et al. Hypoxia-inducible factor 1 regulates vascular endothelial growth factor expression in human pancreatic cancer. Pancreas 2003; 26:56–64.
143. Vaupel P, Mayer A, Hockel M. Tumor hypoxia and malignant progression. Methods Enzymol 2004; 381:335–354.
144. Zhong H, De Marzo AM, Laughner E, et al. Overexpression of hypoxia-inducible factor 1alpha in common human cancers and their metastases. Cancer Res 1999; 59:5830–5835.
145. Biroccio A, Candiloro A, Mottolese M, et al. Bcl-2 overexpression and hypoxia synergistically act to modulate vascular endothelial growth factor expression and in vivo angiogenesis in a breast carcinoma line. FASEB J 2000; 14:652–660.
146. Dachs GU, Tozer GM. Hypoxia modulated gene expression: angiogenesis, metastasis and therapeutic exploitation. Eur J Cancer 2000; 36:1649–1660.
147. Semenza GL. HIF-1: using two hands to flip the angiogenic switch. Cancer Metastasis Rev 2000; 19:59–65.
148. Giatromanolaki A, Harris AL. Tumour hypoxia, hypoxia signaling pathways and hypoxia inducible factor expression in human cancer. Anticancer Res 2001; 21:4317–4324.
149. Oikawa M, Abe M, Kurosawa H, et al. Hypoxia induces transcription factor ETS-1 via the activity of hypoxia-inducible factor-1. Biochem Biophys Res Commun 2001; 289:39–43.
150. Pilch H, Schlenger K, Steiner E, et al. Hypoxia-stimulated expression of angiogenic growth factors in cervical cancer cells and cervical cancer-derived fibroblasts. Int J Gynecol Cancer 2001; 11:137–142.
151. Harris AL. Hypoxia: a key regulatory factor in tumour growth. Nature Rev Cancer 2002; 2:38–47.
152. Rofstad EK, Halsor EF. Hypoxia-associated spontaneous pulmonary metastasis in human melanoma xenografts: involvement of microvascular hot spots induced in hypoxic foci by interleukin 8. Br J Cancer 2002; 86:301–308.
153. Brizel DM, Sibley GS, Prosnitz LR, et al. Tumor hypoxia adversely affects the prognosis of carcinoma of the head and neck. Int J Radiat Oncol Biol Phys 1997; 38:285–289.
154. Fyles AW, Milosevic M, Wong R, et al. Oxygenation predicts radiation response and survival in patients with cervix cancer. Radiother Oncol 1998; 48:149–156.
155. Brizel DM, Dodge RK, Clough RW, et al. Oxygenation of head and neck cancer: changes during radiotherapy and impact on treatment outcome. Radiother Oncol 1999; 53:113–117.
156. Dunst J, Kuhnt T, Strauss HG, et al. Anemia in cervical cancers: impact on survival, patterns of relapse, and association with hypoxia and angiogenesis. Int J Radiat Oncol Biol Phys 2003; 56:778–787.

157. Semenza GL. Intratumoral hypoxia, radiation resistance, and HIF-1. Cancer Cell 2004; 5:405–406.
158. Thews O, Koenig R, Kelleher DK, et al. Enhanced radiosensitivity in experimental tumours following erythropoietin treatment of chemotherapy-induced anaemia. Br J Cancer 1998; 78:752–756.
159. Thews O, Kelleher DK, Vaupel P. Erythropoietin restores the anemia-induced reduction in cyclophosphamide cytotoxicity in rat tumors. Cancer Res 2001; 61: 1358–1361.
160. Teicher BA, Holden SA, al-Achi A, et al. Classification of antineoplastic treatments by their differential toxicity toward putative oxygenated and hypoxic tumor subpopulations in vivo in the FSaIIC murine fibrosarcoma. Cancer Res 1990; 50:3339–3344.
161. Van Belle SJ, Cocquyt V. Impact of haemoglobin levels on the outcome of cancers treated with chemotherapy. Crit Rev Oncol Hematol 2003; 47:1–11.
162. Caro JJ, Salas M, Ward A, et al. Anemia as an independent prognostic factor for survival in patients with cancer: a systemic, quantitative review. Cancer 2001; 91: 2214–2221.
163. Kallinowski F, Zander R, Hoeckel M, et al. Tumor tissue oxygenation as evaluated by computerized-pO_2-histography. Int J Radiat Oncol Biol Phys 1990; 19:953–961.
164. Vaupel P, Briest S, Hockel M. Hypoxia in breast cancer: pathogenesis, characterization and biological/therapeutic implications. Wien Med Wochenschr 2002; 152: 334–342.
165. Vaupel P, Mayer A, Hockel M. Impact of hemoglobin levels on tumor oxygenation: the higher, the better? Strahlenther Onkol 2006; 182:63–71.
166. Leyland-Jones B, Semiglazov V, Pawlicki M, et al. Maintaining normal hemoglobin levels with epoetin alfa in mainly nonanemic patients with metastatic breast cancer receiving first-line chemotherapy: a survival study. J Clin Oncol 2005; 23:5960–5972.
167. Henke M, Laszig R, Rube C, et al. Erythropoietin to treat head and neck cancer patients with anaemia undergoing radiotherapy: randomised, double-blind, placebo-controlled trial. Lancet 2003; 362:1255–1260.
168. Wright JR, Ung YC, Julian JA, et al. Randomized, double-blind, placebo-controlled trial of erythropoietin in non-small-cell lung cancer with disease-related anemia. J Clin Oncol 2007; 25:1027–1032.
169. Grote T, Yeilding AL, Castillo R, et al. Efficacy and safety analysis of epoetin alfa in patients with small-cell lung cancer: a randomized, double-blind, placebo-controlled trial. J Clin Oncol 2005; 23:9377–9386.
170. Bohlius J, Langensiepen S, Schwarzer G, et al. Recombinant human erythropoietin and overall survival in cancer patients: results of a comprehensive meta-analysis. J Natl Cancer Inst 2005; 97:489–498.
171. Bohlius J, Wilson J, Seidenfeld J, et al. Recombinant human erythropoietins and cancer patients: updated meta-analysis of 57 studies including 9353 patients. J Natl Cancer Inst 2006; 98:708–714.
172. Hedenus M, Vansteenkiste J, Kotasek D, et al. Darbepoetin alfa for the treatment of chemotherapy-induced anemia: disease progression and survival analysis from four randomized, double-blind, placebo-controlled trials. J Clin Oncol 2005; 23:6941–6948.
173. Aapro M, Coiffier B, Dunst J, et al. Effect of treatment with epoetin beta on short-term tumour progression and survival in anaemic patients with cancer: a meta-analysis. Br J Cancer 2006; 95:1467–1473.

174. Acs G, Acs P, Beckwith SM, et al. Erythropoietin and erythropoietin receptor expression in human cancer. Cancer Res 2001; 61:3561–3565.
175. Arcasoy MO, Amin K, Karayal AF, et al. Functional significance of erythropoietin receptor expression in breast cancer. Lab Invest 2002; 82:911–918.
176. Acs G, Zhang PJ, Rebbeck TR, et al. Immunohistochemical expression of erythropoietin and erythropoietin receptor in breast carcinoma. Cancer 2002; 95:969–981.
177. Henke M, Mattern D, Pepe M, et al. Do erythropoietin receptors on cancer cells explain unexpected clinical findings? J Clin Oncol 2006; 24:4708–4713.
178. Elliott S, Busse L, Bass MB, et al. Anti-Epo receptor antibodies do not predict Epo receptor expression. Blood 2006; 107:1892–1895.
179. Hardee ME, Kirkpatrick JP, Shan S, et al. Human recombinant erythropoietin (rEpo) has no effect on tumour growth or angiogenesis. Br J Cancer 2005; 93:1350–1355.
180. Shannon AM, Bouchier-Hayes DJ, Condron CM, et al. Correction of anaemia through the use of darbepoetin alfa improves chemotherapeutic outcome in a murine model of Lewis lung carcinoma. Br J Cancer 2005; 93:224–232.
181. Rak J, Yu JL, Luyendyk J, et al. Oncogenes, trousseau syndrome, and cancer-related changes in the coagulome of mice and humans. Cancer Res 2006; 66:10643–10646.
182. Akl EA, Kamath G, Kim SY, et al. Oral anticoagulation for prolonging survival in patients with cancer. Cochrane Database Syst Rev 2007; CD006466.
183. Akl E, van Doormaal F, Barba M, et al. Parenteral anticoagulation for prolonging survival in patients with cancer who have no other indication for anticoagulation. Cochrane Database Syst Rev 2007; CD006652.
184. Piccioli A, Falanga A, Prandoni P. Anticoagulants and cancer survival. Semin Thromb Hemost 2006; 32:810–813.

4

Neutropenia and Its Complications

David C. Dale
*Department of Medicine, University of
Washington, Seattle, Washington, U.S.A.*

Jeffrey Crawford and Gary H. Lyman
*Department of Medicine, Duke University School
of Medicine and the Duke Comprehensive
Cancer Center, Durham, North Carolina, U.S.A.*

INTRODUCTION

Neutrophils form the first line of host defense from infections by bacterial and fungal pathogens. Whenever there is any break in the integrity of a body surface, it is the capacity to generate an acute inflammatory response with rapid accumulation of neutrophils at a site of injury that provides the body's first defense against infections. Maintenance of this protective force requires the steady production of neutrophils for killing and removing microorganisms and destroying their toxic products (1,2).

Neutrophils are produced in the bone marrow from hematopoietic stem cells; the production of a mature neutrophil from its early progenitor takes approximately 10 to 14 days. With infections, this process is accelerated by enhanced production of endogenous myeloid growth factors. Similarly, administration of exogenous growth factors such as granulocyte colony stimulating factor (G-CSF) or granulocyte macrophage colony stimulating factor (GM-CSF) will accelerate neutrophil production and increase blood neutrophil count (3–6).

Neutrophils and monocytes have a common early developmental pathway that branches to produce these distinctive types of phagocytic cells, which share many functional properties. Neutrophils develop primary, secondary, and tertiary granules containing numerous enzymes and antibacterial factors that account for their broad capacity to kill microorganisms. Simultaneously with the synthesis of these specialized proteins, neutrophils acquire a rich supply of glycogen in the cytoplasm as a source of energy, and a wide array of surface glycoproteins to facilitate their movement from the bone marrow to the blood and to the tissues. Monocytes also have similar granules containing broadly acting antimicrobial proteins, and they share many structural and functional properties with neutrophils. However, in contrast to neutrophils, which are end-stage cells largely devoid of the capacity to divide or synthesize new proteins when they leave the bone marrow, circulating monocytes retain these properties and are much long-lived and multifunctional cells (1,2).

For normal host defense, all the components of the phagocytes, i.e., granule-associated proteins, the capacity to generate an intense "metabolic burst," and the surface glycoproteins to direct their trafficking, must be intact. There are numerous well-defined clinical syndromes associated with deficiencies in these features of phagocytes (7). Transient abnormalities in neutrophil functions can also be detected in the recovery phase from chemotherapy-induced neutropenia, but most of the risks of infectious complications are due to deficiencies of cell numbers and are not specifically related to abnormalities of their function. It is important to keep in mind that recovery from chemotherapy involves rebuilding the elaborate system for stable production of neutrophils, and the initial cells entering the blood in the recovery phase are produced by a perturbed system. It may take days or even weeks for the system to recover fully (8–10).

The quantitative aspects of neutrophil production are also very important in relationship to the effects of cancer chemotherapy. Normally, adults produce about 1×10^9 neutrophils per kilogram of body weight per day (1,2). Blood neutrophils have a short lifespan; the half-life of the mature neutrophil is only about 6 to 10 hours. This means that each day the body must produce essentially a fresh population of these cells. Probably no other cell type has such a high production and rapid turnover. The high turnover rate of blood neutrophils necessitates a high mitotic activity of their myeloid precursors in the marrow to maintain the neutrophil supply. Myelopoiesis and the supply of blood neutrophils is maintained by a renewable supply of myeloid progenitor cells derived from hematopoietic stem cells. The myeloid growth factors, most prominently G-CSF, are the key regulators of this component of hematopoiesis. Experimentally, deficiencies of G-CSF or it receptor cause neutropenia, and G-CSF administration stimulates neutrophil production in a dose-dependent manner (4,5). These hallmarks of myelopoiesis and the critical role of neutrophils in the response to infection make neutropenia the dose-limiting toxicity of myelosuppressive cancer chemotherapy (11). The short life span of neutrophils also accounts for the difficulties encountered in the development of neutrophil transfusions as a therapy for neutropenia (12,13).

NEUTROPENIA AND FEBRILE NEUTROPENIA

Neutropenia is defined as a blood neutrophil count below the lower limit of normal, i.e., $<2.0 \times 10^9$ per liter. The term *granulocytopenia* is sometimes used synonymously with neutropenia. *Leukopenia* refers to a reduction in the total white blood cell (WBC) count to less than normal, i.e., less than 3.0×10^9 per liter. Neutropenia is the most common cause for leukopenia. In general, it is preferable to refer to absolute counts (WBC × percentage of cells in differential count) of neutrophils, monocytes, lymphocytes, or eosinophils in making inferences about a patient's risk of infection or other complication from chemotherapy (14).

In healthy individuals, blood neutrophil counts vary modestly from day to day, without a discernible pattern of this variation (15). Many factors affect the circulating neutrophil level, including exercise, anxiety, stress, drugs, infections, and all types of inflammatory conditions (14). In patients who have recently received myelosuppressive chemotherapy, the circulating neutrophil count may not fully reflect the body's capacity to generate neutrophils, because there is often a lag between damage to the marrow and changes in blood neutrophil counts. For these reasons, blood neutrophil counts should always be interpreted on the basis of the patient's history and the setting in which the measurement is made.

Neutropenia is usually subdivided into mild (neutrophil counts above 1.0×10^9 per liter), moderate (neutrophil counts between 0.5×10^9 per liter and 1.0×10^9 per liter), and severe (counts below 0.5×10^9 per liter). These subdivisions are arbitrary, but they are very important (11).

In patients with neutropenia, the risk of fever (usually a temperature greater than 101°F or 38.2°C), febrile neutropenia (fever as just defined with blood neutrophils less that 0.5×10^9 per liter), and infectious complications depends on both the severity of neutropenia and its duration. With counts below 0.5×10^9 per liter the risk of infection increases day by day, and it increases even more rapidly for counts less than 0.1×10^9 per liter. Severe neutropenia lasting no more than one to three days may be associated with fever, but infectious complications are uncommon. However, longer periods of neutropenia are associated with a substantially increased risk; the risk of febrile neutropenia and infections increase at a rate of about 10% per day. Longer durations of severe neutropenia, e.g., after myeloablation for hematopoietic stem cell transplantation, further enhance this risk.

When infections occur in this setting, they are usually due to the resident microorganisms on the skin, mucus membranes, and inhabiting the gastrointestinal tract (16). If the organisms on the surfaces of the body have been altered by local or systemic antibiotic treatments, infections by resistant bacterial and fungal infections are increasingly likely. If neutropenia is accompanied by other alterations of host defenses, e.g., lymphocytopenia, monocytopenia, hypogammaglobulinemia, or malnutrition, a broader array of infectious complications is increasingly likely. Indwelling catheters, implanted devices, and ulceration of the skin or mucus membranes are important factors enhancing the risk of infectious complications (17).

When cancer patients develop febrile neutropenia, they need prompt evaluation, laboratory tests, and imaging studies. Initially it may be difficult to determine the seriousness of the event, but fear of a cascade of serious consequences usually prompts empiric treatment with antibiotics (Fig. 1) (11). Exactly what happens depends on the cause of the fever and risk factors of the patient. Because of uncertainty, hospitalization for observation and antibiotics remain the standard of care in most locales (18). A recent review of discharge data for more than 40,000 patients from 115 U.S. medical centers between 1995 and 2000 showed that patients admitted with febrile neutropenia had an in-hospital mortality rate of 9.5%, rising from 2.6% for patients without any major comorbidities to 21.4% for those with two or more concomitant problems such as congestive heart failure, lung disease or diabetes (19). In this study, 29% of the patients were over 65 years. Risk factors for in-patient mortality were gram-negative sepsis, pneumonia, renal impairment, cerebrovascular disease, liver disease, and lung disease. This study reinforces the seriousness of febrile neutropenia, particularly in older patients with pre-existing chronic illnesses (19).

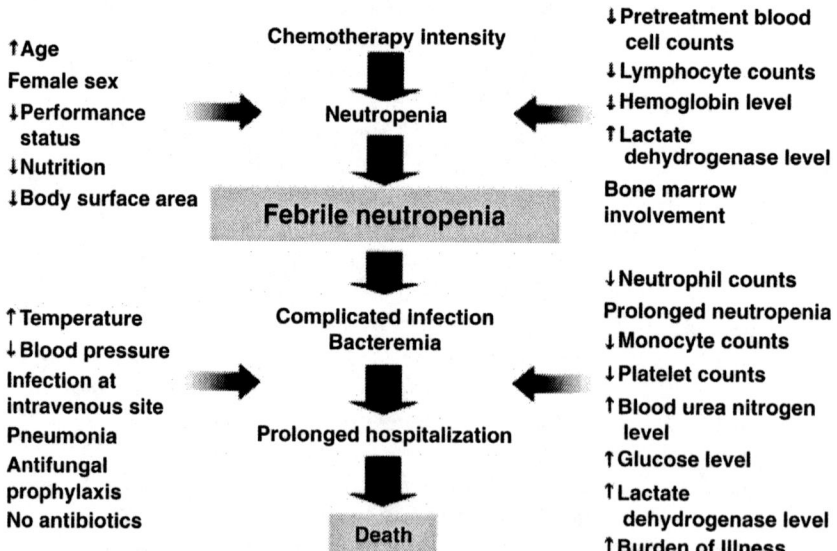

Figure 1 Schematic diagram of the cascade of chemotherapy-induced neutropenia and neutropenic complications including febrile neutropenia, complicated infection, and death, along with some of the associated risk factors reported in previous studies (31).

Neutropenia has other consequences for patients with cancer. Many clinicians hesitate to administer full-dose chemotherapy to patients with pre-existing neutropenia due to previous radiation, chemotherapy, or intrinsic hematological abnormalities, e.g., chronic idiopathic neutropenia. Neutropenia may also be due to ethnicity, e.g., as is often observed in African-Americans and others of African origin (20). Current data indicate that in the absence of other risk factors, persons of African origin can usually receive standard dose chemotherapy (21).

Neutropenia developing after initiation of chemotherapy also often leads to dose reduction or dose delays in cancer treatment (22). The full consequences of such reductions are not known but probably vary with the type and stage of the cancer, the degree and timing of dose reductions, and patient-specific factors (23). Most available data indicate that full doses of standard-dose chemotherapy maximize the likelihood of a favorable response and long-term survival for chemotherapy-sensitive malignancies (24,25). In fact, several recent studies suggest that the development of neutropenia is a biological marker of delivery of adequate doses of chemotherapy to achieve a favorable treatment response, suggesting that the development of neutropenia is a biologic index of sufficient treatment to affect both the normal host cells and the cancer cells in the individual undergoing treatment (26).

CAUSE OF NEUTROPENIA

In addition to cancer chemotherapy, neutropenia has many other causes, including congenital and acquired hematological disorders, inflammatory diseases (e.g., rheumatoid arthritis, sarcoidosis), infectious diseases (e.g., human immunodeficiency virus infection, infectious mononucleosis), and reactions to many drugs (e.g., penicillins, sulfonamides) (1,14). In general, chronic steady-state neutropenia, as occurs in chronic idiopathic neutropenia, is associated with a lesser risk of severe infections than occurs with myelotoxic chemotherapy causing the complete interruption of neutrophil production. Thus, the management of neutropenia always depends on its etiology and the specific circumstances in which it is encountered.

CHEMOTHERAPY-INDUCED NEUTROPENIA

The pattern of neutropenia after myelosuppressive drugs varies substantially from drug to drug, with the dose of each drug and combinations of drugs and within the population of patients treated (27). Some agents, e.g., cyclophosphamide, are well recognized to cause an abrupt drop in neutrophil counts, from which recovery occurs rapidly after single exposure. Other agents, e.g., the taxanes and anthracyclines, predictably cause longer periods of neutropenia. A third class of agents, i.e., busulfan, causes neutropenia that has a slower onset but a longer duration. Biological agents, such as rituximab, may cause neutropenia weeks after the drug is administered (28,29). Our understanding of chemotherapy-induced neutropenia is further complicated by varying doses of drugs used in clinical trials and practice, the overlapping toxicities of these agents, and the limited number of neutrophil counts collected and reported in most studies (30).

Currently a useful approach is to characterize standard chemotherapy regimens based on the likelihood that the regimen causes severe neutropenia. Regimens are then classified as having a 10% to 20% or >20% probability of causing neutropenia in the treatment of specific malignancies (Table 1). Such a scheme has been developed for clinical guidelines by the National Comprehensive Cancer Network (NCCN), the American Society of Clinical Oncology, and the European Organization for Research on Treatment of Cancer (EORTC) with their recent guidelines on the appropriate uses of myeloid growth factors in cancer treatment (31–35).

In addition to these regimen-specific factors, various host factors are also critical in determining the risk of chemotherapy-induced neutropenia. Based on a large registry study of oncology practices in the United States, Lyman et al. qualified the risk and timing of neutropenia, febrile neutropenia, and neutropenia-related events, including the risk of reductions in chemotherapy treatment (31). These studies have shown that across the spectrum of chemotherapy regimens currently used for the treatment of solid tumors and lymphoma, the greatest risk of neutropenia is in the first cycle of treatment (Fig. 2) (31,36,37). About two-third of this risk is in the first cycle, if primary prevention with a myeloid growth factor is not given. Within each tumor type (e.g., patients with breast cancer, non-Hodgkin's lymphoma, lung cancer), there are patient-specific risk factors. The best defined of these factors are the patient's age, performance status, comorbidities (diabetes, liver disease, and renal disease), prior treatments, and pre-existing neutropenia or anemia (31). From a practical basis, definition of these patient-specific risk factors and validation of the value of their use in clinical practice is extremely important for understanding and communicating to the patient the risk of neutropenia and its complications (Table 2).

INFECTIOUS COMPLICATIONS OF NEUTROPENIA

The management of febrile neutropenia and the infectious complications of chemotherapy-induced neutropenia in cancer patients are discussed elsewhere.

PREVENTION OF FEBRILE NEUTROPENIA

Since the advent of modern chemotherapy in the 1950s and the recognition of neutropenia as the dose-limiting toxicity with most chemotherapy regimens, clinicians have sought strategies to prevent febrile neutropenia. In the 1970s, it was thought that oral lithium carbonate might be useful as a stimulus to neutrophil production, but this agent proved to be either too weak to be helpful or too toxic to be safe (38–40). Subsequently, oral antibiotics, particularly the combination of trimethoprim-sulfamethoxazole (TMP-SMZ) and the quinolones

Table 1 Incidence of Febrile Neutropenia for Selected Chemotherapy Regimens: Reported Rates Across Guidelines

Cancer type	Regimen	Myeloid growth factor guideline (% febrile neutropenia)		
		ASCO	EORTC	NCCN
Breast	AC	10	10–20	10–20
	AC-Pac	3	5	
	AC-Pac(dd)	6		>20
	AC-Doc		5–25	
	A-T-C	3	3	
	CEF	8–9	14	
	TAC	24–34	21–24	>20
	Apac		21–32	>20
	Adoc	33	33–48	
	FEC120		9–14	
	FEC100		0–2	
	FAC		5	
	CMFiv		0–3	
	CMFpo		1	
	Doc	21	16–17	10–20
	DocCapec		13	
SCLC	Carbo/VP-16			10–20
	TopC			10–20
	CAE		24–57	>20
	Topotecan		28	>20
	TopT		>20	>20
	ICE		24	
	VICE		70	
NSCLC	VIG		25	>20
	DP	3.7	26	>20
	Cis/Pac	16	16	10–20
	Cis/Gem	4	1–7	
	Cis/Doc	11	5–11	
	Carbo/Pac	4	0–9	
	VP-16/Cis		54	
	Vinor/Cis		1–10	
NHL	ESHAP	30	30–64	>20
	ACOD		11	10–20
	FM		11	10–20
	CHOP		17–50	
	RCHOP	18	19	10–20
	DHAP	48	48	

(*Continued*)

Table 1 Incidence of Febrile Neutropenia for Selected Chemotherapy Regimens: Reported Rates Across Guidelines (*Continued*)

Cancer type	Regimen	Myeloid growth factor guideline (% febrile neutropenia)		
		ASCO	EORTC	NCCN
Colorectal	5-FU/LV		1–15	
	FOLFIRI	9.3	3–14	
	FOLFOX	6	0–8	
	IFL	7.1	3–7	
	Irinotecan	5.8	2–7	
Germ Cell	VIP			>20
	EC		10	10–20
	BEP→EP		13	
	BOP→VIP-B		46	
Ovary	Top	18	10–18	>20
	Pac		22	>20
	Doc		33	>20
	Cis/Pac	Rare		
	Carbo/Pac		3–8	
	Gem/Cis		9	
Sarcoma	MAID		58	>20
	Doxorubicin			>20
	Dox/Ifos			>20

Source: From Ref. 35.
Abbreviations: AC, doxorubicin/cyclophosphamide; AC-Pac, doxorubicin/cyclophosphamide/pacli taxel; AC-Pac(dd), doxorubicin/cyclophosphamide/paclitaxel (dose dense); AC-Doc, doxorubicin/cyclophosphamide/docetaxel; A-T-C, doxorubicin/paclitaxel/ cyclophosphamide; CAE, cyclophospha mide/doxorubicin/VP-16; CEF, cyclophosphamide/epirubicin/fluorouracil; TAC, docetaxel/doxorubicin/cyclophosphamide; APac, doxorubicin/paclitaxel; ADoc, doxorubicin/docetaxel; FEC120, cyclophosphamide/epirubicin/fluorouracil; FEC100, cyclophosphamide/epirubicin/fluorouracil; FAC, fluorouracil/doxorubicin/cyclophosphamide; CMFiv, cyclophosphamide/methotrexate/fluorouracil—intravenous; CMFpo, cyclophosphamide/methotrexate/fluorouracil—oral; Doc, docetaxel; DocCapec, doc etaxel/capecitabine; Carbo/VP-16, carboplatin/etoposide; TopC, topotecan/cisplatin; TopT, topotecan/paclitaxel; ICE, ifosfamide/carboplatin/etoposide; VICE, vincristine/ifosfamide/carboplatin/etoposide; VIG, gemcitabine/ifosfamide/dacarbazine; DP, docetaxel/carboplatin; Cis/Pac, cisplatin/paclitaxel; Cis/Gem, cisplatin/gemcitabine; Cis/Doc, cisplatin/docetaxel; Carbo/Pac, carboplatin/paclitaxel; VP-16/Cis, etoposide/cisplatin; Vinor/Cis, vinorelbine/cisplatin; ESHAP, etoposide/methylprednisolone/cisplatin/cytarabine; ACOD, doxorubicin/cyclophosphamide/vincristine/prednisone; FM, fludarabine/mitoxantrone; CHOP, cyclophosphamide/doxorubicin/vincristine/prednisone; RCHOP, cyclophosphamide/doxorubicin/vincristine/prednisone/rituximab; DHAP, cisplatin/cytarabine/dexamethasone; 5-FU/LV, 5-FU/leucovorin; FOLFIRI, 5-FU/leucovorin/irinotecan; FOLFOX, 5-FU/leucovorin/oxaliplatin; IFL, irinotecan/fluorouracil/lecucovorin; VIP, vinblastine/ifosfamide/cisplatin; EC, etoposide/cisplatin; BEP→EP, bleomycin/etoposide/cisplatinis→etoposide/cisplatin; BOP→VIP-B, bleomycin/vincristine/cisplatin→cisplatin/ifosfamide/etoposide/bleomycin; Top, topotecan; Pac, paclitaxel; MAID, mesna/adriamycin/ifosfamide/dacarbazine Dox/Ifos, doxorubicin/ifosfamide.

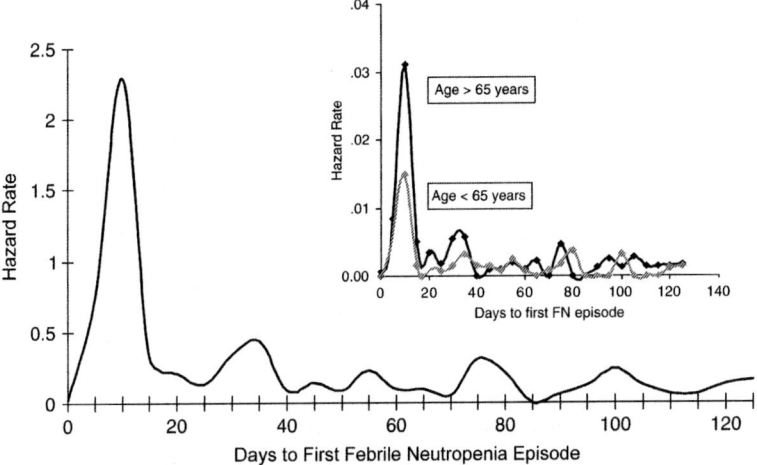

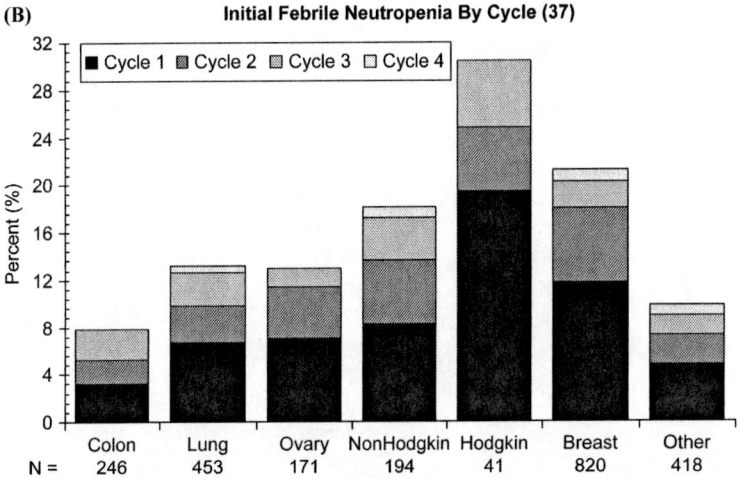

Figure 2 (**A**) Hazard function of the time to the initial episode of febrile neutropenia among 577 patients with diffuse large-cell non-Hodgkin's lymphoma treated with CHOP chemotherapy demonstrating the greatest risk of febrile neutropenia occurs in the initial cycle of treatment (31,36). The insert represents the hazard function of the initial episode of febrile neutropenia within the same population split on the basis of age, demonstrating that the patients ≥65 years of age experience nearly twice the risk of febrile neutropenia in cycle 1 than younger patients. (**B**) Graph of the proportion of patients experiencing febrile neutropenia in each of the first four cycles of chemotherapy derived from a prospective study of unselected patients treated in 112 community oncology practices from throughout the United States, demonstrating that the preponderance of episodes of febrile neutropenia occurs in the initial cycles of treatment across most major cancer types studied (37).

Table 2 Risk Factors for Febrile Neutropenia and Its Complications

Category	ASCO	EORTC	NCCN
Disease-related	Advanced stage disease	Advanced disease/ metastasis	Advanced stage disease; bone marrow involvement; elevated LDH (lymphoma); leukemia; lung cancer
Treatment-related	Previous episode of febrile neutropenia; extensive prior chemotherapy; concurrent XRT or large prior radiation ports	Previous episode of febrile neutropenia; no antibiotic prophylaxis;* no GCSF use; planned dose intensity >80%	Prior history of severe neutropenia; planned dose intensity >80%; extensive prior chemotherapy; concurrent/prior radiation
Patient-related age gender ethnicity performance status comorbidities laboratory	≥65; poor performance status; poor nutritional status; open or infected wounds; serious comorbidities; cytopenia secondary to bone marrow involvement	≥65; female Asian origin; poor performance status; poor nutritional status; cardiovascular, renal disease; ≥1 comorbidity; body surface area < 2.0 m^2; abnormal liver transaminases; Hb < 12 gm/dL; serum albumin ≤ 3.5g/dL; pretreatment ANC < 1500	≥65; female poor performance status (ECOG ≥ 2); poor nutritional, immune status; open or infected wounds; COPD; cardiovascular disease; diabetes mellitus; elevated bilirubin or alkaline phosphatase; low hg; preexisting ANC < 1000 or lymphocytopenia

*Indiscriminant use of antibiotic prophylaxis is not recommended.
Source: From Ref. 35.

have been well studied, as well as the myeloid growth factors G-CSF and GM-CSF. The uses of G-CSF and GM-CSF for prevention of febrile neutropenia are considered elsewhere.

There are several extensive reviews, meta-analyses, and recent editorials on the use of antibiotics to prevent febrile neutropenia after cancer chemotherapy (41–45). The initial trials of antibiotic prophylaxis with TMP-SMZ were relatively small and suggested a large benefit (46–47). A recent meta-analysis indicates that 14 randomized, controlled trials were conducted over a 15-year period; 6 favored the treatment and 8 favored the controls. The summarized data on 870 patients (total events: controls 58, treated patients 40) failed to show a significant effect ($p = 0.06$). From a clinical perspective, the additional problem was the occurrence of yeast infections, if the treatment with TMP-SMZ was prolonged (42).

Randomized controlled trials with the quinolones, e.g., ciprofloxacin, norfloxacin, ofloxacin, and levofloxacin, began in the early 1980s. Fifty-two randomized controlled trials were included in a recent meta-analysis that clearly reported a positive treatment effect (42). The results of the test for an overall effect were $Z = 3.25$, $p = 0.001$ in placebo-controlled trials. Other meta-analyses have given similar results (41). The available data also showed that quinolones were more effective and better tolerated than TMP-SMZ (41). The quinolones are readily absorbed and are effective agents against a wide range of gram-negative bacilli as well as gram-positive cocci. The clinical trials, however, are not uniform in enrollment criteria. Only some reports included results of surveillance cultures, to determine if resistant microorganisms emerged on the patients' body surfaces during the trial or in the environment. The major concern of most specialists in microbiology and infectious diseases is that wide use of the quinolones for prophylaxis will lead to progressively more resistant bacteria in the environment, including the environment of cancer treatment centers where there are many patients who are highly susceptible to bacterial and fungal infections (16,18,44,45). Those experts therefore have usually recommended against the wide use of quinolone prophylaxis.

Antibiotic therapy for febrile neutropenia is covered in separate chapters and the uses of myeloid growth factors for prophylaxis and treatment of infections in this setting is covered elsewhere.

SUMMARY

Neutropenia has been a critical toxicity limiting the treatment of malignancies for more than half a century. Over this period, our understanding of the problem has increased enormously. The major risk factors for neutropenia and its complications with common chemotherapy regimens are the type of cancer (hematological or nonhematological malignancy), treatment regimen (drugs, dose, and schedule), and host factors (age, comorbidities, hematological status, and previous treatments). Basic and clinical research have also improved our understanding of the regulation of neutrophil and monocyte production and function and led to the development of the myeloid growth factors, particularly G-CSF as an effective agent to stimulate myeloid recovery after chemotherapy. The quinolone family of antibiotics is the most effective alternate agent to reduce the occurrence of febrile neutropenia in this setting. This information, if properly applied, promises to continue improvement in cancer treatment and outcomes.

REFERENCES

1. Dale DC, Liles WC. Neutrophils and monocytes: normal physiology and disorders of neutrophil and monocyte production. In: Handin RI, Lux SE, Stossel TP, eds. Blood: Principles and Practice of Hematology. Philadelphia, PA: Lippincott, Williams and Wilkins, 2003:455–482.
2. Dale DC. Nonmalignant Disorders of Leukocytes. In: Dale DC, Federman DD, eds. ACP Medicine 2006, vol 1. New York, NY: WebMD, Inc., 2006:1030–1037.
3. Hübel K, Dale DC, Liles WC. Therapeutic use of cytokines to modulate phagocyte function for the treatment of infectious diseases: current status of G-CSF, GM-CSF, M-CSF, and IFNg. J Infect Dis 2002; 185:1490–1501.
4. Chatta GS, Price TH, Allen RC, et al. The effects of *in vivo* recombinant methionyl human granulocyte colony stimulating factor (rhG-CSF) on the neutrophil response and peripheral blood colony-forming cells in healthy young and elderly volunteers. Blood 1994; 84:2923–2929.
5. Price TH, Chatta GS, Dale DC. The effect of recombinant granulocyte colony-stimulating factor on neutrophil kinetics in normal young and elderly humans. Blood 1996; 88:335–340.
6. Dale DC, Liles WC, Llewellyn C, et al. The effects of granulocyte macrophage colony-stimulating factor (GM-CSF) on neutrophil kinetics and function in normal human volunteers. Am J Hematol 1998; 57:7–15.
7. Boxer, LA. Neutrophil abnormalities. Pediatr Rev 2003; 24:52–62.
8. Lejeune M, Sariban E, Cantinieaux B, et al. Granulocyte functions in children with cancer are differentially sensitive to the toxic effect of chemotherapy. Pediatr Res 1996; 39:835–842.
9. Lejeune M, Ferster A, Cantinieaux B, et al. Prolonged but reversible neutrophil dysfunction differentially sensitive to granulocyte colony-stimulating factor in children with acute lymphoblastic leukaemia. Br J Haematol 1998; 102: 1284–1291.
10. Levy O, Sisson RB, Fryer HE, et al. Neutrophil defense in patients undergoing bone marrow transplantation: bactericidal/permeability-increasing protein (BPI) and defensins in graft-derived neutrophils. Transplantation 2002; 73:1522–1526.
11. Pizzo PA. Fever in immunocompromised patients. N Engl J Med 1999; 341:893–900.
12. Dale DC, Liles WC, Llewellyn C, et al. Neutrophil transfusions: kinetics and functions of neutrophils mobilized with granulocyte-colony stimulating factor and dexamethasone. Transplantation 1998; 38:713–721.
13. Atallah E, Schiffer CA. Granulocyte transfusion. Curr Opin Hematol 2006; 13:45–49.
14. Dale DC. Neutropenia and Neutrophilia. In: Lichtman MA, Beutler E, Kipps TJ, Seligsohn U, Kaushansky K, Prchal JT, eds. Williams Hematology. 7th ed. New York, NY: McGraw-Hill Co, Inc., 2006:907–919.
15. Dale DC, Alling DW, Wolff SM. Application of time series analysis to serial blood neutrophil counts in normal individuals and patients receiving cyclophosphamide. Br J Hematol 1973; 24:57–64.
16. Hughes WT, Armstrong D, Bodey GP, et al. 2002 guidelines for the use of antimicrobial agents in neutropenic patients with cancer. Clin Infect Dis 2002; 35:891–895.
17. Raad I, Hachem R, Hanna H, et al. Sources and outcomes of bloodstream infections in cancer patients: the role of central venous catheters. Eur J Clin Microbiol Infect Dis 2007 Jun 21; [epub ahead of print].

18. Sepkowitz KA. Treatment of patients with hematologic neoplasm, fever, and neutropenia. Clin Infect Dis 2005; 40(suppl 4):S253–S256.
19. Kuderer NM, Dale DC, Crawford J, et al. Mortality, morbidity, and cost associated with febrile neutropenia in adult cancer patients. Cancer 2006; 106:2258–2266.
20. Hershman D, Weinberg M, Rosner Z, et al. Ethnic neutropenia and treatment delay in African American women undergoing chemotherapy for early-stage breast cancer. Natl Cancer Inst 2003; 95:1545–1548.
21. Smith K, Wray L, Klein-Cabral M, et al. Ethnic disparities in adjuvant chemotherapy for breast cancer are not caused by excess toxicity in black patients. Clin Breast Cancer 2005; 6:260–266; discussion 267–269.
22. Lyman GH, Dale DC, Crawford J. Incidence and predictors of low dose-intensity in adjuvant breast cancer chemotherapy: a nationwide study of community practices. J Clin Oncol 2003; 21:4524–4531.
23. Shayne M, Crawford J, Dale DC, et al, for the ANC Study Group. Predictors of reduced dose intensity in patients with early-stage breast cancer receiving adjuvant chemotherapy. Breast Cancer Res Treat 2006; 100:255–262.
24. Piccart MJ, Biganzoli L, Di Leo A. The impact of chemotherapy dose density and dose intensity on breast cancer outcome: what have we learned? Eur J Cancer 2000; 36(suppl 1):S4–S10.
25. Chang J. Chemotherapy dose reduction and delay in clinical practice: evaluating the risk to patient outcome in adjuvant chemotherapy for breast cancer. Eur J Cancer 2000; 36(suppl 1):S11–S14.
26. Banerji U, Ashley S, Coward J, et al. The association of chemotherapy induced neutropenia on treatment outcomes in small cell lung cancer. Lung Cancer 2006; 54:371–377.
27. Milokovich G. Adverse events associated with commonly used cancer regimens. In: Scheife R, Milkovich G, guest eds. Pharmacotherapy. Lexington, KY: University of Kentucky, 2000; 20(suppl); 7(2):955–964.
28. Fukuno K, Tsurumi H, Ando N, et al. Late-onset neutropenia in patients treated with rituximab for non-Hodgkin's lymphoma. Int J Hematol 2006; 242–247.
29. Terrier B, Ittah M, Tourneur L, et al. Late-onsert neutropenia following tituximab results from a hematopoietic lineage competition due to an excessive BAFF-induced B-cell recovery. Haematologica 2007; 92(3 suppl):ECR10.
30. Dale DC, McCarter GC, Crawford J, et al. Myelotoxicity and dose intensity of chemotherapy: reporting practices from randomized clinical trials. J Natl Compr Canc Netw 2003; 1:440–454.
31. Lyman GH. Guidelines of the National Comprehensive Cancer Network on the use of myeloid growth factors with cancer chemotherapy: a review of the evidence. J Natl Compr Canc Netw 2005; 3:557–571.
32. Crawford J, Althaus B, Armitage J, et al. Myeloid growth factors. NCCN Clinical Practice Guidelines on Oncology. Jenkintown, PA: NCCN, 2007.
33. Smith TJ, Khatcheressian J, Lyman GH, et al. 2006 update of recommendations for the use of white blood cell growth factors: an evidence-based clinical practice guideline. J Clin Oncol 2006; 24:3187–3205.
34. Aapro MS, Cameron DA, Pettengell R, et al. EORTC guidelines for the use of granulocyte-colony stimulating factor to reduce the incidence of chemotherapy-induced febrile neutropenia in adult patients with lymphomas and solid tumours. Eur J Cancer 2006; 42:2433–2453.

35. Lyman GH, Kleiner JM. Summary and Comparison of Myeloid Growth Factor Guidelines in Patients Receiving Cancer Chemotherapy. J Natl Compr Cancer Netw 2007; 5: 217–228.
36. Lyman GH, Morrison VA, Dale DC, et al. Risk of febrile neutropenia among patients with intermediate-grade non-Hodgkin's lymphoma receiving CHOP chemotherapy. Leukem Lymphoma 2003; 44: 2069–2076.
37. Crawford J, Dale DC, Kuderer NM, et al. Risk and timing of neutropenic events in adult cancer patients receiving chemotherapy: the results of a prospective nationwide study of oncology practice. J Natl Comp Canc Netw 2008 (in press).
38. Richman CM, Makii MM, Weiser PA, et al. The effect of lithium carbonate on chemotherapy-induced neutropenia and thrombocytopenia. Am J Hematol 1984; 16:313–323.
39. Lyman GH, Williams CC, Preston D: The use of lithium carbonate to reduce infection and leukopenia during systemic chemotherapy. N Engl J Med 1980; 302: 257–260.
40. Lyman GH, Williams CC, Dinwoodie WR, et al. Sudden death in cancer patients receiving lithium. J Clin Oncology 1984; 2:1270–1276.
41. Engels EA, Lau J, Barza M. Efficacy of quinolone prophylaxis in neutropenic cancer patients: a meta-analysis. J Clin Oncol 1998; 16:1179–1187.
42. Gafter-Gvili A, Fraser A, Paul M, et al. Meta-analysis: antibiotic prophylaxis reduces mortality in neutropenic patients. Ann Intern Med 2005; 142:979.
43. Timmer-Bonte J, Tjan-Heijnen V. Febrile neutropenia: Highlighting the role of prophylactic antibiotics and granulocyte colony-stimulating factor during standard dose chemotherapy for solid tumors. Anti-Cancer Drugs 2006; 17:881–889.
44. Gafter-Gvili A, Fraser A, Paul M, et al. Antibiotic prophylaxis for bacterial infections in afebrile neutropenic patients following chemotherapy. Cochrane Database Syst Rev 2005; 4:CD004386.
45. Baden LR. Prophylactic antimicrobial agents and the importance of fitness. N Engl J Med 2005; 353:1052–1054.
46. Enno A, Catovsky D, Darrell J, et al. Co-trimoxazole for prevention of infection in acute leukemia. Lancet 1978; 2:395–397.
47. Gurwith MJ, Brunton JL, Lank BA, et al. A prospective controlled investigation of prophylactic trimethoprim/sulfamethoxazole in hospitalized granulocytopenic patients. Am J Med 1979; 66:248–256.

5

Bacterial Infections in Cancer Patients

Kenneth V. I. Rolston and Gerald P. Bodey
Department of Infectious Diseases, Infection Control and Employee Health, Division of Internal Medicine, The University of Texas M.D. Anderson Cancer Center, Houston, Texas, U.S.A.

INTRODUCTION

The use of intensive chemotherapeutic regimens, hematopoietic stem cell transplantation, and other therapeutic modalities, has increased the remission and cure rates of many cancer patients. These modalities have also been associated with more severe myelosuppression and immunosuppression, increasing the frequency of severe, sometimes fatal, infection. Although substantial progress has been made in prevention, early diagnosis, and treatment of infections, the spectrum of organisms causing these infections undergoes periodic changes, new opportunistic pathogens emerge, and common organisms develop multiple mechanisms of resistance. Also, patients today are less restricted in their activities and may be exposed to human, plant, or animal pathogens more frequently than in the past, leading to an increasing proportion of infections originating outside the hospital. Additionally, the usual signs and symptoms of infection including fever may be minimal or absent, especially among severely neutropenic patients and those receiving adrenal corticosteroids. Consequently, patients must be monitored carefully, especially during periods of increased risk. The availability of sophisticated technology such as CT scan, antigen detection, and molecular techniques (PCR) have assisted in the diagnosis of some infections and offers promise for greater success in the future. Nevertheless, a specific diagnosis of infection is often not possible, and empiric therapy must be administered on the basis of local epidemiology and susceptibility/resistance patterns. In recent years, it has become possible to stratify patients into categories such as high-risk and low-risk for the development of severe infections and associated complications. Treatment strategies such as early discharge, outpatient management, and orally administered drugs are now commonplace in low-risk patients.

PREDISPOSING FACTORS

Malignant diseases often interfere with host defense mechanisms, and specific deficiencies are associated with a unique set of infections (Table 1). However, multiple defects may be present in the same patient making infection with a wide variety of pathogens likely. These deficiencies include neutropenia, impaired cellular immunity, impaired humoral immunity, and other immunological deficits, local factors such as necrotic tumors, obstruction, and breaches of natural barriers such as the skin and mucosal surfaces due to the increasing use of catheters and other medical devices, chemoradiation, and following extensive surgery. All these factors need to be considered when making diagnostic and therapeutic decisions in a timely manner, so that the most appropriate therapy is administered promptly.

CURRENT SPECTRUM OF BACTERIAL INFECTION

Several epidemiological surveys have documented a recent predominance of gram-positive organisms particularly in patients with bacteremia (1–3). However, bacteremias occur in only 15% to 20% of patients with documented infections.

Table 1 Common Bacterial Infections Associated with Various Defects in Host Defense Mechanisms

Defect[a]	Common infections
Neutropenia (ANC $\leq$ 500/mm^3)	Gram-positive cocci, gram-negative bacilli
Impaired cellular immunity	*Listeria monocytogenes, Rhodococcus equi, Nocardia* spp., mycobacteria, *Salmonella* spp.
Hypogammaglobulinemia	Encapsulated organisms, *Streptococcus pneumoniae, Haemophilus influenzae, Neisseria meningitis*
Tissue necrosis/local obstruction	Gram-positive cocci, gram-negative bacilli, anaerobes
Catheter/other devices	Gram-positive cocci, other skin organisms (*Bacillus* spp., *Corynebacterium* spp.), mycobacteria, gram-negative bacilli

Abbreviation: ANC, absolute neutrophil count.
[a]Multiple defects are often present in the same patient.

Infections at most other sites (respiratory tract, gastrointestinal tract, urinary tract, skin, and skin structure) are frequently caused by gram-negative bacilli or are polymicrobial (4–6). Unfortunately, most surveys include only single-organism bacteremias, with very little data on infections at other sites and polymicrobial infections, leading to an incomplete and inaccurate description of the true spectrum of bacterial infection. This may partly be due to a lack of widely accepted definitions for various infections in severely neutropenic/immunocompromised patients (7). Such definitions need to be developed so that more accurate epidemiological data can be captured and reported (6).

The most commonly isolated gram-positive organisms colonize the skin and gain entry into the bloodstream when breaches of the integument occur. These include coagulase-negative staphylococci, *Staphylococcus aureus*, *Corynebacterium* spp., and *Bacillus* spp. Most infections caused by these organisms are associated with the use of central venous catheters (CVCs), and an important, often controversial, management decision is whether or not the offending catheter should be removed. Catheter removal is almost always necessary when *S. aureus* is the causative pathogen. Gram-positive organisms also colonize in the oropharynx and intestinal tract and can cause infection in the setting of mucosal erosion at these sites (8–12). These include viridans group streptococci, other (beta hemolytic) streptococci, *Stomatococcus mucilaginosus*, *Streptococcus pneumoniae*, and *Enterococcus* spp. Gram-positive pathogens associated with defects in cellular immunity include *Listeria monocytogenes* and *Rhodococcus equi*, and excessive vancomycin usage has been associated with the selection of vancomycin-resistant organisms such as *Lactobacilli*, *Leuconstoc* spp., *Pediococcus* spp., and vancomycin-resistant enterococci (VRE) (13–16).

Many gram-positive organisms have developed resistance to antimicrobial agents frequently used for the prevention and/or treatment of infections in cancer patients. At many institutions, more than 50% of *S. aureus* and more than 90% of coagulase-negative staphylococci are methicillin resistant, approximately 17% to 20% of enterococci are vancomycin resistant, and many streptococci (VGS and *S. pneumoniae*) are penicillin resistant. These developments represent new challenges and highlight the need for infection prevention, infection control, antibiotic stewardship, and new drug development (16–18).

Gram-negative bacilli currently account for 15% to 20% of documented bacterial infections in cancer patients (2). The most commonly isolated organisms are *Escherichia coli*, *Klebsiella* spp., and *Pseudomonas aeruginosa* (19). Other enterobacteriaceae (*Enterobacter*, *Citrobacter*, *Serratia*, and *Proteus* spp.) and nonfermentative gram-negative bacilli (*Acinetobacter* spp., nonaeruginosa *Pseudomonas* spp., and *Stenotrophomonas maltophilia*) account for the remainder of gram-negative infections (Table 2). Although the use of antimicrobial (predominantly quinolone) prophylaxis has reduced the frequency of microbiologically documented gram-negative infections, it has also led to the emergence/selection of resistant gram-negative organisms (20,21). Some

Table 2 Nature and Spectrum of Bacterial Infections in Patients with Cancer

Common infections
    Bacteremia
    Pneumonia
    Urinary tract infection
    Skin and skin structure infection
    Abdominal/intestinal infection
Frequently isolated gram-positive pathogens
    Coagulase-negative staphylococci
    Staphylococcus aureus (including MRSA)
    Viridans group streptococci
    Enterococcus species (including VRE)
    Streptococcus pneumoniae and other streptococcus species
    Corynebacterium species
    Bacillus species
    Stomatococcus mucilaginosus
    Listeria monocytogenes
    Rhodococcus equi
Frequently isolated gram-negative pathogens
    Escherichia coli
    Klebsiella species
    Pseudomonas aeurginosa
    Enterobacter species
    Citrobacter species
    Serratia species
    Acinetobacter species
    Stenotrophomonas maltophilia
    Alcaligenes/Achromobacter species
    Proteus species
    Salmonella species
Anaerobic organisms
    Bacteroides species
    Clostridium species

organisms have developed multiple resistance mechanisms making them resistant to virtually all classes of antimicrobial agents currently in use, resulting in the reemergence of agents such as colistin and polymyxin B for treatment (17,18). Unfortunately, these agents are not optimal in patients with neutropenia (22).

    Infections with substantial tissue involvement (pneumonia, skin and skin structure infections, hepatobiliary and gastrointestinal infections) are often polymicrobial (6), and approximately 80% have a gram-negative component (23). The morbidity and mortality associated with polymicrobial infections appear to be greater than with monomicrobial infections (6,23). Anaerobes are isolated infrequently, even from polymicrobial infections.

PROBLEM INFECTIONS IN NEUTROPENIC PATIENTS

Abdominal Infections

Acute abdominal infection is a difficult management problem, especially in neutropenic patients who are unable to mount an adequate inflammatory response. These infections include cholecystitis, appendicitis, and diverticulitis, and those associated with complications of their diseases such as tumor lysis syndrome, neutropenic enterocolitis (typhlitis), splenic infarcts, or Vinca alkaloid neuropathy.

Neutropenic enterocolitis is a necrotizing infection more common in children with acute leukemia. It may be limited to the cecum (typhlitis) but more often involves the entire intestine. The cause is unknown, but neutropenia is a major predisposing factor and some chemotherapeutic agents may play a role. Common clinical manifestations are fever, abdominal distention, tenderness, and decreased bowel sounds (24). Computerized tomography often reveals paralytic ileus with the absence of gas in the right lower quadrant, and bowel wall thickening. Bacteremia, if present, is generally caused by enteric gram-negative bacilli and *Clostridium septicum*. Therapy consists of nasogastric suction, intravenous fluids, and broad-spectrum antibiotics with coverage against *P. aeruginosa* and anaerobic organisms. Surgery should be avoided unless there is a clear lack of response to supportive measures and/or complications such as perforation or hemorrhage occur.

Perianal Infections

Perianal infections are more common in patients with monocytic or myelomonocytic leukemia, but can occur in patients undergoing chemotherapy for other malignancies (25). Most patients have severe neutropenia, and recurrent episodes occur in patients with hemorrhoids, anal fissures, or other local lesions. Manifestations include fever and pain that is aggravated by defecation. Local lesions are tender, erythematous, and indurated, and can progress to ulceration and necrosis, which may extend to the genitalia or into the rectum. Cloudy, watery fluid containing numerous organisms is often present, but true abscess formation is rare due to the frequent presence of severe neutropenia. Cultures generally reveal an average of three organisms, usually gram-negative bacilli and Enterococcus species. Lesions should be incised and drained promptly. Therapy consists of analgesics, sitz baths and warm compresses, and stool softeners or antidiarrheal medications depending on symptoms. Antibiotic regimens should be broad spectrum with activity against *P. aeruginosa* and anaerobes (25).

Pneumonitis

Pneumonitis is the most common clinically documented infection among cancer patients. A microbiologic diagnosis is often not possible, as many neutropenic patients often fail to produce sputum. Moreover, sputum cultures are often misleading due to contamination by organisms residing in the oral cavity. Bronchoalveolar lavage and even open lung biopsy often fails to identify a pathogen in these patients.

Pneumonitis is generally a polymicrobial infection. Uncommon pathogens such as *S. epidermidis, Acinetobacter* spp., *S. maltophilia,* and *Pseudomonas putida* can cause serious infections in neutropenic/immunocompromised patients. Fungal, viral, or mycobacterial infections are not uncommon, particularly in patients with impaired cellular immunity. The chest roentgenogram can provide useful clues to the cause of pneumonitis, and CT scans are especially useful in some cases. Empiric therapy with broad-spectrum antimicrobial agents is indicated and aggressive efforts should be made to establish a specific diagnosis. Knowing the pathogens likely to cause infection associated with specific host deficiencies can help focus on appropriate diagnostic procedures.

INITIAL MANAGEMENT OF THE FEBRILE NEUTROPENIC PATIENT

Standard management of the febrile neutropenic patient includes the administration of empiric broad-spectrum antibiotic therapy based on local epidemiology and susceptibility/resistance patterns (26). Recent advances have made it possible to identify low-risk subsets among such patients. Consequently, the first step in the management of the febrile neutropenic patient consists of establishing which risk group the patient belongs to. Several risk prediction rules have been developed and validated (27–29). The most widely accepted and used model is the one developed by the Multinational Association of Supportive Care in Cancer (MASCC risk index), which ascribes weighted points to various clinical characteristics including age, clinical status, comorbidity, severity of disease, etc. A cumulative score of >20 is predictive of low-risk status with <5% chance of developing serious medical complications during an episode of fever and neutropenia (Table 3) (29). Once patients have been identified as being "low-risk" or "not low-risk," various risk-adapted treatment strategies are available based on institutional infrastructure and local expertise (Fig. 1). These include early discharge (24–72 hr) or treatment of the entire febrile episode in the outpatient/clinical setting in low-risk patients, using parenteral, sequential (IV → PO), or oral regimens (30). Commonly used regimens for outpatient therapy are listed in Table 4. Some patients who are classified as "not low-risk" might also be eligible for early discharge on outpatient regimens, if they are clinically stable and are responding to the initial empiric regimen after a few days of hospitalization (31). Most truly high-risk patients will need hospital-based therapy for the entire febrile episode, with close monitoring for response, the development of complications, drug-related toxicity, or multidrug-resistant superinfections (26). Commonly used regimens for hospital-based empiric therapy are also listed in Table 4.

Outpatient antibiotic therapy using oral regimens became feasible once quinolones such as ciprofloxacin became available for clinical use. Almost all

Table 3 Details of the MASCC Risk Index Scoring System

Patient or clinical characteristic	Numerical weight
Burden of illness	
No or mild symptoms	5
No hypotension (systolic BP > 90 mmHg)	5
No chronic obstructive pulmonary disease (COPD)	4
Solid tumor/no previous fungal infection	4
No dehydration (requiring parenteral fluid administration)	3
Burden of illness	
Moderate symptoms	3
Outpatient status on development of neutropenic fever	3
Age < 60 years	2

Note: A cumulative score of >20 is considered to be predictive of low-risk (<5%) for the development of serious medical complications and <1% for death, during an episode of neutropenic fever (29).

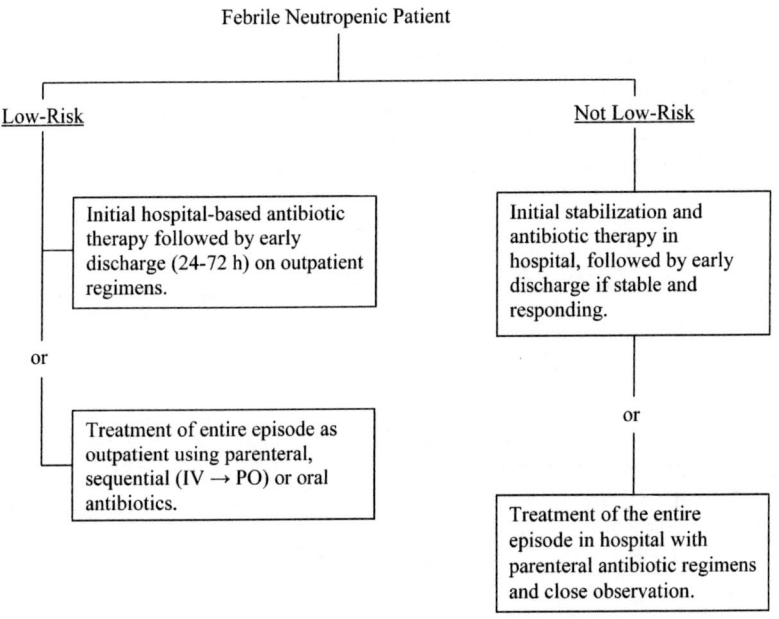

Figure 1 Risk-based strategies for the management of febrile neutropenic patients.

oral regimens are quinolone-based combinations with agents such as amoxicillin/clavulanate, clindamycin, or azithromycin (Table 4). Response rates with such regimens are generally >95% (32,33). Monotherapy using newer generation quinolones (moxifloxacin and levofloxacin) is still under investigation and early results are quite promising (34,35). Low-risk patients who are unable to take oral

Table 4 Antibiotic Regimens Commonly Used for Empiric Therapy in Febrile Neutropenic Patients

Regimens used in low-risk patients
   Oral regimens
      Ciprofloxacin[a] + amoxicillin/clavulanate
      Ciprofloxacin + clindamycin or azithromycin
      Moxifloxacin or levofloxacin[b]
   Parenteral regimens
      Ceftriazone (±) amikacin
      Aztreonam + clindamycin or quinolone
      Ceftazidime[c] (or other cephalosporins)
Regimens used in non-low-risk patients
   Monotherapy
      Extended-spectrum cephalosporins (cefepime, ceftazidime[c])
      Carbapenems (imipenem, meropenem)
      Other agents (piperacillin/tazobactam)
Combination regimens
      Aminoglycoside[d] + extended spectrum cephalosporins
      Aminoglycoside + carbapenem or piperacillin/tazobactam
      Vancomycin (or linezolid) + extended spectrum cephalosporin, or
         carbapenem, or piperacillin/tazobactam, or aztreonam
      Vancomycin + quinolone[e]

[a] Other quinolones (moxifloxacin, levofloxacin) may be substituted for ciprofloxacin.
[b] Quinolone monotherapy (moxifloxacin, levofloxacin) is still under investigation.
[c] Ceftazidime may not be adequate for empiric monotherapy based on current resistance patterns.
[d] Usually amikacin, but tobramycin or gentamicin can also be used based on local susceptibility patterns.
[e] Quinolones should not be used in empiric regimens in patients who have received quinolone prophylaxis.

antibiotics due to the presence of low-grade mucositis or nausea may still be safely treated with parenteral outpatient regimens (Table 4). The advantages and disadvantages of outpatient management of febrile neutropenic patients are outlined in Table 5. There needs to be considerable institutional investment in infrastructure/multidisciplinary teams in order to have a successful program of outpatient management (Table 6).

Several choices are available for hospital-based parenteral therapy as well. These include monotherapy with extended spectrum cephalosporins, carbapenem, or agents such as piperacillin/tazobactam (Table 4). Patients with complicated infections or infections involving deep tissues (perianal infections, neutropenic enterocolitis, pneumonia, extensive skin/skin structure infections) might respond better if they receive antimicrobial combinations (generally an aminoglycoside with a beta lactam) (36). Patients colonized with resistant gram-positive organisms such as MRSA, or those strongly suspected to have a

Table 5 Advantages and Disadvantages of Early Discharge/Outpatient Antibiotic Therapy of Febrile Neutropenic Patients

Advantages
- Avoidance of iatrogenic/logistic/environmental hazards of hospitalization
- Lower overall cost of care
- Lower frequency of "healthcare-associated" infection
- Increased convenience (patient, family, or other caregivers)
- Enhanced quality of life (patient)
- More efficient resource utilization (hospital or other healthcare organization)

Disadvantages
- Potential for development of serious complications/morbidity in an unsupervised setting (e.g., septic shock)
- Need to develop and maintain expensive infrastructure, multidisciplinary teams, and monitoring capability (e.g., 24 hr hotline)
- Potential for noncompliance with therapy

Table 6 Requirements for a Successful Program of Outpatient Antibiotic Therapy for Febrile Neutropenic Patients

- Institutional support of adequate infrastructure (ER, infusion services, outpatient pharmacy, etc.)
- Dedicated, multidisciplinary team of healthcare providers
- Availability of real-time, local epidemiologic, and susceptibility/resistance data
- Selection of microbiologically appropriate (not merely convenient) treatment regimens
- Motivated, compliant patients supported by family or other caregivers
- Adequate transportation and communication
- Adequate outpatient monitoring for response/failure, development of complications, or toxicity
- Access 24 hr a day to emergency management team (hotline, ER, or ambulatory center)

gram-positive infection should probably receive empiric regimens, which contain vancomycin with the caveat that this agent be discontinued if microbiological data reveal the absence of gram-positive pathogens.

The length of therapy remains the subject of debate. There are two schools of thought with some evidence to support both points of view. Some experts recommend the continuation of antibiotic therapy until the resolution of all signs and symptoms of infection and recovery from neutropenia (26,37). While successful, this approach might lead to unnecessary antibiotic therapy in a substantial number of patients, particularly those without a documented infection (4). The other approach is to discontinue antibiotic therapy once fever and other manifestations of infection have resolved, even if the patient is still neutropenic (4). This approach might be better suited to today's healthcare environment in which antimicrobial stewardship is of utmost importance (4,37,38).

MANAGEMENT OF THE PERSISTENTLY FEBRILE PATIENT

Persistence of fever despite adequate empiric antibiotic therapy can be due to one of several causes including (1) retention of an infected foreign object, most commonly a CVC, (2) an undrained focus such as an abdominal, pelvic, or perianal abscess, (3) the development of a bacterial superinfection with an organism not susceptible to the coverage being provided, or (4) the development of an occult fungal infection, especially in patients with hematologic malignancies or recipients of hematopoietic stem cell transplants (39). Making a specific diagnosis as to the cause of persistent fever is paramount in these patients. Removal of the offending foreign body if present, drainage of an abscess or debridement of necrotic tissue when indicated, and additional antibacterial coverage (gram-positive, gram-negative, anaerobic) as necessary are important options in the management of these patients. Persistently neutropenic patients with documented infections who are not responding to adequate antibiotic therapy might benefit from granulocyte transfusions and/or hematopoietic growth factors (e.g., G-CSF) (40). Investigative studies (serology, radiographic imaging, tissue biopsy) particularly to document fungal infections need to be undertaken, and empiric preemptive antifungal therapy is recommended.

INFECTION PREVENTION

Infection prevention is an extremely important aspect in the management of the cancer patients, particularly with the emergence of many multidrug-resistant organisms. Detailed discussion of the use of protected environments with laminar air flow, specialized diets, immunoglobulins, and hematopoeitc growth factors (G-CSF, GM-CSF) is beyond the scope of this chapter. Nevertheless, these modalities have been used by themselves or in combination, with some success in high-risk patients (26). At the present time the quinolones (ciprofloxacin, levofloxacin, moxifloxacin) are considered the agents of choice for antibacterial prophylaxis due to their availability for oral administration, and their activity against many gram-positive and gram-negative pathogens (41,42).

Two recent large studies of levofloxacin prophylaxis in patients with leukemias, lymphomas, and solid tumors found statistically lower frequencies of microbiologically documented infections, bacteremias, and reduced frequency of fever and hospitalization among patients receiving prophylaxis (43,44). However, there was no discernable difference in mortality, and the emergence of quinolone resistance was a concern (45). In contrast, the discontinuation of quinolone prophylaxis was associated with an increase in gram-negative bacteremic episodes and associated mortality at one institution, necessitating the reintroduction of quinolone prophylaxis (20). This occurred despite a significant increase in quinolone resistance among strains of $E.$ $coli$ (>50% vs. 15%) during periods of prophylaxis. The Infectious Diseases Society of America (IDSA) and many other experts caution against routine prophylaxis in patients with chemotherapy-induced neutropenia, and recommend it only for high-risk patients who are expected to have severe and prolonged neutropenia (21,26,41,45).

RESISTANCE, INFECTION CONTROL, AND ANTIMICROBIAL STEWARDSHIP

During the course of their illness, many cancer patients are exposed to multiple courses of antibiotic therapy for a variety of reasons (prophylaxis, empiric therapy, preemptive therapy, specific or targeted therapy). This heavy antibiotic usage has led to the selection of microorganisms that are resistant to many antibiotics commonly used in cancer patients (37). Other reasons for the development of resistance include the use (misuse?) of antimicrobial agents in agriculture, animal husbandry, household products, and other nonmedical settings, and the ability of microorganisms to mutate and develop multiple mechanisms or resistance that render several classes of antimicrobial agents ineffective (46–49). Additionally, widespread and swift global travel facilitates the spread of resistant clones across international borders. Many cancer patients today are less restricted in their activities and are exposed to human, plant, or animal pathogens, including multidrug-resistant organisms, more often than in the past, with an increasing proportion of infections being acquired outside the hospital. Bacterial organisms that are particularly problematic in cancer patients include methicillin-resistant staphylococci, VRE, penicillin-resistant *Streptococcus* spp., multidrug-resistant *P. aeruginosa*, *Stenotrophomonas maltophilia*, and occasionally, resistant *Acinetobacter* spp. (50,51). One of the mechanisms of combating resistant organisms is developing new pharmaceutical agents. Unfortunately, the costs associated with new drug development are exorbitant, and many pharmaceutical houses have suppressed or abandoned their anti-infective development programs. These issues have been highlighted in several recent publications from the IDSA (17,18). Consequently, judicious use of currently available agents, and adherence to appropriate infection control guidelines and policies are very important tools in preventing the emergence and spread of multidrug-resistant pathogens. The IDSA and the Society for Healthcare Epidemiology of America (SHEA) have recently published guidelines for developing institutional programs to enhance antimicrobial stewardship (38). Salient features of such programs are listed in Table 7. All institutions caring for cancer patients and other patients at high risk for developing infectious complications are strongly encouraged to develop and implement such programs.

SUMMARY

Infections remain the most common complications in patients with cancer, due to the immunological defects associated with the underlying disease and its treatment. Environmental factors, the increasing use of foreign medical devices, and the widespread and frequent use of antimicrobial agents in these high-risk

Table 7 Antimicrobial Stewardship: Strategies to Reduce Drug Resistance and the Spread of Resistant Organisms

- Education (physician, mid-level providers, pharmacists, etc.)
- Formulary restriction
- Prior approval requirements
- Limited antibacterial prophylaxis
- Targeted therapy (when possible)
- Streamlining (de-escalation) of empiric regimen
- Antibiotic cycling vs. antibiotic heterogeneity
- Computer-assisted program
- Strict adherence to infection control policies
- New drug development

Source: Adapted from: Refs. 17, 18, 37, 38.

patients have altered the epidemiology of bacterial infections in such patients, and led to the emergence of multidrug-resistant organisms. Nevertheless, the majority of patients with bacterial infections respond to empiric or targeted therapy. With the emergence of multidrug-resistant organisms, the importance of infection prevention, infection control, antimicrobial stewardship, and new drug development has come into sharper focus. Programs and guidelines in all these areas have been developed, and hopefully these will result in better supportive care of the cancer patient.

REFERENCES

1. Wisplinghoff H, Seifert H, Wenzel RP, et al. Current trends in the epidemiology of nosocomial bloodstream infections in patients with hematological malignancies and solid neoplasms in hospitals in the United States. Clin Infect Dis 2003; 36:1103–1110.
2. Yadegarynia D, Tarrand J, Raad I, et al. Current spectrum of bacterial infections in cancer patients. Clin Infect Dis 2003; 37:1144,1145.
3. Zinner SH. Changing epidemiology of infections in patients with neutropenia and cancer: emphasis on gram-positive and resistant bacteria. Clin Infect Dis 1999; 29:490–494.
4. Rolston KVI, Bodey GP. Infections in patients with cancer. In: Kufe DW, Bast Jr, RC, Hait WN, Hong WK, Pollock RE, Weichselbaum RR, Holland JF, Frei, III E, eds. Cancer Medicine. 7th ed. Ontario, Canada: BC Decker, Hamilton, 2006:2222–2245.
5. Adachi JA, Yadegarynia D, Rolston K. Spectrum of polymicrobial bacterial infection in patients with cancer, 1975–2002. American Society for Microbiology. Polymicrobial Diseases, Lake Tahoe, NV, 2003, October 19–23 (abstr 4).
6. Rolston KVI, Bodey GP, Safdar A. Polymicrobial infections in cancer patients: an underappreciated/underreported entity. Clin Infect Dis 2007; 45:228–233.

7. Hughes WT, Pizzo PA, Wade JA, et al. Evaluation of new anti-infective drugs for the treatment of febrile episodes in neutropenic patients. Clin Infect Dis 1992; 15 (suppl 1):206–215.
8. Han XY, Kamana M, Rolston KVI. Viridans streptococci isolated by culture from blood of cancer patients: clinical and microbiologic analysis of 50 cases. J Clin Microbiol 2006; 44:160–165.
9. Kumashi P, Girgawy E, Tarrand J, et al. Streptococcus pneumoniae bacteremia in patients with cancer: disease characteristics and outcomes in the era of escalating drug resistance (1998–2002). Medicine 2005; 84:303–312.
10. Youssef S. Rodriguez G, Rolston KV, et al. Streptococcus pneumoniae infections in 47 hematopoietic stem cell transplantation recipients. Clinical characteristics of infections and vaccine-breakthrough infections, 1989–2005. Medicine 2007; 86:69–77.
11. Fanourgiakis P, Georgala A, Vekemans M, et al. Bacteremia due to *Stomatococcus mucilaginosus* in neutropenic patients in the setting of a cancer institute.Clin Micriobiol Infect 2003; 9:1068–1072.
12. Matar MJ, Tarrand J, Raad I, et al. Colonization and infection with vancomycin-resistant Enterococcus among patients with cancer. Amer J Infect Control 2006; 34:534–536.
13. Rivero GA, Torres HA, Rolston KVI, et al. *Listeria monocytogenes* infection in patient with cancer. Diag Microbiol Infect Dis 2003; 47:393–398.
14. Weinstock DM, Brown AE. Rodococcus equi: an emerging pathogen. Clin Infect Dis 2002; 15:1379–1385.
15. Chatzinikolaou I, Dholakia NA, Kontoyiannis D, et al. *Rhodococcus* spp. infection in cancer patients. Proceedings, 37th Annual Infectious Diseases Society of America, Philadelphia, PA, 1999, November 18–21 (abstr 128).
16. Prince R, Coyle E, Rolston K, et al. In vitro activity of daptomycin and linezolid against vancomycin-resistant gram-positive pathogens from cancer patients. Proceedings, 17th European Congress of Clinical Microbiology and Infectious Diseases (ECCMID) and 25th International Congress of Chemotherapy (ICC), Munich, Germany, 2007, March 31–April 3 (abstr P697).
17. Infectious Diseases Society of America. Bad Bugs, No Drugs, July 2004 (http://www.idsociety.org/pa/IDSA_Paper4_final_web.pdf)
18. Talbot GH, Bradley J, Edwards Jr, JE, et al. Bad bugs need drugs: an update on the development pipeline from the antimicrobial availability task force of the Infectious Diseases Society of America. Clin Infect Dis 2006; 42:657–668.
19. Rolston KVI, Tarrand JJ. *Pseudomonas aeruginosa*—Still a frequent pathogen in patients with cancer: 11-year experience from a comprehensive cancer center. Clin Infect Dis 1999; 29:463,464.
20. Reuter S, Kern WV, Sigge A, et al. Impact of fluoroquinolone prophylaxis on reduced infection-related mortality among patients with neutropenia and hematologic malignancies. Clin Infect Dis 2005; 40:1087–1093.
21. Zinner SH. Fluoroquinolone prophylaxis in patients with neutropenia. Clin Infect Dis 2005; 40:1094,1095.
22. Bodey GP. Antibiotics in patients with neutropenia. Arch Intern Med 1984; 144:1845–1851.
23. Elting LS, Bodey GP, Fainstein V. Polymicrobial septicemia in the cancer patient. Medicine 1986; 65:218–225.

24. Gomez L, Martino R, Rolston KV. Neutropenic enterocolitis: spectrum of the disease and comparison of definite and possible cases. Clin Infect Dis 1998; 27:695–699.
25. Rolston KVI, Bodey GP. Diagnosis and management of perianal and perirectal infection in the granulocytopenic patient. In: Remington J, Swartz MN, eds. Current Clinical Topics in Infectious Diseases. Boston: Blackwell Scientific Publications, 1993:164–171.
26. Hughes WT, Armstrong D, Bodey GP, et al. 2002 Guidelines for the use of antimicrobial agents in neutropenic patients with cancer. Clin Infect Dis 2002; 34:730–751.
27. Talcott JA, Siegel RD, Finberg R, et al. Risk assessment in cancer patients with fever and neutropenia: a prospective, two-center validation of a prediction rule. J Clin Oncol 1992; 10:316–322.
28. Talcott JA, Whalen A, Clark J, et al. Home antibiotic therapy for low-risk patients with fever and neutropenia: a pilot study of 30 patients based on a validated prediction rule. J Clin Oncol 1994; 12:107–114.
29. Klastersky J, Paesmans M, Rubenstein E, et al. The MASCC Risk Index: a multinational scoring system to predict low-risk febrile neutropenic cancer patients. J Clin Oncol 2000; 18:3038–3051.
30. Rolston KVI. The Infectious Diseases Society of America 2002 Guidelines for the use of antimicrobial agents in patients with cancer and neutropenia: salient features and comments. Clin Infect Dis 2004; 39(suppl 1):44–48.
31. Quezada G, Sunderland T, Chan KW, et al. Medical and non-medical barriers to outpatient treatment of fever and neutropenia in children with cancer. Pediatr Blood Cancer 2007; 48:273–277.
32. Rolston K, Rubenstein EB, Elting L, et al. Ambulatory management of febrile episodes in low-risk neutropenic patients. Proceedings, 35th Interscience Conference on Antimicrobial Agents and Chemotherapy, San Francisco, California, 1995, September 17–20 (abstr 2235).
33. Klastersky J, Paesman M, Georgala A, et al. Outpatient oral antibiotics for febrile neutropenic cancer patients using a score predictive for complications. J Clin Oncol 2006; 24:4129–4134.
34. Rolston KVI, Manzullo EF, Elting LS, et al. Once daily, oral, outpatient quinolone monotherapy for low-risk cancer patients with fever and neutropenia. Cancer 2006; 106:2489–2494.
35. Chamilos G, Bamias A, Efstathiou E, et al. Outpatient treatment of low-risk neutropenic fever in cancer patients using oral moxifloxacin. Cancer 2005; 103:2629–2935.
36. Elting LS, Rubenstein EB, Rolston KVI, Bodey GP. Outcomes of bacteremia in patients with cancer and neutropenia: observations from two decades of epidemiological and clinical trials. Clin Infect Dis 1997; 25:247–259.
37. Rolston KVI. Challenges in the treatment of infections caused by gram-positive and gram-negative bacteria in patients with cancer and neutropenia. Clin Infect Dis 2005; 40, S246–S252.
38. Dellit TH, Owens RC, McGowan Jr., JE, et al. Infectious Diseases Society of America and the Society for Healthcare Epidemiology of America Guidelines for developing an institutional program to enhance antimicrobial stewardship. Clin Infect Dis 2007; 44:159–176.
39. Klastersky J, Paesman M. Risk-adapted strategy for the management of febrile neutropenia in cancer patients. Support Care Cancer 2007; 15:477–482.

40. Smith TH, Khatcheressian J, Lyman GH, et al. 2006 Update of recommendations for the use of white blood cell growth factors: an evidence-based clinical practice guideline. J Clin Oncol 2006; 24:3187–3205.
41. Segal BH, Freifeld A. Antibacterial prophylaxis in patients with neutropenia. J Natl Compr Canc Netw 2007; 5:235–242.
42. Leibovici L, Paul M, Cullen M. Antibiotic prophylaxis in neutropenic patients. New evidence, practical decisions. Cancer 2006; 107:1743–1751.
43. Bucaneve G, Micozzi A, Menichetti F, et al. Levofloxacin to prevent bacterial infection in patients with cancer neutropenia. N Engl J Med 2005; 353:977–987.
44. Cullen M, Steven N, Billingham L, et al. Antibacterial prophylaxis after chemotherapy for solid tumors and lymphomas. N Engl J Med 2007; 353:988–998.
45. Baden LR. Prophylactic antimicrobial agents and the importance of fitness. N Engl J Med 2005; 353:1052–1054.
46. Toleman MA, Rolston K, Jones RN, et al. Molecular and biochemical characterization of OXA-45, an extended-spectrum class 2d', β-lactamase in *Pseudomonas aeurginosa*. Antimicrob Agents Chemother 2004; 347:2859–2863.
47. Toleman MA, Rolston K, Jones RN, Walsh TR. bla_{VIM-7}, an evolutionarily distinct metallo-β-lactamase gene in a *Pseudomonas aeruginosa* isolate from the United States. Antimicrob Agents Chemother 2004; 48:329–332.
48. Ohmagari N, Hanna H, Graviss L, Hackett B, Perego C, Gonzalez V, Dvorak T, Hogan H, Hachem R, Rolston K, Raad I. Risk factors for infections with multidrug-resistant *Pseudomonas aeruginosa* in patients with cancer. Cancer 2005; 104:205–212.
49. Aboufaycal H, Sader HS, Rolston K, et al. bla_{VIM-2} and bla_{VIM-7} carbapenemase-producing *Pseudomonas aeruginosa* isolates detected in a Tertiary Care Medical Center in the United States: report from the MYSTIC program. J Clin Microbiol 2007; 45:614,615.
50. Rolston KVI, Kontoyiannis DP, Yadegarynia D, et al. Nonfermentative gram-negative bacilli in cancer patients: increasing frequency of infection and antimicrobial susceptibility of clinical isolates to fluoroquinolones. Diag Microbiol Infect Dis 2005; 51:215–218.
51. Rolston KVI, Yadegarynia D, Kontoyiannis DP, et al. The spectrum of gram-positive bloodstream infections in patients with hematologic malignancies, and the in-vitro activity of various quinolones against gram-positive bacteria isolated from cancer patients. Int J Infect Dis 2006; 10:223–230.

6

Management of Fungal Infections in Cancer Patients

Mickael Aoun and Jean Klastersky
Institut Jules Bordet, Université Libre de Bruxelles, Brussels, Belgium

Kristel Buvé and Johan Maertens
Department of Hematology, University Hospital Gasthuisberg, Acute Leukemia and Transplantation Unit, Leuven, Belgium

INTRODUCTION

Antifungal therapy has undergone a tremendous development over the last two decades. Three major classes of antifungals are now available, with different mechanisms of action, different spectrum of activity, specific pharmacokinetic parameters, individual toxicity profiles, and variable routes of administration (Table 1).

The management of invasive fungal infections (IFI) in immunocompromised patients has implicated different strategies including prophylaxis, empiric (E) or preemptive (PE) treatment, and specific therapy of established infections. The selection of a particular molecule among the expanding list of antifungals is the result of a complex process. In fact, this chapter is influenced by several key elements, among which the epidemiology, the host risk factors, the relative lack of sensitivity of diagnostic tools, and the usual paucity of characteristic clinical manifestations all play an important role.

Table 1 Major classes of antifungals

	Mode of action	Routes of administration	Limiting toxicity	Limiting pharmacokinetic parameters	Common resistance
Polyenes					
Amphotericin B-deoxycholate	Pore formation in cell membranes through affinity to ergosterol	IV	Immediate reactions nephrotoxicity	Bioavailability Penetration into eyes, CNS	*C. lusitaniae*, *Trichosporon* sp., *Fusarium* sp, *Scedosporium* sp., *A. terreus*
Liposomal amphotericin B					
Amphotericin-B lipid complex					
Amphotericin B colloidal dispersion					
5-fluorocytosinefluorocytosine	Inhibition of DNA synthesis	IV, oral	Myelotoxicity Skin rash	—	Zygomycetes, *Scedosporium* sp. *Fusarium* sp., 5–10% of Cryptococcus and *Candida* sp.
Triazoles					
Fluconazole	Inhibition of C14-demethylase	IV, oral	Increase of LFTs Skin rash	—	*Aspergillus* sp., *C. krusei*, *C. glabrata*, Zygomycetes
Itraconazole	Inhibition of ergosterol synthesis	IV,[a] oral	QT prolongation Increase of LFTs Drug interactions	Oral bioavailability Urine excretion <1%	Zygomycetes *Sisyrinchium inflatum*

Drug	Route	Mechanism	Side effects	Pharmacokinetics	Notes/Spectrum
Voriconazole	IV, oral		Increase of LFTs QT prolongation Drug interactions CNS toxicity	Polymorphism of metabolizing enzyme 2C19 Urine excretion <1%	S. inflatum
Posaconazole	Oral, IV[b]		Skin rash Increase of LFTs, QT prolongation Drug interaction	Oral bioavailability Urine excretion <1%	
Echinocandins					
Caspofungin	IV	Inhibition of 1,3-β-D-glucan synthesis	Histamine-like reactions Interaction with cyclosporin	High protein binding Poor penetration into CNS, eye Urine excretion <1%	Cryptococcus, Zygomycetes, Fusarium sp., Paecilomyces lilacinus, S. prolificans, S. inflatum, C. parapsilosis?
Micafungin			Histamine-like reactions Interaction with sirolimus and nifedipine		
Anidulafungin			Histamine-like reactions		

Abbreviation: LFTs, liver function tests.
[a]Not registered in all countries.
[b]Still under investigation.

The epidemiology of infectious complications in cancer patients continues to show a high incidence of IFI, varying between 5% and 25%, and an important associated mortality of 40% to 50%. However, the true incidence of IFI is difficult to estimate. On one hand, failure to microbiologically diagnose IFI, because of antifungal prophylaxis or E therapy and low sensitivity of culture, will result in underestimation. On the other hand, postmortem studies have the potential for both overestimation and underestimation.

EPIDEMIOLOGY

Candida species, Aspergillus species, and *Cryptococcosis neoformans* are responsible for more than 90% of IFI in cancer patients. However, most IFI are caused by Candida species in solid tumor patients and by Aspergillus species in patients with hematological malignancies. Recent trends in the incidence of invasive candidiasis (IC) have shown a steady rate among patients with solid tumors, while a marked decrease has occurred in hematology patients since the 1990s, after the generalization of fluconazole antifungal prophylaxis. In fact, among the patients with acute leukemia and hematopoietic stem cell transplants (HSCT), previously associated with 11% to 12% risk of IC, the introduction of azole antifungal prophylaxis reduced the risk to less than 1% (1). The most important decline was reported for *Candida albicans* and *Candida tropicalis,* paralleled by an increase of *Candida glabrata* and *Candida krusei*. Although, the causal association with fluconazole use in hematological malignancies has been pointed out, other factors have been implicated in the emergence of these two more resistant Candida species. In the case of *C. glabrata*, age older than 60 years and the severity of the underlying disease, and for both *C. glabrata* and *C. krusei*, exposure to antibiotics such as piperacillin-tazobactam and vancomycin, have been identified as additional risk factors (2). *Candida parapsilosis* has been strongly associated with intravascular catheters and parenteral nutrition and has the potential for nosocomial transmission by hand carriage (3).

Despite the highly variable incidence of invasive aspergillosis (IA), there is a general perception of an increase of Aspergillus infections in patients with hematological malignancies (4). In a large retrospective study on patients with hematological malignancy admitted between 1999 and 2003, 4.6% developed IFI, although the overall incidence of IA was only 2.6%, patients with acute lymphoid leukemia (ALL) and acute myeloid leukemia (AML) had a higher risk with 4.3% and 7.9%, respectively. Other studies in HSCT recipients have shown the predominance of IA with an incidence varying between 5% and 25% and up to 38% in a very high-risk group of patients with chronic graft versus host disease (GVHD). More disturbing is the recent increase of nonfumigatus species such *Aspergillus flavus* and *Aspergillus terreus* (4,5). Moreover, data suggesting an increase in the incidence of non-Aspergillus molds are accumulating (4,6). Zygomycetes and Fusarium species have emerged recently as significant pathogens and are reported increasingly in hematological malignancy patients. Patients who had previously undergone splenectomy seem to be at increased risk for these uncommon moulds. Other reports have indicated an association with the selective pressure of voriconazole prophylaxis. Scedosporium species, Trichosporon species, Cryptococcus species, and dematiaceous fungi remain so far uncommon.

RISK FACTORS

A number of risk factors for the development of IFI have been identified. In general, these include prior fungal exposure or colonization, severe state of immunosuppression (e.g., older age, active cancer, prolonged and profound neutropenia), nature of the underlying hematologic disease (AML/myelodysplasic syndromes (MDS) > ALL > lymphoma and myeloma), GVHD/graft rejection in HSCT recipients (especially for those receiving corticosteroids), organ dysfunction (e.g., renal, hepatic or pulmonary dysfunction, mucositis), and prior exposure to antifungals (7–13).

With respect to allogeneic HSCT recipients, several factors, such as the underlying disease of the recipient, the HLA match of the graft, and the stem cell source, can also influence the incidence, timing, and type of mould infection. For example, zygomycosis is more frequently reported late (i.e., >90 days after transplantation), corresponding with the onset of GVHD, while infection with Scedosporium species typically occurs within the first 30 days after transplantation (14). The risk of early-onset aspergillosis is higher among patients with aplastic anemia and among recipients of cord blood stem cells, who typically have a long pre-engraftment period. In contrast, late-onset aspergillosis is more likely among patients with multiple myeloma and among those receiving peripheral blood stem cells from mismatched or HLA-unrelated donors (15). Risk factors for zygomycosis overlap those for IA (i.e., corticosteroid exposure, GVHD, allogeneic BMT, cytomegalovirus reactivation, prolonged neutropenia); however, initial presentation with sinusitis and the development of a breakthrough infection while on voriconazole prophylaxis are factors that suggest a diagnosis of zygomycosis over aspergillosis (16).

In general, patients with acute leukemia, those undergoing allogeneic transplantation, and those with multiple risk factors carry the highest risk, whereas younger patients, patients with lymphoma, and those undergoing autologous transplantation are at a lower risk (7,9). Changing therapeutic practices, however, may alter risk factor patterns in the future. In particular, the increased use of monoclonal antibodies such as alemtuzumab and anti-TNF antibodies such as infliximab might result in an increased frequency of IFI in "nonclassical" risk groups (i.e., chronic lymphocytic leukemia, end-stage lymphoma, low-risk MDS) (17–19).

DIAGNOSIS

Early diagnosis, early adequate therapy, and rapid recovery from immunosuppression constitute the tripod of successful management of IFI. However, due to the decreased inflammatory response in immunocompromised patients, the clinical symptoms and signs may not develop until the fungal infection is in an advanced stage. In addition, blood cultures may be negative in about 50% of disseminated disease. In fact, in a recent review of autopsy-proven IFI in patients with hematological malignancy, only 25% were diagnosed antemortem (4).

Which fungi can be detected in blood cultures? Candida species, Trichosporon species, *C. neoformans,* Malassezia species, Fusarium species, Scedosporium species, *A. terreus,* and many dematiaceous fungi can be isolated from blood, although the type of blood culture systems employed may impact on the yield of detection (20).

By contrast, the interpretation of culture results of respiratory tract specimens is more problematic since many fungi are ubiquitous in the environment. The distinction between contamination, colonization, and genuine infection based on culture of such specimens is simply impossible. Nevertheless, in high-risk patients, as those with allogeneic HSCT recipients and prolonged neutropenica hematology patients, the positive predictive value for an invasive infection of a sputum or bronchoalveolar lavage culture yielding an Aspergillus species is high. Therefore, the histopathological demonstration of fungal elements in tissue biopsy remains the most reliable proof of the occurrence of an IFI, although hampered on many instances by the invasive procedures needed and the risk of complications. By contrast, detection of polysaccharide antigens shedded by *C. neoformans* and *Histoplasmosis capsulatum* in serum proved to be a rapid and noninvasive method for early diagnosis. Likewise, a major advance in the management of fungal infections in hematological malignancies has been achieved by the recent development of the galactomannan immunoassay for the diagnosis of IA, and $(1\rightarrow3)$-β-D-glucan test for both IA and IC and other fungal infections except zygomycosis and cryptococcosis. Although not validated for body fluids other than serum, the detection of positive galactomannan test in CSF is indicative of CNS aspergillosis, and when performed on BAL fluid and combined with high-resolution chest CT scan, the positive and negative predictive values are 100% (21). Interestingly, the serial serum samples testing for β-D-glucan in patients with AML or MDS showed a 100% negative predictive value, a specificity of 90% and 96% for a single and two sequential positive results, respectively. The use of PCR for the diagnosis of IFI is still limited to some institutions despite several promising reports; more trials in clinical settings in patients at risk are needed in order to establish their potential for early diagnosis in comparison with the immunological tests.

TRENDS IN ANTIFUNGAL SUSCEPTIBILITY

A huge effort has been accomplished in order to bring the antifungal susceptibility testing to the same level as that of antibacterial testing in providing clinically useful information for guiding therapy. Standardization of methods for both yeasts and moulds are available and breakpoints for interpretation are being developed for many antifungal agents.

Although the interpretive breakpoint values for amphotericin B have been difficult to establish, MICs higher than 1 μg/mL indicate probable resistance and should prompt either higher doses or a choice of another antifungal. Based on this finding, the previous uniform activity of amphotericin B against Candida species has been questioned. Indeed, *C. glabrata* with a MIC of 2 μg/mL and *C. krusei* with a MIC of 4 μg/mL are less susceptible to amphotericin B (22,23). More recently, a South African clade of *C. albicans* with MIC $\geq$ 2 μg/mL has been identified, indicating that some geographic differences in susceptibility may be discovered in parallel to the extension of epidemiologic studies of fungal infections (24). Secondary resistance to amphotericin B has been described in *Candida lusitaniae* where initial isolation appears susceptible but resistance develops upon exposure to amphotericin B (25). The same phenomenon has been reported for *Candida rugosa* (26). Surprisingly, the global resistance rate to fluconazole is less than 3% among all Candida species causing invasive infection. However, there are some exceptions, with *C. glabrata* being resistant in 14.3% to 22.8% and *C. krusei* in 40% (27), and thus the resistance rate of fluconazole in a given institution will be driven by the frequency of these species. Variable resistance rates to fluconazole have been reported for *Candida guilliermondii* (6.3–26.1%), *Candida famata* (9.8–47.4%), and *C. rugosa* (14.3–66.1%). Triazoles including fluconazole, itraconazole, voriconazole, and posaconazole share the same mechanism of activity and are affected by the same mechanisms of resistance. The best example for this phenomenon is *C. glabrata*, where cross-resistance among triazoles has been reported. A similar finding has been described for *C. rugosa*. An exception to this is *C. krusei*, which remains susceptible to voriconazole and has been treated successfully with this agent.

All three available echinocandins possess the same mechanism of action—they are fungicidal against Candida species, including those resistant to triazoles, with the exception of *C. parapsilosis* and *C. guilliermondii*, with MIC $\geq$ 2 μg/mL being reported for all three echinocandins. Emergence of resistance to echinocandins during prolonged treatment with caspofungin or micafungin has been reported but remains very uncommon. *C. parapsilosis* endocarditis, *C. glabrata* candidemia, and *C. albicans* esophagitis are illustrative examples (28–30).

Although standardized methods have been developed for MIC testing of filamentous fungi, we still lack good correlation evaluation between in vitro susceptibility and in vivo outcome, and interpretive MIC breakpoints are lacking for many of the filamentous fungi. Moreover, the microbiologcal identification and culture of the filamentous fungi are necessary for the antifungal selection based on species; because of these limitations, the antifungal susceptibility testing in filamentous fungi is not routinely used at present for selection or modification of antifungal therapy.

MANAGEMENT STRATEGIES

Prophylaxis

Before adopting a prophylactic approach, several factors should be considered. In general, (1) if an infection is severe, (2) if the infection cannot easily be diagnosed or treated, and (3) if prophylaxis does not incur clinically significant adverse events, there might be a bias toward prophylaxis, provided that the number needed to treat is relatively low. For instance, the routine use of broad-spectrum antifungals for the prevention of Zygomycetes or Scedosporium infections, although these infections are often severe and difficult to diagnose and treat, cannot be recommended given the current low incidence. In addition, national and even local epidemiological findings remain key factors for the final decision making. For instance, the unusual low frequency of candidemia (1.3%) in adult allogeneic HSCT recipients not receiving antifungal prophylaxis in Finland argues against the use of antifungal prophylaxis (31).

If, however, the infection can easily be treated and diagnosed and prophylaxis is not safe or not well tolerated, then there is a bias against general prophylaxis, irrespective of the number needed to treat.

Although primary antifungal prophylaxis has been extensively evaluated in high-risk hematology patients, the jury is still out regarding its optimal use, primarily because a conclusive reduction in overall mortality has not been demonstrated, except for the use of fluconazole in HSCT recipients (data only from a single center), and because most studies are flawed by shortcomings in their design (32). Because of this, antifungal prophylaxis practice patterns vary considerably between different centers, both in Europe and the United States (33).

There remains debate as to whether and when to initiate antifungal prophylaxis in hematology patients at risk for IFI. Although a large number of studies have evaluated IFI prophylaxis regimens, results have been mixed with respect to outcomes (e.g., incidence of proven and probable IFI, overall and attributable mortality, need for parenteral antifungal therapy). Inconsistent results have been due to differences in study design, study populations, and variable dosing schedules and/or the use of multiple agents (34). In an effort to increase the statistical power, meta-analyses have been performed to pool the results of similar trials. Overall, these meta-analyses have shown that antifungal prophylaxis results in a reduced overall incidence of IFI (though mainly driven by fewer noninvasive mucosal infections and invasive *Candida* infections) and fungal infection-related mortality.

The early meta-analysis performed by Kanda et al. involved 16 studies evaluating oral fluconazole prophylaxis versus placebo among patients with neutropenia. Use of fluconazole was associated with a decreased overall incidence of IFI and fungal-related death, but only in bone marrow transplant recipients and when fluconazole was used at a dose of 400 mg/day (35). As might be expected, fluconazole prophylaxis was not associated with a reduction in the rate of proven IA or systemic infections due to non-*albicans Candida* species (35).

The meta-analysis conducted by Bow et al. included 38 randomized, controlled trials involving azoles and amphotericin B compared with either placebo or no treatment in severely neutropenic patients receiving chemotherapy. Fluconazole, itraconazole, ketoconazole, and amphotericin B reduced the incidence of IFI. However, only fluconazole was associated with a decreased risk of IFI-related mortality. In a regression analysis, HSCT, prolonged neutropenia, acute leukemia with prolonged neutropenia, and higher azole dose were predictors of treatment effect (34).

Glasmacher et al. performed a meta-analysis of 13 trials involving itraconazole use in neutropenic heamatology patients and found that itraconazole prophylaxis was associated with a reduction in the rate of IFI and IFI-related mortality. However, a subgroup analysis displayed a very significant dose-response relationship; bioavailable doses of at least 200 mg/day (equivalent to oral doses $\geq$400 mg/day or intravenous doses $\geq$200 mg/day) were superior to bioavailable doses <110 mg/day (usually obtained with the capsule formulation). Overall itraconazole was effective in reducing the incidence of proven invasive yeast infections and infections caused by non-*albicans Candida* species, but not IA infection (36). However, at a bioavailable dose of 200 mg/day or higher, itraconazole prophylaxis significantly reduced the incidence of IA, as well as aspergillosis-related mortality.

The most updated systematic review, including 49 randomized trials (until 2006) and only presented in abstract form, showed that the prophylactic use of azoles (itraconazole, fluconazole, ketoconazole) or intravenous polyenes significantly reduced documented IFI, fungal-related mortality, as well as 30 day all-cause mortality. Overall mortality was significantly reduced in HSCT recipients and there was a strong trend toward reduced mortality in leukemia patients (37).

Several studies have directly compared agents for IFI prophylaxis among patients with hematologic malignancies. In five prophylaxis studies comparing oral formulations of fluconazole and itraconazole, the IFI risk was similar or lower for itraconazole-treated patients (38–42). Two other studies compared intravenous followed by oral itraconazole with intravenous or oral fluconazole in patients receiving allogeneic HSCT (43–44). One study found that IFI were significantly more frequent in patients receiving at least one dose of fluconazole prophylactically compared with those receiving at least one dose of itraconazole prophylactically (44). However, the study was hampered by significant imbalances in risk factors for IFI between study arms (favoring itraconazole). In addition, the rate of IFI in the fluconazole study arm was unusually high compared to historical series. The other study found itraconazole to be superior to fluconazole in preventing IFI in the on-treatment analysis but not in the intention-to-treat analysis (43). Moreover, this study had a high drop-out rate in the itraconazole arm and revealed unexpected hepatotoxicity due to the interaction of itraconazole with cyclophosphamide. A meta-analysis of fluconazole versus itraconazole prophylaxis trials that included five of these seven trials found that there was no significant difference between these agents for IFI development or all-cause mortality (45). However, a more detailed reanalysis according to itraconazole formulation (bioavailability) subgroups showed a significantly superior outcome in those receiving itraconazole oral solution (46).

In patients undergoing autologous or allogeneic HSCT, micafungin prophylaxis during the neutropenic phase was associated with greater treatment success (defined as the absence of proven, probable, or suspected IFI through the end of therapy and the absence of a proven or probable IFI in the four-week follow-up period) compared with fluconazole prophylaxis but there was no difference in overall mortality (47). In a single-center trial in patients with hematologic malignancies, caspofungin, and itraconazole, prophylaxis was associated with similar rates of IFI and mortality (48). Prophylaxis studies comparing the azoles, itraconazole, and fluconazole with amphotericin B (including liposomal formulations) have revealed no significant difference between agents with respect to the development of IFI or all-cause mortality (49,50).

Two recent trials have demonstrated that posaconazole reduces the incidence of IFI and decreases mortality in neutropenic AML/MDS patients. The first study involved patients with newly diagnosed or relapsed acute myelogenous leukemia or myelodysplastic syndrome who were treated with intensive chemotherapy. Posaconazole 200 mg three times daily or a standard azole regimen (either fluconazole 400 mg once daily or itraconazole 200 mg twice daily) was given with each cycle of chemotherapy until complete remission or for up to 12 weeks. Posaconazole treatment was associated with significantly fewer total IFI during the treatment phase and fewer infections due to Aspergillus. Analysis of time to death within 100 days post-randomization showed a survival benefit in favor of posaconazole in terms of all-cause and IFI-related death (51). The other study involved allogeneic HSCT recipients with severe, acute, or chronic GVHD. Patients were randomized to receive posaconazole 200 mg three times daily or fluconazole 400 mg once daily for up to 16 weeks. The incidence of total IFI during the 16-week study period was similar in the posaconazole and fluconazole groups, but the incidence of total breakthrough infections while on treatment was significantly lower in posaconazole-treated patients. Aspergillus infections were significantly reduced among patients receiving posaconazole during the 16-week study period and as breakthrough infections while on treatment. Although IFI-related mortality was significantly lower in the posaconazole group, overall survival was not different in both treatment arms (52). Posaconazole was well tolerated in both study populations.

In September 2005, the first European Conference of Infections in Leukemia (ECIL) proposed recommendations regarding antifungal prophylaxis in patients with acute leukemia, including HSCT recipients (Fig. 1). Based on the Centre for Disease Control grading system, each recommendation was assigned a strength of recommendation category (A, B, C, D, E), with A indicating strongly recommended, C indicating optional, and E indicating not recommended. A quality of evidence grade (I, II, III) is also assigned with I indicating evidence from at least one

Management of Fungal Infections in Cancer Patients

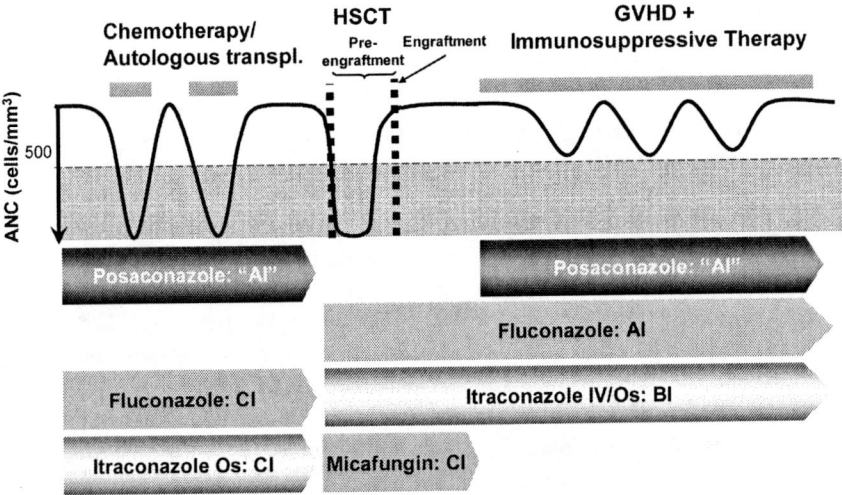

Figure 1 Antifungal prophylaxis in leukemia patients: ECIL recommendations. *Abbreviations*: Os, oral solution; HSCT, hematopoietic stem cell transplant; GVHD, graft versus host disease, ANC, absolute neutrophil count.

well-executed randomized clinical trial and II indicating that the evidence is from at least one well-designed clinical trial without randomization, from cohort or case-controlled studies, multiple time-series studies, or dramatic results from uncontrolled studies, and III indicating evidence from respected opinions based on clinical experience, descriptive studies, or expert committee reports.

Based on data from full reports demonstrating a reduction in IFI, IFI-related mortality, and overall mortality, fluconazole 400 mg/day received an AI recommendation in patients undergoing allogeneic HSCT. In patients with autologous transplant or acute leukemia, fluconazole 50 to 400 mg/day received a CI recommendation. Itraconazole (oral solution 2.5 mg/kg twice a day and intravenous injection 200 mg/day) use is recommended in patients undergoing allogeneic HSCT who can tolerate the drug and who are not at increased risk for significant drug interactions (BI). Itraconazole capsules were deemed unsuitable for prophylaxis because they have poor bioavailability, producing adequate serum plasma concentrations only after several days or weeks of treatment. Micafungin 50 mg/day received a CI recommendation in HSCT recipients. Based on the insufficient power of available studies and the risk of toxicity, amphotericin B (in any formulation) is not recommended for antifungal prophylaxis. Posaconazole received a provisional AI recommendation in AML/MDS patients and in allogeneic HSCT recipients during acute (≥grade II) or extensive chronic GVHD. The recommendation is provisional because the study results had not yet been published in full (in September 2005) and have yet not been discussed with or approved by the plenary ECIL group.

Empiric and Preemptive Approaches

The justification of E therapy of presumed IFI in persistently neutropenic patients comes basically from three considerations: first, the undisputed success of E antibacterial therapy for febrile neutropenia; second, the observation that delayed treatment of IFI increases mortality and, finally, the fact that early diagnosis of IFI, namely of IA infection, is difficult. The E approach with antifungal agents in persistently neutropenic patients is based on two small pivotal trials (53,54) but has been endorsed since by consensus guidelines (55). Most of what we know in that area stems from three prospective randomized controlled studies by Walsh et al. (56–58). These studies have been performed under the same leadership and have used identical criteria for patient inclusion and evaluation, making comparisons possible between them.

Recently, these three studies have been comprehensively reviewed (59); as indicated in Table 2, the overall success of E therapy, as estimated from the analysis of a composite evaluation score, was not clearly different between the therapeutic modalities used. However, one can question the intrinsic value of a composite score that uses endpoints such as resolution of fever, no breakthrough infection, resolution of baseline infection, survival for seven days and no discontinuation for toxic effects or lack of efficacy for the evaluation of the overall success of an E approach in patients with febrile neutropenia not responding to

Table 2 Measures of the Success (%) of Empiric Antifungal Therapy with Conventional or Liposomal Amphotericin B, Voriconazole or Caspofungin

	Ampho B	Liposomal ampho B			Voriconazole	Caspofungin
		Ampho B	Vorico	Caspo		
No. patients	344	343	422	539	415	556
Overall success	49.4	50.1	30.6	33.7	26.0	33.9
Resolution of fever	58.1	58.0	36.5	41.4	32.5	41.2
No. breakthrough fungal infections	89.2	90.1	95.0	95.5	98.1	94.8
Resolution of baseline infection	72.7	81.8	66.7	25.9	46.2	51.9
Survival for 7 days	89.5	92.7	94.1	89.2	92.0	92.6
No discontinuation for toxic effects or lack of efficacy	81.4	85.7	93.4	85.5	90.1	89.7

Source: Adapted from Ref. 59 review paper.

Table 3 Outcome of Empiric Antifungal Therapy in Microbiologically Demonstrated Fungal Infections

	Liposomal ampho B (961)	Voriconazole (415)	Caspofungin (556)
Breakthrough FI	45 (4.6)	8 (1.9)	29 (5.2)
No cure of baseline FI	22 (2.2)	7 (1.6)	13 (2.3)
Total failures*	67 (6.9%)	15 (3.6%)	42 (7.7%)

Source: Adapted from Ref. 59.
Abbreviation: FI, fungal infections.
*$p = 0.03$.

empiric broad-spectrum antibiotics. Therefore, the hypothesis was made that microbiologically proven fungal infections detected after the initiation of an E regimen (the so-called baseline and breakthrough infections) actually represented the significant failures of the E strategy. If one accepts that way of analyzing these three large controlled E trials (56–58), the results with various regimens (liposomal amphotericin B, voriconazole, and caspofungin) can be compared using the large numbers of patients as a common denominator. In addition, it is quite obvious from Table 2 that the first E trial, comparing conventional and liposomal amphotericin B as an E therapy for possible IFI, reports results that are in deep contrast with those from the two other series, namely, in terms of overall success. These differences are due mainly to discordance in the rates of resolution of fever and cure of baseline infection. With respect to resolution of baseline infection, one has to stress that we are dealing here with very small numbers of patients. Indeed, the 72.7% of cure of baseline infection with conventional amphotericin B is derived from eight favorable responses in 11 patients and the 81.8% of cure with liposomal amphotericin B stems from nine favorable results in 11 patients. This is the reason why we decided to focus the rest of our analysis to the data from the two latest trials (57,58) where the reported results are more uniform in terms of overall success, as well as for each of the parameters used to build the composite evaluation score. With these considerations in mind, the analysis of the two latest Walsh's trials (56–58), with strict emphasis on microbiologically demonstrated infections, is summarized in Table 3. It can be seen that the total number of failures (breakthrough infections plus absence of cure of baseline infections) is 6.9%, 3.6%, and 7.7% for liposomal amphotericin B, voriconazole, and caspofungin, respectively; a statistically significant difference ($p = 0.03$). As far as IAs are concerned, the total numbers of failures were 24/961 (2.4%) for liposomal amphotericin B, 8/415 (1.9) for voriconazole and 7/556 (3.0%) for caspofungin. It is also noteworthy that, in the study comparing liposomal amphotericin B and voriconazole (57), voriconazole was superior to liposomal amphotericin B in preventing breakthrough aspergillar infections that were documented, respectively, in 4/415 (0.95%) and 13/422 (3.30%) of the patients.

The significance of these observations must be put into perspective with respect to the prevalence of IFI in persistently neutropenic and febrile patients not receiving E therapy but who might have been candidates for it. The prevalence of IFI, derived from a series of studies (53,54,60–62), is probably in the range of 20% to 30%.

If all these speculations are correct, it would mean that E therapy eradicates 90% of the IFI present in persistently febrile and neutropenic patients, since we observe a ±2.5% failure rate of the E approach in a population with a ±25% prevalence of occult IFI.

Of course, to achieve these results, one has to treat empirically, with expensive and/or potentially toxic drugs, all the patients with persistent febrile neutropenia, knowing that the risk of occult IFI is present only in 25% of them. This is the reason why another strategy, the "preemptive approach" has been proposed to fill the gap between over- and undertreatment of IFI (63). Basically, PE approach is based on the belief that one could safely predict probable IFI on clinical and microbiological grounds (64) and thus limit antifungal therapy only to patients very likely to present IFI. The first study to prospectively address the issue of PE therapy of IFI in persistently febrile neutropenic patients was conducted by Maertens et al. (62). In that study, liposomal amphotericin B was administered to eligible patients only if two consecutive EIA assay for galactomannan, with an optimal density ≥0.5, had been obtained or if a CT scan of the chest was suggestive of IFI, supported by microbiology.

The study population consisted of 117 febrile episodes, among which 35 (29%) failed to respond to E antibacterial therapy; the prevalence of IFI was 22% with a mortality of 36% in patients with proven or probable IFI (most often aspergillosis). The main positive findings in that study were the followings: (1) no aspergillar infection was missed; (2) early therapy could be initiated in clinically nonsuspect cases; (3) there has been a significant (78%) reduction in the use of antifungal drugs.

Does it validate the PE approach and make it the new standard? Probably, at this point, the concept needs more investigation (65). Actually, if one focuses the analysis on the 35 patients who remained febrile after initiation of E antibacterial therapy, it appears that 10 episodes of IAI have been documented in that group, with 2 (20%) deaths. If those 35 patients would have been treated empirically with an active antifungal agent, according to our earlier speculations, only one episode (2.4%) of IA would have been detected.

Thus, although there are several important positive aspects associated with the PE approach, its efficacy remains to be clearly demonstrated. In addition, it should be stressed that the Maertens' approach is quite demanding in terms of clinical and biological surveillance of the patients as well as in microbiological and radiological examinations; this high level of medical care probably cannot be implemented in many centers without additional substantial expenses in terms of personal, laboratory, and radiology investments.

Table 4 Empiric (E) vs Preemptive Approach (PE)

		Results	
	E 150 patients	PE 143 patients	
Diagnosed IFI	4 (2.6%)	13 (9.0%)	$p < 0.02$
Overall survival	147 (98%)	136 (95%)	NS
IFI-related mortality	0 (0%)	3 (2.1%)	$p = 0.12$
Mean cost (Euros)	3595	3745	NS

Source: Adapted from Ref. 66.

Recently, a prospective randomized study comparing E versus PE antifungal therapy in high-risk febrile neutropenic patients has been reported by Cordonnier et al. (66). In that study, 293 adult patients with hematological malignancies were randomized between E and PE strategy, using polyenes. E patients were given antifungal therapy in case of persistent or recurrent fever, whatever the accompanying symptoms may be, while PE patients were given therapy only in case of pneumonia, mucositis, shock, sinusitis, or skin lesions evocative of IFI; or in case of a positive galactomannan, antigen test. Survival was not inferior in the PE group (136/143) as compared to the E group (147/150). The IFI-related mortality was not significantly different in the E (0/150, 0%) group and the PE group (3/143, 2.1%), and there were significantly more IFI diagnosed in the PE group (13/143) when compared to the E group (4/150); a significant difference ($p < 0.02$) was observed. The PE patients received significantly less antifungal therapy than E patients (46% vs. 66%), but the median medication costs did not differ significantly between the two study groups (67).

Thus, as summarized in Table 4, this controlled study does not indicate a superiority of the PE approach as compared to the E strategy, neither in terms of efficacy or cost effectiveness.

The experience with the PE approach is still limited; although demanding in terms of diagnostic procedures, it reduces the rate of overtreatment. However, there is no evidence so far that PE therapy is superior or more cost effective that the E approach.

Treatment of Established Infections

Invasive Candidiasis

An array of clinical presentations with different severity and prognosis are gathered under the umbrella of IC. Between a transient candidemia, a candidemia with signs of sepsis, and a disseminated candidiasis, variable burden of the disease and consequently different response rates to therapy are expected. However, all these various entities are not apparent in many reports. In fact, several large randomized comparative trials in the treatment of candidemia and IC have assessed the role of fluconazole, itraconazole, voriconazole, amphotericin B-deoxycholate,

Table 5 Comparative Trials of Antifungal Agents in Candidemia and Invasive Candidiasis

Trials	Response rate[a]	Overall mortality
Fluconazole vs. amphotericin B-d	70% vs. 79%[b]	33% vs. 40%
Itraconazole vs. amphotericin B-d	35% vs. 41%[c]	40%
ABLC vs. amphotericin B-d	63% vs. 68%	41% vs. 49%
Caspofugin vs. amphotericin B-d	73% vs. 62%	30% vs. 34%
Voriconazole vs. amphotericin B-d/fluconazole	41% vs. 41%[c] 65% vs. 71%[b]	36% vs. 42%
Micafungin vs. Ambisome®	89.6% vs. 89.5%[b]	–
Anidulafungin vs. fluconazole	75% vs. 60.2%[b]	26% vs. 31%

[a]Cure + improved. End point assessment:
[b]variable: up to 12-week follow-up;
[c]fixed: 12-week follow up;
[d]fixed: end of therapy.

lipid formulations of amphotericin B, and three echinocandins: caspofungin, anidulafungin, and micafugin.

Table 5 summarizes the response rates and crude mortality in candidemia and IC. What can be drawn from all these studies is that the efficacy is comparable among these antifungals and the crude mortality as well as attributable mortality rates are not different. Nevertheless, there are differences in tolerance and toxicity. Moreover, a huge difference in costs exists between amphotericin B, fluconazole, oral itraconazole, and oral voriconazole on one side and the lipid formulations of amphotericin B, the IV voriconazole, and the echinocandins on the other side.

Taking into account the specific properties of each of the antifungals, their safety profiles, and different costs several recommendations can be made for first-line therapy and modifications according to laboratory tests and clinical evolution. Among the parameters that influence the initial antifungal therapy in IC, immunosuppression such as neutropenia, epidemiology with the risk of *C. glabrata* or *C. krusei,* and signs of sepsis shock, are the most important.

A study by Rex et al. (68) compared fluconazole with fluconazole plus amphotericin B-deoxycholate and found higher response rates in the combination arm (69% vs. 57%), with more rapid negativation of blood culture; the mortality rates were similar. Another recent study compared lipid formulation of amphotericin B plus placebo with lipid formulations plus mycograb in a double-blind manner (69); higher complete response rates (84% vs. 48%, $p < 0.001$), higher rates of infections clearance (hazard ratio, 2.3; 95% CI, 1.4–3.8, $p = 0.001$), and less Candida attributable mortality (18% vs. 4%, $p = 0.025$) were observed in the mycograb arm.

Invasive Aspergillosis

Until recently, the clinical experience in the treatment of IA was limited to one agent, that is, amphotericin B-deoxycholate. In contrast with the treatment of IC, the nephrotoxicity of amphotericin B-deoxycholate was more frequent due to the higher daily dosage and longer duration needed to treat IA. Lipid formulations of amphotericin B were developed as an alternative in case of intolerance, toxicity, or failure, and were tested in open nonrandomized trials and shown to be less nephrotoxic than amphotericin B-deoxycholate and equally effective.

During the recent years, two randomized comparative trials addressing the first-line therapy of IA have been achieved. The first one compared voriconazole with amphotericin B-deoxycholate and included a substantial number of patients with probable or proven IA. Switch to another antifungal in case of toxicity was allowed in both arms and occurred more frequently with amphotericin B-deoxycholate being shifted to a lipid formulation. Voriconazole was found to be superior to amphotericin B deoxycholate with a success rate of 53% versus 32%. Survival benefit from voriconazole therapy appeared early, reporting the crucial role of initial effective therapy for IA (70). A second study for first-line therapy of IA compared 3 and 10 mg/kg of liposomal amphotericin B (71). A favorable response was achieved in 50% and 46% of patients, respectively, which indicated that high doses do not improve the outcome. Moreover, higher rates of nephrotoxicity and hypokalemia, as well as a higher overall mortality rate, were observed in the 10 mg/kg group.

Salvage therapy in IA, given either for intolerance of or refractoriness to previous antifungals, has been the subject of several open nonrandomized trials, including a relatively limited number of patients. Surprisingly, the response rate was quite similar, turning around 40%, irrespective of the class or molecule used (72–78). However, not all studies had included an equivalent proportion of refractory cases, neither an equivalent proportion of probable or proven IA. In fact, the caspofungin study differs from the others by a high rate of refractoriness (>80%) and a high percentage of proven cases (>40%) although the total number of patients enrolled is small.

Combination antifungal therapy is an attractive track to explore in order to further improve outcome of IA. Polyenes and azoles act through the same target, which is ergosterol, while echinocandins, with their different target and their good safety profile, offer a more convenient combination with either class of polyenes or azoles. Many of the studies on combination antifungal therapy have been retrospective and included few patients with probable or proven cases. One of the most illustrative is the study by Marr et al. (79), which evaluated retrospectively the outcome of patients with hematological malignancy and refractory IA to amphotericin B who received either voriconazole (31 cases) or a combination of voriconazole and caspofungin (16 cases). Reduced mortality was obtained with the combination as compared with voriconazole alone. There is only one prospective nonrandomized trial where caspofungin was combined with either amphotericin B formulations or with a triazole as a salvage therapy for IA. Among the 53 patients included, the success rate was 55% (80). However, in order to draw firm conclusions concerning the exact potential of combined therapy, we still need a randomized comparative trial.

A. terreus, which is by far less frequent than *Aspergillus fumigatus* and *A. flavus*, is associated with a high rate of failure and mortality when treated with amphotericin B. This has been paralleled by the recent finding that Aspergillus is resistant in vitro to amphotericin B with MIC $\geq$ 2 µg/mL. A retrospective review of 87 cases of IA caused by *A. terreus* and treated with voriconazole, showed a reduction in mortality as compared to historical control of patients treated with amphotericin B (50% vs. 72%, respectively) (81). The dissemination of IA to the central nervous systems is a major complication with a mortality rate close to 100%. Few antifungal agents, voriconazole and posaconazole, penetrate well into the cerebral parenchyma, while echinocandins and polyenes penetrate poorly into the brain. Among the 86 cases of CNS aspergillosis treated with voriconazole and analyzed retrospectively (82), the response rate was 34%, which is quite high considering the almost constant fatal nature of this complication.

Zygomycosis

The combination of antifungal therapy and repeated surgical debridement is determinant for the outcome of this severe infection characterized by infarction of infection tissues. Zygomycetes are resistant to many antifungals including fluconazole, voriconazole, flucytosine, and echinocandins. Variable susceptibility has been reported for itraconazole and terbinafine. Among the available antifungals, two have shown in vitro activity against zygomycetes. The first one is amphotericin B with MIC 90 values of 0.5 µg/mL and the second one is posaconazole with MIC 90 values of 1 µg/mL. *Rhizopus* spp. seems to be less susceptible to both agents. Amphotericin B and posaconazole were able to prolong survival in animal models of zygomycosis. Amphotericin B improved survival in 90% to 100% of mice infected by *F. microsporus*, *Absidia corymbifera*, and *A. elegans* (83), while posaconazole improved the survival and reduced tissue burden of *Mucor* spp. in neutropenic mice (84). In another study of immunocompromised mice with disseminated zygomycosis, posaconazole was active against *Rhizopus microsporus* and *A. corymbifera*, but not against *Rhizopus oryzae*.

For several decades, the clinical experience in the treatment of zygomycosis has been limited to amphotericin B-deoxycholate, with high daily doses up to 1.5 mg/kg being recommended. However, renal toxicity was constantly a limiting factor and the mortality was high (85). Lipid formulations of amphotericin B offer the possibility of higher daily dose administration with less nephrotoxicity and have been used successfully in this indication. The largest clinical experience in the treatment of zygomycosis with lipid formulations of amphotericin B has been achieved with ABLC and included 64 patients with an overall response rate of 72% and among disseminated cases a success rate of 64% (86). The clinical experience with posaconazole in the treatment of zygomycosis is growing progressively. Retrospective review of cases treated with the oral suspension of posaconazole showed a success rate of 70% in refractory zygomycosis (87). The availability of a new intravenous formulation of this drug will undoubtedly increase its potential in the management of zygomycosis. Concomitant to antifungal therapy, early and repeated surgical debridement of necrotic lesions is an essential adjunctive measure. However, with the better control of the disease offered by lipid formulations of amphotericin B and posaconazole, extensive surgical debridement with enucleation and other dysfigurating are less needed.

Among the complementary important measures, discontinuation or decrease of immunosuppressive therapy whenever possible, control of hyperglycemia and acidosis, and discontinuation of desferroxamine therapy are all-important decisions that can help for a successful management. Although not recommended routinely because of the lack of randomized trials, colony-stimulating factors, leukocyte transfusions, and hyperbaric oxygen therapy should be discussed in selected refractory cases.

Fusariosis and Scedosporiosis

Fusarium species and *Scedosporium apiospermum* have variable in vitro susceptibility to amphotericin B and echinocandins, but are susceptible to triazoles, while *Scedosporium prolificans* demonstrates in vitro resistance to all antifungals. Because, fusariosis and scedosporiosis are uncommon, no randomized trials have been undertaken. Only single-arm small series of patients treated with voriconazole (88) and posaconazole (89) have allowed the approval of these two drugs for this indication. Both have demonstrated good clinical efficacy and decreased the mortality in these refractory infections usually associated with high fatality rate.

Cryptococcal Infections

Most of the strategies regarding the management of cryptococcal infections derive from large controlled trials in AIDS patients before the availability of effective antiretroviral therapy. The main evidence from these trials suggested that combination of amphotericin B at 1 mg/kg/day with flucytosine 150 mg/kg/day in four divided doses is the best initial treatment, given for 2 or 3 weeks, with more rapid clearance of the fungus from the cerebrospinal fluid (90,91). The lipid formulations of amphotericin B have not demonstrated a higher response rate in cryptococcal meningitis, but have better tolerance and less nephrotoxicity than amphotericin B-deoxycholate. Maintenance therapy with fluconazole 400 mg daily for the whole duration of immunosuppression is recommended. Ventriculoperitoneal shunt may be inserted in case of cyptococcal meningitis with hydrocephalus.

Pheohyphomycosis

This infection is caused by fungi that produce melanin pigment in their cell wall and typical dark colonies on culture. The main sites of infection are the sinuses, the lungs, and the skin with a predilection for CNS dissemination. The treatment has commonly involved flucytosine in combination with amphotericin B and resulted in high rates of failure or relapse, and the mortality in disseminated cases could be very high. Since the introduction of triazoles, itraconazole and voriconazole have demonstrated high response rates in a limited number of patients (92,93). Posaconazole has shown excellent in vitro and in vivo activity in animal models (94) and has been used successfully in few cases (95).

CONCLUSIONS

Facing in patients with fungal infections difficult early diagnosis and high mortality rates, several strategies have been developed. These include prophylaxis for patients at high risk, E and PE antifungal therapy for those with persisting fever, and of course specifically adapted treatment for the established infections. Several classes of antifungals exist nowadays and new molecules are continuously developed within each class, expanding markedly our choice and the possibility of combination. Cost is a major issue and there is a huge difference in prices between the old and new agents. It is our duty to put the balance right and our responsibility to use these molecules appropriately with the adequate drug in the best indication.

REFERENCES

1. Pfaller MA, Diekema DJ. Epidemiology of invasive Candidiasis: a persistent public health problem. Clin Microbiol Rev 2007; 20:133–163.
2. Malani L, Hmous J, Chiu L, et al. *Candida glabrata* fungemia: experience in a tertiary care center. Clin Infect Dis 2005; 41:975–981.
3. Sarvikivi E, Lyytikainen O, Soll DR, et al. Emergence of fluconazole resistance in a *Candida parapsilosis* strain that caused infections in a neonatal intensive care unit. J Clin Microbiol 2005; 43:2729–2735.
4. Chamilos G, Luna M, Lewis RE, et al. Invasive fungal infections in patients with hematologic malignancies in a tertiary car cancer center: an autopsy study over a 15-year period (1989–2003). Haematologica 2006; 91:986–989.
5. Baddley JW, Pappas PG, Smith AC, et al. Epidemiology of *Aspergillus terreus* at a University Hospital. J Clin Microbiol 2003; 41:5525–5529.
6. Singh N. Trends in the epidemiology of opportunistic fungal infections: predisposing factors and the impact of antimicrobial use practices. Clin Infect Dis 2001; 33:1692–1696.
7. O'Brien SN, Blijlevens NMA, Mahfouz TH, et al. Infections in patients with hematological cancer: recent developments. Hematology Am Soc Hematol Edu Program 2003; 438–472.
8. Bow EJ, Loewen R, Cheang MS, et al. Invasive fungal disease in adults undergoing remission-induction therapy for acute myeloid leukemia: the pathogenetic role of the antileukemic regimen. Clin Infect Dis 1995; 21:361–369.
9. Prentice HG, Kibbler CC, Prentice AG. Towards a targeted, risk-based, antifungal strategy in neutropenic patients. Br J Haematol 2000; 110:273–284.

10. Lionakis MS, Lewis RE, Torres HA, et al. Increased frequency of non-*fumigatus* *Aspergillus* species in amphotericin B- or triazole-pre-exposed cancer patients with positive cultures for aspergilli. Diagn Microbiol Infect Dis 2005; 52: 15–20.
11. Martino R, Subira M, Rovira M et al. Invasive fungal infections after allogeneic peripheral blood stem cell transplantation: incidence and risk factors in 395 patients. Br J Haematol 2002; 116: 475–482.
12. Mahfouz T, Anaissie E. Prevention of fungal infections in the immunocompromised host. Curr Opin Investig Drugs 2003; 4:974–990.
13. Anaissie EJ, Rex JH, Uzun O, et al. Predictors of adverse outcome in cancer patients with candidemia. Am J Med 1998; 104:238–245.
14. Marr KA, Carter RA, Crippa F, et al. Epidemiology and outcome of mould infections in hematopoietic stem cell transplant recipients. Clin Infect Dis 2002; 34: 909–917.
15. Marr KA, Patterson T, Denning D. Aspergillosis: pathogenesis, clinical manifestations, and therapy. Infect Dis Clin North Am 2002; 16:875–894.
16. Kontoyiannis DP, Lionakis MS, Lewis RE et al. Zygomycosis in a tertiary-care cancer center in the era of *Aspergillus*-active antifungal therapy: a case-control observational study of 27 recent cases. J Infect Dis 2005; 91: 1350–1360.
17. Nath DS, Kandaswamy R, Gruessner R, et al. Fungal infections in transplant recipients receiving alemtuzumab. Transplant Proc 2005; 37:934–936.
18. De Rosa FG, Shaz D, Campagna AC, et al. Invasive pulmonary aspergillosis soon after therapy with infliximab, a tumor necrosis factor-alpha-neutralizing antibody: a possible healthcare-associated case? Infect Control Hosp Epidemiol 2003; 24:477–482.
19. Warris A, Bjorneklett A, Gaustad P. Invasive pulmonary aspergillosis associated with infliximab therapy. N Engl J Med 2001; 344:1099–1100.
20. Horvath LL, George BJ, Murray CK et al. Direct comparison of the BACTEC 9320 and BacT/ALERT 3D automated blood culture systems for Candida growth detection. J Clin Microbiol 2004; 42:115–118.
21. Becker MJ, Lugtenburg EL, Cornelissen JJ, et al. Galactomannan detection in computerized tomography-based broncho-alveolar lavage fluid and serum in haematological patients at risk for invasive pulmonary aspergillosis. B J Haematol 2003; 121:448–457.
22. Pfaller MA, Messer SA, Boyken S, et al. Evaluation of E-test method using Mueller-Hinton agar with glucose and methylene blue for determining amphotericin B MICs for 4,936 clinical isolates of Candida species. J Clin Microbiol 2004; 42:4977–4979.
23. Pfaller MA, Messer SA, Boyken S, et al. Geographic variation in the susceptibilities of invasive isolates of *Candida glabrata* to seven systemically active antifungal agents: a global assessment from the ARTEMIS Antifungal Surveillance Program conducted in 2001 and 2002. J Clin Microbiol 2004; 42:3142–3146.
24. Blignaut E, Molepo J, Pujot C, et al. Clade-related amphotericin B resistance among South African *Candida albicans* isolates. Diagn Microbiol Infect Dis 2005; 53:29–31.
25. Miller NS, Dick JD, Merz DG. Phenotypic switching in *Candida lusitaniae* on copper sulfate indicator agar: association with amphotericin B resistance and filamentation. J Clin Microbiol 2006; 44:1536–1539.
26. Colombo AL, Melo ASA, Rosas RFC, et al. Outbreak of *Candida rugosa* candidemia: an emerging pathogen that may be refractory to amphotericin B therapy. Diagn Microbiol Infect Dis 2003; 46:263–257.

27. Pfaller MA, Diekema DJ, Sheehan DJ. Interpretative breakpoints for fluconazole and Candida revisited: a blueprint for the future of antifungal susceptibility testing. Clin Microbiol Rev 2006; 19:435–447.
28. Moudgal V, Kittle T, Boikov D, et al. Multiechinocandin and multiazole-resistant *Candida parapsilosis* isolates serially obtained during therapy for prosthetic valve endocarditis. Antimicrob Agents Chemother 2005; 49:767–769.
29. Dodgson KJ, Dodgson AR, Pujol C, et al. Caspofungin-resistant *C. glabrata*. Clin Microbiol Infect 2005; 11(suppl 2): 364.
30. Hernandez S, Lopez-Ribot JL, Najvar LK, et al. Caspofungin resistant to *Candida albicans*: correlating clinical outcome with laboratory susceptibility testing of three isogenic isolates serially obtained from a patient with progressive *Candida esophagitis*. Antimicrob Agents Chemother 2004; 48:1382–1383.
31. Jantunen E, Nihtinen A, Volin L, et al. Candidaemia in allogeneic stem cell transplant recipients: low risk without fluconazole prophylaxis. Bone Marrow Transplant 2004; 34:891–895.
32. Glasmacher A, Prentice AG. Evidence-based review of antifungal prophylaxis in neutropenic patients with haematological malignancies. J Antimicrob Chemother 2005; 56:i23–i32.
33. Trifilio S, Verma A, Mehta J. Antimicrobial prophylaxis in hematopoietic stem cell transplant recipients: heterogeneity of current clinical practice. Bone Marrow Transplant 2004; 33:735–739.
34. Bow EJ, Laverdiere M, Lussier N, et al. Antifungal prophylaxis for severely neutropenic chemotherapy recipients: a meta-analysis of randomized-controlled clinical trials. Cancer 2002; 94:3230–3246.
35. Kanda Y, Yamamoto R, Chizuka A et al. Prophylactic action of oral fluconazole against fungal infection in neutropenic patients: a meta-analysis of 16 randomized, controlled trials. Cancer 2000; 89:1611–1625.
36. Glasmacher A, Prentice A, Gorschluter M et al. Itraconazole prevents invasive fungal infections in neutropenic patients treated for hematologic malignancies: evidence from a meta-analysis of 3,597 patients. J Clin Oncol 2003; 21:4615–4626.
37. Robenshtok E, Gafter-Gvili A, Paul M, et al. Antifungal prophylaxis for patients with chemotherapy or haematopoietic stem cell transplantation-meta-analysis. Proceedings, 17th European Congress of clinical Microbiology and Infectious Diseases (ECCMID) and 25th international Congress of Chemotherapy (ICC); Munich, Germany, 2007.
38. Morgenstern GR, Prentice AG, Prentice HG et al. A randomized controlled trial of itraconazole versus fluconazole for the prevention of fungal infections in patients with haematological malignancies. Br J Haematol 1999; 105:901–911.
39. Glasmacher A, Cornely O, Ullmann AJ et al. An open-label randomized trial comparing itraconazole oral solution with fluconazole oral solution for primary prophylaxis of fungal infections in patients with hematological malignancy and profound neutropenia. J Antimicrob Chemother 2006; 57:317–325.
40. Oren I, Rowe JM, Sprecher H et al. A prospective randomized trial of itraconazole vs fluconazole for the prevention of fungal infections in patients with acute leukemia and hematopoietic stem cell transplant recipients. Bone Marrow Transplant 2006; 38:127–134.
41. Annaloro C, Oriani A, Tagliaferri E et al. Efficacy of different prophylactic antifungal regimens in bone marrow transplantation. Haematologica 1995; 80:512–517.

42. Huijgens PC, Simoons-Smit AM, van Loenen AC et al. Fluconazole versus itraconazole for the prevention of fungal infections in hemato-oncology. J Clin Pathol. 1999; 52:376–380.
43. Marr KA, Crippa F, Leisenring W et al. Itraconazole versus fluconazole for prevention of fungal infections in patients receiving allogeneic stem cell transplants. Blood 2004; 103:1527–1533.
44. Winston DJ, Maziarz RT, Chandrasekar PH et al. Intravenous and oral itraconazole versus intravenous and oral fluconazole for long-term antifungal prophylaxis in allogeneic hematopoietic stem-cell transplant recipients. A multicenter, randomized trial. Ann Intern Med 2003; 138:705–713.
45. Vardakas KZ, Michalopoulos A, Falagas ME. Fluconazole versus itraconazole for antifungal prophylaxis in neutropenic patients with hematological malignancies: a meta-analysis of randomized-controlled trials. Br J Haematol 2005; 131:22–28.
46. Prentice AG, Glasmacher A, Djulbegovic B. In meta-analysis itraconazole is superior to fluconazole for prophylaxis of systemic fungal infection in the treatment of hematological malignancy. Br J Haematol 2006; 132:656–658.
47. van Burik JA, Ratnatharathorn V, Stepan DE et al. Micafungin versus fluconazole for prophylaxis against invasive fungal infections during neutropenia in patients undergoing hematopoietic stem cell transplantation. Clin Infect Dis 2004; 39:1407–1416.
48. Mattiuzzi GN, Alvarado G, Giles FJ et al. Open-label, randomized comparison of itraconazole versus caspofungin for prophylaxis in patients with hematologic malignancies. Antimicrob Agents Chemother 2006; 50:143–147.
49. Mattiuzzi GN, Estey E, Raad I et al. Liposomal amphotericin B versus the combination of fluconazole and itraconazole as prophylaxis for invasive fungal infections during induction: chemotherapy for patients with acute myelogenous leukemia and myelodysplastic syndrome. Cancer 2003; 97:450–456.
50. Wolff SN, Fay J, Stevens D et al. Fluconazole vs low-dose amphotericin B for the prevention of fungal infections in patients undergoing bone marrow transplantation: a study of the North American Marrow Transplant Group. Bone Marrow Transplant 2000; 25:853–859.
51. Cornely OA, Maertens J, Winston DJ, et al. Posaconazole vs. fluconazole or itraconazole prophylaxis in patients with neutropenia. N Engl J Med 2007; 356:348–359.
52. Ullmann AJ, Lipton JH, Vesole DH, et al. Posaconazole or fluconazole for prophylaxis in severe graft-versus-host disease. N Engl J Med 2007; 356:355–347.
53. Pizzo PA, Robichaud KJ, Gill FA et al. Empiric antibiotic and antifungal therapy for cancer patients with prolonged fever and granulocytopenia. Am J Med 1998; 272: 101–111.
54. EORTC International Antimicrobial Therapy Cooperative Group, . Empiric antifungal therapy in febrile granulocytopenic patients. Am J Med 1989; 86:668–672.
55. Hugues WT, Armstrong D, Cornely OA et al. Guidelines for the use of antimicrobial agents in neutropenic patients with cancer. Clin Infect Dis 2002; 34:730–750.
56. Walsh TJ, Finberg RW, Arndt C et al. Liposomal amphotericin B for empirical therapy in patients with persistent fever and neutropenia. N Engl J Med 1999; 340: 764–771.
57. Walsh TJ, Pappas P, Winston DJ et al. Voriconazole compared with liposomal amphotericin B for empirical antifungal therapy in patients with neutropenia and persistent fever. N Engl J Med 2002; 346:225–234.

58. Walsh TJ, Teppler H, Donowitz GR et al. Caspofungin versus liposomal amphotericin B for empirical antifungal theapy in patients with persistent fever and neutropenia. N Engl J Med 2004; 351:1391–1402.
59. Klastersky J. Antifungal therapy in patients with fever and neutropenia: more rational and less empirical? N Engl J Med 2004; 351:1445–1447.
60. Guiot HFL, Fibbe WE, van't Wout. Risk factors for fungal infection in patients with malignant hematologic disorders: implications for empirical therapy and prophylaxis. Clin Infect Dis 1994; 18:525–532.
61. Corey L, Boeckh M. Persistent fever in patients with neutropenia. N Engl J Med, 2002; 346:222–224.
62. Maertens J, Theunissen K, Verhoef G et al. Galactomannan and computed tomography-based preemptive antifungal therapy in neutropenic patients at high risk for invasive fungal infection: a prospective feasibility study. Clin Infect Dis 2005; 41:1242–1250.
63. de Pauw B. Between over- and undertreatment of invasive fungal disease. Clin Infect Dis 2005; 41:1251–1253.
64. Ascioglu S, Rex H, de Pauw B et al. Defining opportunistic invasive fungal infections in immunocompromized patients with cancer and hematopoietic stem cell transplants: an international consensus. Clin Infect Dis 2002; 37:7–14
65. Maertens J; Deeren D, Dierickx D et al. Preemptive antifungal therapy: still a way to go. Curr Opin Infect Dis 2006; 19:551–556.
66. Cordonnier C, Pautas C, Maury S et al. Empirical versus pre-emptive antifungal therapy in high-risk febrile neutropenic patients: a prospective randomized study. Blood 2006; 108: Abstract 2019.
67. Schwarzinger M, Beauchamp C, Maury S et al. Empirical versus pre-emptive antifungal therapy in high-risk febrile neutropenic patients: ana economic analysis. Blood 2006; 108:Abstract 2021
68. Rex JH, Poppas PG, Karchmer AW, et al. A randomized and blinded multicenter trial of high-dose fluconazole plus placebo versus fluconazole plus amphotericin B as therapy for candidemia and its consequences in nonneutropenic subjects. Clin Infect Dis 2003; 36:1221–1228.
69. Pachl J, Svoboda P, Jacobs F, et al. A randomized, blinded, multicenter trial of lipid-associated amphotericin B alone versus in combination with an antibody-based inhibitor of heat shock protein 90 in patients with invasive candidiasis. Clin Infect Dis 2006; 42:1404–1413.
70. Herbrecht R, Denning DW, Patterson TF, et al. Voriconazole versus amphotericin B for primary therapy of invasive aspergillosis. N Engl J Med 2002; 347, 408–415.
71. Cornely OA, Maertens JA, Bresnik M et al. Liposomal amphotericin B as initial therapy for invasive mold infection: a randomized trial comparing a high-loading dose regimen with standard dosing (ambiload trial). Clin Infect Dis 2007; 44: 1289–1297.
72. Walsh TJ, Hiemenz JW, Seibel NL et al. Amphotericin B lipid complex for invasive fungal infections: analysis of safety and efficacy in 556 cases. Clin Infect Dis 1998; 26:1383–1396.
73. Walsh TJ, Goodman JL, Pappas P et al. Safety, tolerance, and pharmacokinetics of high-dose liposomal amphotericin B (AmBisome) in patients infected with Aspergillus species and other filamentous fungi: maximum tolerated dose study. Antimicrob Agents Chemother 2001; 45:3487–3496.

74. White WJ, Anaissie EJ, Kusne S et al. Amphotericin B colloidal dispersion vs. amphotericin B as therapy for invasive aspergillosis. Clin Infect Dis 1997; 24:635–642.
75. Denning DW, Ribaud P, Milpied N et al. Efficacy and safety of voriconazole in the treatment of acute invasive aspergillosis. Clin Infect Dis 2002; 34:563–571.
76. Denning DW, Lee JY, Hostetler JS et al. NIAID Mycoses Study Group Multicenter Trial of Oral Itraconazole Therapy for Invasive Aspergillosis. Am J Med 1994; 97: 135–144
77. Walsh TJ, Raad I, Patterson TF et al. Treatment of invasive aspergillosis with posaconazole in patients who are refractory to or intolerant of conventional therapy: an externally controlled trial. Clin Infect Dis 2007; 44:2–412.
78. Maertens J, Raad D, Sable CA et al. Multicenter, noncomparative study to evaluate safety and efficacy of caspofungin (CAS) in adults with invasive aspergillosis (IA) refractory (R) or intolerant (I) to amphotericin B (AMB), AMB lipid formulations (Lipid AMB) or azoles. Proceedings, 40th Interscience Conference an Antimicrobial Agents and Chemotherapy, USA, 2000, 371.
79. Marr KA, Boeckh M, Carter RA et al. Combination antifungal therapy for invasive aspergillosis. Clin Infect Dis 2004; 39:797–802.
80. Maertens J, Glashmacher A, Herbrecht R et al. Multicenter, noncomparative study of caspofungin (CAS) combined with other antifungals in adults with invasive aspergillosis (IA) refractory (R) or intolerant (I) to prior therapy (Rx): final data. Proceedings, 45th Interscience Conference on Antimicrobial Agents and Chemotherapy, USA, 2005, M954.
81. Steinbach WJ, Benjamin Jr DK, Kontoyiannis DP et al. Invasive aspergillosis (IA) caused by *Aspergillus terreus*: multicenter retrospective analysis of 87 cases. Proceedings, 43rd Interscience Conference an Antimicrobial Agents and Chemotherapy, USA, 2003, M1753.
82. Troke PF, Schwarz S, Ruhnke M et al. Voriconazole (VRC) therapy (Rx) in 86 patients with CNS Aspergillus (CNSA): a retrospective analysis. Proceedings, 43rd Interscience Conference an Antimicrobial Agents and Chemotherapy, USA, 2003, M1755.
83. Dannaoui F, Mouton JW, Meis JF et al. Efficacy of antifungal therapy in a non-neutropenic murine model of zygomycosis. Antimicrob Agents Chemother 2002; 46: 1953–1959.
84. Sun QN, Najvar LK, Bocanegra R et al. In vivo activity of posaconazole against Mucor sp. In an immunosuppressed-mouse model. Antimicrob Agents Chemother 2002; 46:2310–2312.
85. Roden MM, Zaoutis TE, Buchanan WL et al. Epidemiology and outcome of zygomycosis: a review of 929 reported cases. Clin Infect Dis 2005; 41:634–653.
86. Larkin JA, Montero JA. Efficacy and safety of amphotericin B lipid complex for zygomycosis. Infect Med 2003; 20:201–206.
87. Kontoyiannis DP, Hare R, Solomon H et al. Posaconazole is highly effective as a second-line agents in Zygomycosis: summary of 91 cases. Proceedings, 45th Interscience Conference an Antimicrobial Agents and Chemotherapy, USA, 2005, M974.
88. Perfect JR, Marr KA, Walsh TJ et al. Voriconazole treatment for less-common, emerging, or refractory fungal infections. Clin Infect Dis 2003; 36:1122–1131.
89. Lamaris GA, Chamilos G, Lewis RE et al. Scedosporium infection in a tertiary care cancer center: a review of 25 cases from 1989–2006. Clin Infect Dis 2006; 43: 1580–1584.

90. Saag MS, Graybill RJ, Larsen RA et al. Practice guidelines for the management of cryptococcal disease. Infectious Diseases Society of America. Clin Infect Dis 2000; 30:710–718.
91. Bennett JE, Dismukes WE, Durna RJ et al. A comparison of amphotericin B alone and combined with flucytosine in the treatment of cryptoccal meningitis. N Engl J Med 1979; 301:126–131.
92. Schwinn A, Strohm S, Helgenberger M et al. Phaeohyphomycosis caused by Exophiala jeanselmei treated with itraconazole. Mycoses 1993; 36:445–448.
93. Hanieh S, Miller R, Daveson L et al. Cerebral phaeohyphomycosis caused by Cladophialophora bantiana in a patient with chronic lymphocytic leukemia. Clin Microbiol Newsletter 2006; 28:110–112
94. Graybill JR, Najvar LK, Johnson E et al. Posaconazole therapy of disseminated phaeohyphomycosis in a murine model. Antimicrob Agents Chemother 2004; 48: 2288–2291.
95. Negroni R, Helou SH, Petri N et al. Case study: posaconazole treatment of disseminated phaeohyphomycosis due to exophiala spinifera. Clin Infect Dis 2004; 38: e15–e20.

7

Myeloid Growth Factors

Jeffrey Crawford
*Department of Medicine, Duke University School
of Medicine and the Duke Comprehensive
Cancer Center, Durham, North Carolina, U.S.A.*

INTRODUCTION

The history of the myeloid growth factors parallels the development and evolution of biotechnology over the last several decades. The relationship of neutropenia and infection has been recognized since the advent of myelotoxic chemotherapy and was well described in work by Bodey more than 50 years ago (1). However, it was not until the development of in vitro assays for myeloid precursor cells that we could begin to study myeloid development. These cell culture systems also facilitated the subsequent studies of the myeloid growth factors that were designated at G-CSF (granulocyte colony-stimulating factor) and GM-CSF (granulocyte macrophage colony-stimulating factor) based on their differential stimulatory effects of myeloid colonies in vitro (2). In the 1980s, these colony-stimulating factors were subsequently purified, cloned, and placed into early human clinical trials within a matter of a few years. Likewise, from the onset of the first human trials in the mid to late 1980s to the approval of G-CSF and GM-CSF in 1991 by the FDA was equally rapid. This accelerated timeline can be attributed to a number of factors, including the decades of prior scientific discovery leading to the biotechnology revolution, the pressing need for these agents in the clinic, their relative safety and efficacy, as well as a more streamlined process for drug development compared to our current standards.

Over the last two decades, since myeloid growth factors were introduced into clinical trials and clinical practice, we have learned a great deal about the

Table 1 FDA-Approved Indications for Myeloid Growth Factors

Growth factor/ cytokine	Generic name	Trade name(s)	Distributor(s)/ manufacturer(s)	Indication(s)
G-CSF	Filgrastim Pegfilgrastim	Neupogen Neulasta	Amgen Amgen	Cancer patients receiving myelo-suppressive chemotherapy Patients with nonmyeloid malignancy following BMT Patients with severe chronic neutropenia Following induction chemotherapy in AML
GM-CSF	Sargramostim	Leukine Prokine	Berlex	Following autologous BMT BMT engraftment delay or failure Following induction chemotherapy in older patients with AML Allogeneic BMT for mobilization of PBPCs and for use after PBPC transplantation

Source: Adapted from Ref. 34.

biology and application of these products, but we still have a steep learning curve ahead. Table 1 lists the current FDA-approved indications for the myeloid growth factors G-CSF and GM-CSF. It should be noted that in addition to these agents currently approved in the United States, additional forms of G-CSF (lenograstim) as well as GM-CSF (molgramostim) are approved elsewhere in the world, and appear to have properties similar to their generic counterparts. G-CSF and

GM-CSF share some similar clinical indications, including their roles in management of patients with acute myeloid leukemia, as well as in mobilization of peripheral blood progenitor cells in following bone marrow or peripheral blood stem cell reinfusion. In addition, G-CSF is approved for management of severe, chronic neutropenia, which is discussed elsewhere in the chapter by Dr. Dale.

The major use of the myeloid growth factors has been in the management of cancer patients receiving myelosuppressive chemotherapy. As noted in Table 1, filgrastim and pegfilgrastim have an approved indication in this setting, but sargramostim does not, although it is clearly used in this setting and is included in discussions of the myeloid growth factors in practice guidelines of American Society of Clinical Oncology (ASCO), National Comprehensive Cancer Network (NCCN), and the European Organisation for Research and Treatment of Cancer (EORTC) (3–5).

While other chapters in this book have focused on the problem of neutropenia per se, as well as the epidemiology and patient risk factors associated with chemotherapy-induced neutropenia, this chapter will focus predominantly on the biology of the myeloid growth factors and their potential differences in both biology and clinical application and then focus on the clinical trial development that have lead to current guidelines and clinical practice.

BIOLOGY OF MYELOID GROWTH FACTORS

Granulocyte Colony-Stimulating Factor

The naturally occurring form of endogenous G-CSF is a 174-amino acid glycoprotein that has selected activity for cells of the neutrophil lineage. The recombinant form of G-CSF, filgrastim, is cloned in *Escherichia coli* and differs from native G-CSF by an addition of a methionine at the N-terminus of the molecule, resulting in a lack of glycosylation. By contrast, lenograstim is expressed in mammalian cells and is glycosylated. The biological function of both of these recombinant molecules seem to be similar suggesting that glycosylation does not significantly effect structure or function (2). Endogenous G-CSF is produced by a number of cells in the body including macrophages, fibroblasts, endothelial cells, and stromal cells from the bone marrow. Neutropenia results in release of G-CSF from these cells in a process that is not completely understood, but involves a cascade of multiple other cytokines, including tumor necrosis factor, Interleukin-1, and other cytokines. The G-CSF ligand binds to a receptor that is distinct from the receptors for GM-CSF, although there is a common conserved domain recognized by other CSFs. The G-CSF receptor is present on the surface of cells of neutrophil lineage as well as endothelial cells, and in humans it appears to be most heavily expressed on promyelocytes. As will be discussed subsequently in the pharmacology of this agent, G-CSF binds to the receptor and then is internalized and degraded. This represents a mechanism of clearance for G-CSF, as well as downregulation of the receptor.

While the mechanisms of signaling at the cellular level are still being defined for G-CSF, the net effect of G-CSF ligand receptor interaction is multifold, including an increase in the proliferative rate of neutrophil-specific myeloid precursors, a shortened time course for maturation of neutrophils within the postmitotic compartment, and enhancement of neutrophil function. From a wealth of preclinical and clinical information, it appears that endogenous G-CSF plays an important role both in maintaining normal myelopoiesis and as a biological response agent for neutropenia, infection and other stress responses to the myeloid compartment.

Because of its low molecular weight, both endogenous G-CSF, as well as the recombinant versions of this myeloid growth factor are freely filtered at the level of the kidney, resulting in a very short half-life of the molecule measured in hours. Pegfilgrastim is a recombinant form of G-CSF in which a polyethylene glycol moiety has been added to the N-terminus of the G-CSF molecule (7). The polyethylene glycol moiety adds 20 kDa in size to the 18 kDa filgrastim molecule, essentially eliminating the renal clearance of the molecule, with neutrophil-mediated clearance as a major mode of elimination of pegfilgrastim. This will be discussed further in the clinical trials section, but it appears that in studies of pegfilgrastim compared to filgrastim, the addition of polyethylene glycol does not alter the biological effects of pegfilgrastim on neutrophil production and function compared to filgrastim.

Granulocyte Macrophage Colony-Stimulating Factor

GM-CSF is a 127-amino acid glycoprotein with a molecular weight of approximately 22 kDa. As noted in Table 1, sargramostim is a recombinant glycosylated protein in yeast, produced in the United States. Molgramostim is a nonglycosylated formulation produced from *E. coli* in Europe. Unlike G-CSF, GM-CSF is produced in a wide number of different cells in the body, including lymphocytes, macrophages, esinophils, endothelial cells, fibroblasts, osteoblasts, bone marrow stromal cells, karatinocytes, thymic epithelial cells, mesothelial cells, among others (2). GM-CSF production is increased in response to a variety of cytokines and the response to these cytokines appears to be different in different cell types. For example, tumor necrosis factor and Interleukin-1 induces GM-CSF production by fibroblasts and endothelial cells while lipopolysaccharide stimulates production in macrophages. GM-CSF then interacts with cells that have surface receptors for a unique GM-CSF receptor distinct from the G-CSF receptor. In addition to mature neutrophils, eosinophils, monocytes, and endothelial cells have GM-CSF receptors. The receptor for GM-CSF is a heterodimer with both an alpha and a beta chain, with the alpha chain thought to be the primary binding site of GM-CSF. The beta subunit is a member of the cytokine receptor family common to Interleukin-3 and 5. Binding of the receptor to the ligand leads to dimerization of the two subunits, internalization and degradation, of the complex. Unlike G-CSF, the intercellular signaling appears to occur through the Janus kinase (JAK-2) pathway.

Although GM-CSF does affect hematopoietic precursors, it is not necessary for normal hematopoiesis. Knock out models in mice demonstrate a marked reduction in neutrophil numbers when G-CSF is knocked out, but not with GM-CSF. By contrast, GM-CSF knock out mice do experience pulmonary abnormalities and altered immune function.

It is evident that the biology of G-CSF and GM-CSF are distinct and while there may be overlapping and redundant functions in some areas of the hematopoietic system, there are clearly distinctive actions for both cytokines within and outside the myeloid compartment (8). It is hoped that future studies that exploit these biological differences will result in unique clinical applications for both agents. For example, studies of sargramostim in the management of Crohn's disease have suggested that this agent may decrease disease severity and improve quality of life, perhaps mediated through receptors in the intestinal epithelium and/or immune-mediated effects (9). For the purpose of this chapter, we will focus on the use of myeloid growth factors G-CSF and GM-CSF in supportive care of the cancer patient and specifically focus on cancer chemotherapy.

TREATMENT STRATEGIES FOR CHEMOTHERAPY-INDUCED NEUTROPENIA

The topic of neutropenia and its clinical impact have been well discussed by Dr. Dale in an accompanying chapter of this textbook. Table 2 outlines potential strategies for management of chemotherapy-induced neutropenia. These strategies can be further divided into those involving prevention of chemotherapy-induced neutropenia and treatment of the neutropenic event.

In terms of treatment, studies have demonstrated that patients with asymptomatic neutropenia, in the absence of fever or infection, are not benefited by the use of myeloid growth factors (3). However, for neutropenia, in the setting of fever and/or infection, urgent and immediate treatment with antibiotics is warranted. The strategies for antibiotics are well outlined by Drs. Rolston and Bodey in their chapter on management of febrile neutropenia.

Table 2 Strategies for Management of Chemotherapy-Induced Neutropenia

- Prevention
  - Dose reduction/delay
  - Hematopoietic growth factors
    - G-CSF (filgrastim, lenograstim)
    - GM-CSF (sargramostim, molgramostim)
    - Pegfilgrastim
  - Antibiotics
- Treatment
  - Observation if afebrile
  - Antibiotics
  - Myeloid growth factors

The use of myeloid growth factors in this treatment setting has not been routinely endorsed, but rather the recommendation is that the use of these agents be limited to high-risk patients with documented tissue infections, sepsis, prolonged neutropenia, or other high-risk settings (3). The lower evidence of benefit of these agents in this setting has a biological basis. The impact of myeloid growth factors on neutrophil production requires several days in the postchemotherapy setting in order to increase the number of neutrophil progenitors, shorten the neutrophil maturation time and therefore enhance neutrophil recovery. In addition, at the time the patient develops neutropenia with fever, endogenous G-CSF production has already increased, thus lessening the likely additional benefit of pharmacologic doses of recombinant colony-stimulating factors.

A meta-analysis of randomized controlled trials of the use of colony-stimulating factors for the treatment of chemotherapy-induced febrile neutropenia identified 13 studies (10). While there was no difference in overall mortality, a borderline significant result was noted in the reduction of infection-related mortality (OR = 0.51 (0.26–1.00); $p = 0.05$). More substantial effects of CSF were noted in shorter length of hospitalization (hazard ratio (HR) = 0.63 (0.49–0.82; $p = 0.006$) and a shorter time to neutrophil recovery (HR = 0.32 (0.23–0.46); $p < 0.0001$). Included in these meta-analysis were studies involving either G- or GM-CSF. Both of these agents demonstrated clinical benefits in terms of shortening of hospitalization and reduction in duration of neutropenia in the studies reported. Subset analyses of these individual studies have suggested greater likelihood of benefit in patients with more prolonged neutropenia or complications of neutropenia.

In addition, a clinical prediction score has been developed that may assist in identification of patients likely to have either low or high-risk febrile neutropenia (11). Application of a clinical prediction rule to select patients for a prospective trial may help better define the potential benefits of myeloid growth factors in this setting. In the meantime, the ASCO guidelines do not recommend routine use of myeloid growth factors in the treatment of febrile neutropenia (3). However, they feel that CSFs should be considered in patients who are at high risk for infection-associated complications and have prognostic factors predictive of poor clinical outcomes, which would include expected prolonged neutropenia, age greater than 65 years, uncontrolled primary disease, pneumonia, hypotension and multiorgan dysfunction, invasive fungal infection, or being hospitalized at the time of development of fever (3).

PREVENTION STRATEGIES FOR CHEMOTHERAPY-INDUCED NEUTROPENIA

In most arenas of supportive care, the goal is prevention of the complication rather than management. As outlined in Table 2, the initial approach for prevention of neutropenia and its complications prior to the advent of myeloid growth factors was chemotherapy dose reduction and/or delay. Even in the current era of myeloid growth factors, this strategy remains one that is commonly employed and is discussed further in the chapter by Dr. Lyman. While reducing the amount of chemotherapy being delivered can certainly reduce the toxicity of the chemotherapy, formal studies evaluating the impact of chemotherapy reduction on treatment outcome have rarely been performed. Preclinical studies of cancer pharmacology, as well as dose-finding studies from phase I and II trials have suggested that chemotherapy benefit is optimized when delivered at the maximum tolerated dose (MTD). Unfortunately, MTD is most commonly limited by neutropenia and its complications for most cytotoxic chemotherapy agents alone and in combination.

Furthermore, chemotherapy dose escalation clinical trials, as well as their subsequent phase III counterparts are generally performed in younger patients with less comorbid disease as dictated by the clinical trial eligibility. When these studies are then translated into clinical practice in the clinical setting, the potential for toxicity in an older population with more comorbid disease is substantially elevated. The end result is a much higher frequency of neutropenia and febrile neutropenia in the community setting with standard chemotherapy regimens compared to the published results in the literature. As further discussed by Dr. Lyman, these rates of neutropenia and febrile neutropenia are occurring despite planned dose reduction as well as subsequent dose reduction for toxicity in this population.

Ultimately, the overall benefits of our treatment strategies must combine the use of chemotherapy agents at effective doses with appropriate supportive care to minimize potential toxicities. Although we have learned much from clinical trials, it is clear that prospective studies in community populations that have both short-term toxicity and longer term response and survival and quality-of-life outcomes will be critical to helping oncologists determine the best strategies for their patients.

To further emphasize this point, several studies suggest that neutropenia can be considered a pharmacodynamic endpoint for clinical benefit. For example, in a large retrospective review of 4000 patients with Hodgkin's lymphoma treated on German Hodgkin's Study Group trials, the outcome for women was better than men (12). While this gender difference has been known for some time, the authors were able to relate this difference to an increase in the amount of grade 3 and 4 leukopenia in females compared to males. In a multivariate analysis of freedom from treatment failure the hazard ratio was 0.58 with 95% confidence intervals of 0.46 to 0.73 for women. The hypothesis of the authors was that the better outcome for female patients with Hodgkin's lymphoma is due to greater systemic chemotherapy exposure as measured by the surrogate endpoint of neutropenia.

While many clinicians could appreciate that this could be the case in a highly chemotherapy sensitive and potentially curable setting of Hodgkin's lymphoma, it is quite interesting to see similar results from an analysis of patients with advanced stage non–small cell lung cancer (13). In this study, an analysis of survival was performed from three randomized trials of over 1200 patients with advanced stage non–small cell lung cancer, treated with chemotherapy, including the ELVIS, MILES, and GEMVEN trials, the majority of which were focused in elderly lung cancer patients. In a landmark analysis of 436 of these patients who received all six planned cycles of treatment and were alive at 180 days, the variables of age, gender, performance status, stage, and histologic subtype were not significant determinants of survival. However, the development of either grade 1 or 2 neutropenia (hazard ratio of 0.74) or grade 3 or 4 neutropenia (hazard ratio 0.65) was significantly associated with better survival. For patients with no neutropenia, the survival was 31 weeks, compared to 42 or 43.7 weeks for patients with grade 1 or 2 or grade 3 or 4 neutropenia ($p = 0.01$). Obviously, this landmark analysis eliminates the patients who had disease progression and/or chemotherapy toxicity and did not complete 6 cycles of treatment. However, it does suggest an association between chemotherapy delivery as measured by the pharmacodynamics endpoint of neutropenia, and clinical benefit, even in an incurable setting such as lung cancer.

It is in this clinical setting in which the practitioner caring for patients receiving chemotherapy must decide the best therapeutic strategy from Table 2. Another alternative or complementary approach to reduce neutropenic complications would be the use of prophylactic antibiotics. These are discussed in detail by Dr. Friefeld in an accompanying chapter. In brief, however, a meta-analysis of antibiotic prophylaxis that looked at 95 randomized controlled trials did demonstrate benefit in terms of reduction of fever, documented infection, infection-related death, and all cause mortality in studies using fluoroquinolones (14). However, the majority of these studies were focused on patients with hematologic malignancies and/or undergoing peripheral blood stem cell transplants limiting the applicability of these results to patients with solid tumors and/or lymphoma undergoing standard-dose chemotherapy. In addition, adverse event rates were increased and, in particular, concern was raised in terms of development of resistant bacteria. Because of the latter concern, the Infectious Disease Society of America, as well as other guideline groups does not recommend the routine use of prophylactic antibiotics as a prevention strategy for chemotherapy-induced neutropenia. More recently, the SIGNIFICANT trial was published by Dr. Cullen, looking at solid tumor and lymphoma patients receiving standard-dose multicycle chemotherapy (15). Patients were randomized to levofloxacin or placebo. In this study, substantial reduction was seen in febrile episodes, probable infection, and hospitalization, but no significant difference was seen in this one study in terms of severe infection or death.

Thus, both the meta-analysis (14) and this large trial (15) suggest the potential for prophylactic antibiotics to reduce infection complications, but because of consequences, the results have not yet led to change in guideline recommendations. Moreover, while prophylactic antibiotics may reduce infectious complications, they do not primarily impact the depth or duration of neutropenia, which is a primary determinant of risk. In addition to resulting in infectious complications of neutropenia per se, delayed neutrophil recovery, even in the absence of infection, also may impact subsequent cycles of chemotherapy, both in the ability to continue chemotherapy as well as exposing the patient to even greater risk of complications. Thus, the use of antibiotics alone may not change the dynamics between trying to maintain relative chemotherapy treatment dose intensity to optimize treatment benefit while trying to minimize risk and toxicity of myelosuppression.

CLINICAL TRIALS OF MYELOID GROWTH FACTORS TO PREVENT CHEMOTHERAPY-INDUCED NEUTROPENIA

As noted in Table 1, G-CSF in the form of both filgrastim and pegfilgrastim are approved by the FDA for use in preventive strategies to reduce myelosuppression in the cancer chemotherapy patient. Although GM-CSF does not have the same FDA indication, it is included in guideline recommendations, but with a lower level of evidence to support its use for this indication (3,4). In the initial registration trials for filgrastim, three studies were performed including two in patients receiving chemotherapy with small cell lung cancer and one trial in patients with non-Hodgkin's lymphoma. In all three studies, the reduction in days of grade 4 neutropenia was substantial with an overall reduction by 50% in the first cycle of treatment and continued reduction across all cycles. This resulted in reduction of incidence of febrile neutropenia by approximately 50% in all three studies. The use of intravenous antibiotics and the incidence of hospitalization were also reduced in the G-CSF patients in the two small cell studies (16–18). However, in common for all three studies were chemotherapy schedules associated with a very high risk of febrile neutropenia in the control group. This ranged from 44% in the lymphoma study (18) to 77% in the U.S. small cell trial (16). Based on these studies, filgrastim was approved for clinical use, but the guideline recommendations by ASCO suggested that its use should be limited to high-risk settings where the risk of febrile neutropenia was in excess of 40%, consistent with the available clinical trial data. This coincided with a threshold for cost minimization where modeling suggested that the reduction in hospitalization would offset the cost of G-CSF (19). From subsequent studies by Dr. Lyman, discussed in his chapter elsewhere in this book, the hospitalization costs have substantially increased over the last decade, lowering this cost threshold substantially (20).

These early clinical trials of G-CSF demonstrated several important pharmacodynamic outcomes that are important from a clinical perspective to the present. First, in the setting of substantial neutropenia of several days in these studies, the use of G-CSF did not eliminate neutropenia, but reduced its duration. After the institution of G-CSF 24 hours after chemotherapy, there is an initial rise in the neutrophil count due to the effects on the marginal neutrophil population, as well as a more rapid differentiation of more mature neutrophils and egress from the bone marrow. This is followed by the development of neutropenia, and then subsequent recovery of the neutrophil count. This recovery occurs days before neutrophil recovery would happen in the control group. The latter wave of neutrophil recovery is thought to be related to proliferation of early myeloid progenitors and more rapid differentiation of neutrophils within the bone marrow compartment, under the influence of G-CSF. The net effect is an overall reduction in days of neutropenia, but not generally elimination of neutropenia.

It is important to understand these kinetics when measuring blood counts in patients post-chemotherapy while receiving a colony-stimulating factor. First, an elevated neutrophil count within a few days of chemotherapy is not likely to represent recovery, but rather a shift in the neutrophil pool. It is very important to continue daily G-CSF until the post-nadir neutrophil recovery occurs. Secondly, at the time of neutropenia, there is no evidence that additional myeloid growth factor will be beneficial overall and above that already being administered. This question is commonly asked and will be further elucidated in the discussion of pegfilgrastim. Thirdly, the post-neutrophil recovery often leads to an "overshoot" in neutrophil count for a matter of several days, even after the growth factor is discontinued. Thus, it is difficult to fully interpret the neutrophil count in this setting with regard to concern around infection or other clinical causes of leukocytosis.

From the original U.S. registration trial of G-CSF (16) modeling was done on the potential benefit of filgrastim in reducing the risk of febrile neutropenia (21). In this analysis, the probability of developing febrile neutropenia was analyzed with relation to the days of neutropenia for both the placebo and filgrastim groups. While the relationship is not totally linear, in general the risk of developing febrile neutropenia was approximately 10% for each one day of grade 4 neutropenia. Thus, the placebo group in the very first cycle of treatment had nearly six days of neutropenia, and also had nearly 60% rate of febrile neutropenia. Use of filgrastim proportionally reduced the days of neutropenia and incidence of febrile neutropenia by 50%. Interestingly, this risk of febrile neutropenia, although demonstrated in a solid tumor population treated with combination chemotherapy in the 1990s, closely parallels the same observations made by Dr. Bodey in his original description of the relationship of neutropenia to fever and infection in patients with acute leukemia in the late 1960s (1).

Another commonly asked question concerns the benefits of myeloid growth factors compared to or in combination with prophylactic antibiotics. Unfortunately, in the meta-analysis of antibiotics (14) only a handful of trials explore this question, so no definitive statement can be made about the comparative or additive benefits. However, one randomized trial in this setting was particularly instructive. Based on previous data suggesting benefit of prophylactic antibiotics in patients receiving chemotherapy in small cell lung cancer, a randomized trial was performed of prophylactic antibiotics with or without filgrastim in patients with small cell lung cancer receiving cyclophosphamide, doxorubicin, and etoposide chemotherapy (22). In this study, the incidence of grade 4 neutropenia was reduced in the filgrastim group, along with a reduction in febrile neutropenia in the first cycle, across all cycles of chemotherapy. There was also a trend toward a reduction in febrile neutropenia related to mortality, but this did not reach significance in this study of less than 200 patients. Furthermore, when the investigators evaluated the relationship of febrile neutropenia to age, the risk increased in both groups of patients, particularly above the age of 60, but the additional benefit of G-CSF was seen across all age groups. Thus, this one study would suggest that prophylactic antibiotics alone are inferior to prophylactic antibiotics and G-CSF. Whether or not prophylactic antibiotics add to myeloid growth factor in reducing febrile neutropenia remains to be clarified.

CLINICAL TRIALS OF PEGFILGRASTIM

The biology of pegfilgrastim was briefly discussed at the beginning of this chapter. In the presence of normal renal function, filgrastim is cleared with a half life of the order of three to four hours. In the setting of nephrectomized rats, the clearance of filgrastim is quite similar to pegfilgrastim with the major remaining mechanism of clearance related to neutrophil-mediated receptor ligand internalization and clearance. Early human trials demonstrated that a single injection of pegfilgrastim had a sustained half life of the order of days related to the lack of renal clearance. Furthermore, a number of studies that looked at the biological properties of pegfilgrastim compared to filgrastim showed no difference in proliferation assays, receptor binding, neutrophil response, or neutrophil function studies (22).

The first human trial of pegfilgrastim was performed in patients with non–small cell lung cancer (23). This instructive phase I/II trial looked at a single dose of pegfilgrastim in three different dose cohorts compared to daily filgrastim at the standard 5 µg/kg subsequent daily dosing. An initial stage treated patients two weeks prior to chemotherapy with a single dose of pegfilgrastim or filgrastim given for five daily doses. In the post-chemotherapy setting, the same dose of pegfilgrastim was given 24 hours after chemotherapy and compared to daily dosing of filgrastim at 5 µg/kg daily until neutrophil recovery. In the pre-chemotherapy setting, all patients demonstrated G-CSF-related increases in their neutrophil counts. The increase in the neutrophil counts with pegfilgrastim was dose dependent with a single dose of 100 µg/kg achieving neutrophil effect similar to daily dosing with filgrastim. In the post-chemotherapy setting, the dose of 100 µg/kg of pegfilgrastim again achieved comparable neutrophil recovery, compared to daily dosing with filgrastim over 10 days.

Furthermore, in pharmacokinetic analyses, the single dose of pegfilgrastim post-chemotherapy resulted in elevated and sustained level of G-CSF that was superior to the daily dosing with G-CSF, presumably related to the differences in renal clearance between the two molecules and the levels achieved by a single dose of pegfilgrastim. The elevated serum concentration of pegfilgrastim remained constant after administration post-chemotherapy through the nadir, but as the neutrophil count recovered, the serum levels of pegfilgrastim fell presumably related to neutrophil-mediated clearance and returned to undetectable levels within a few days.

This pharmacokinetic/pharmacodynamic modeling demonstrates the "self-regulating" properties of pegfilgrastim. The administration of a dose of pegfilgrastim leads to saturation of all G-CSF receptors in the body and achievement of a steady-state concentration. That steady state concentration is maintained and drives the production of early myeloid progenitor cells as they recover from myelotoxic chemotherapy, leading to production of new neutrophils, and as new neutrophils are generated, their G-CSF receptors clear the molecule from the circulation. Further pharmacodynamic support for this is that a single injection of pegfilgrastim restores neutrophil counts to normal, with less "overshoot" of the neutrophil count as compared to daily dosing of G-CSF.

A number of other trials were performed with pegfilgrastim in the phase I/II setting in breast cancer and lymphoma, leading to phase III trials that were done in breast cancer. Two pivotal studies were performed in women with breast cancer receiving doxorubicin and docetaxel chemotherapy. Patients were randomized to receive either daily filgrastim or pegfilgrastim on a single day, followed by daily placebo. The pegfilgrastim was administered either on a weight basis (24) or a fixed dose of 6 mg (25). Both studies demonstrated comparable neutrophil recovery, compared to daily filgrastim. There were no gender or age-related differences noted. The incidence of adverse events, particularly bone pain, the most common side effect of G-CSF, was similar in both studies and in both arms of both studies, with a range of 29% to 34% in one trial and 37% to 42% in the second study. Furthermore, the study that looked at fix dose pegfilgrastim at 6 mg as a single dose showed comparable duration of severe neutropenia over a range of body weights from 46 to 125 kg.

As in other trials of myeloid growth factors, the duration of severe neutropenia was longest in the first cycle and shorter in cycles 2 through 4, consistent with a "priming" effect on the bone marrow by the myeloid growth factors. While the primary endpoint of these trials was to look at the noninferiority of pegfilgrastim compared to filgrastim in terms of duration of neutropenia, an interesting observation was made in the rates of febrile neutropenia. In the regimen of docetaxel and doxorubicin used, the historical rate of febrile neutropenia had been approximately 38%. In the filgrastim arms of the two studies, the febrile neutropenia rate was 18% to 20%. Of interest was that despite a comparable degree of neutropenia, there was a lower rate of febrile neutropenia in the pegfilgrastim arms at 9% and 13%. This general observation has been seen across a range of studies and in a recent meta-analysis of randomized controlled trials, it was concluded that a single dose of pegfilgrastim performed better in reducing febrile neutropenia rates, compared to a median of 10 to 14 days of filgrastim (26). Based on the comparability of these studies, a fixed dose of 6 mg of pegfilgrastim became the approved dose of administration.

When pegfilgrastim was initially approved, the drug was recommended for use 24 hours after chemotherapy, similar to other myeloid growth factors.

Furthermore, the drug was not recommended to be administered for a period of at least 14 days before the next chemotherapy. This was based on the phase I data showing safety with the prechemotherapy dosing at that interval. Subsequent analyses of plasma levels of pegfilgrastim from the pivotal trials have clearly demonstrated that the drug was cleared in virtually 100% of patients by day 12. In subsequent trials with q2week dosing chemotherapy, including ABVD and R-CHOP, have demonstrated both efficacy and safety with q2week chemotherapy regimens (27).

A subsequent trial of pegfilgrastim had a major impact on the eventual recommendations for clinical use of myeloid growth factors. In this study, women with breast cancer received docetaxel at 100 mg/m^2 every three weeks. This regimen had been associated with an approximate risk of febrile neutropenia of 20%, which was below the recommended level for prophylactic use of myeloid growth factors at that time. Patients were randomized to receive pegfilgrastim or placebo in the largest clinical trial of myeloid growth factors to date with over 900 women enrolled. The control group had a rate of febrile neutropenia at 17%, consistent with historical experience. However, the surprising result was that the pegfilgrastim patients had a rate of febrile neutropenia of only 1%. This corresponded also with differences in febrile neutropenia–related hospitalizations from 14% in the control group to 1% in the pegfilgrastim group and the use of intravenous antibiotics from 10% in the placebo group to 2% in the pegfilgrastim group, all highly statistical differences (28). This was a surprising reduction in the duration of febrile neutropenia in view of the generally accepted 50% reduction in febrile neutropenia with myeloid growth factors seen in settings with prolonged neutropenia. One explanation may be that the duration of neutropenia with docetaxel is relatively brief. In an analysis of the rates of neutropenia in control and pegfilgrastim groups, the incidence of neutropenia fell from nearly 80% in the placebo group compared to less than 10% in the pegfilgrastim group in the first cycle of treatment. Thus, the conventional wisdom that myeloid growth factors would be less effective with shorter duration of neutropenia was disproven.

META-ANALYSIS OF PRIMARY PROPHYLAXIS WITH G-CSF

The impact of primary prophylaxis with G-CSF on febrile neutropenia and mortality in adult cancer patients receiving chemotherapy was recently reported (29). Seventeen randomized control trials were identified, including nearly 3500 patients. Studies included trials of filgrastim, lenograstim, and pegfilgrastim. As expected from the previous reported studies, the relative risk of febrile neutropenia across all studies was 0.538 with 95% confidence intervals of 0.43–0.67, and it was highly statistically significant for all three myeloid growth factors individually, and collectively.

Figure 1 outlines an additional analysis that evaluated the relationship of the risk of febrile neutropenia in the studies. As noted, all of the trials showed benefit with a risk reduction in the G-CSF compared to the control group.

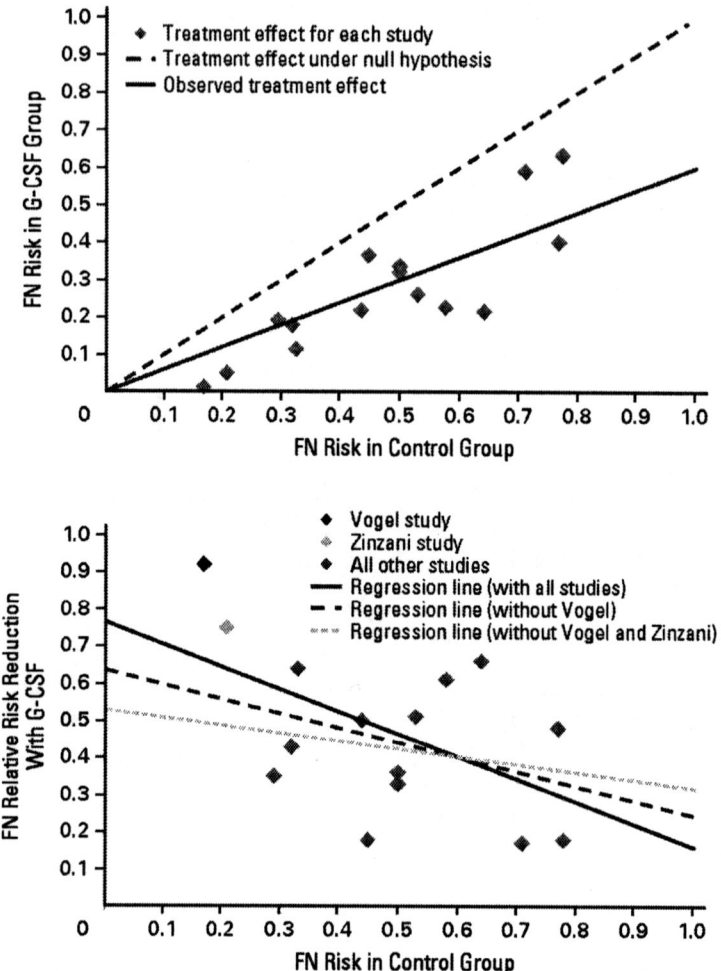

Figure 1 Risk of Febrile Neutropenia (FN) among controls and G-CSF treated patients across studies. The upper panel demonstrates the risk reduction in FN in G-CSF treated groups. The lower panel outlines the linear regression lines, demonstrated greater risk reduction of FN in groups with lower risk of FN. *Source*: From Ref. 29.

However, it is of interest to note that while the overall benefit in reduction may be approximately 50% in settings with very high rates of febrile neutropenia, there is a suggestion that the benefit may be somewhat less. This may be due to the more modest impact of G-CSF in patients without adequate myeloid precursors to achieve neutrophil recovery except after prolonged periods of time compared with patients at relatively low risk of febrile neutropenia, where the duration of neutropenia may be only 1 or 2 days. In this case, the studies suggest almost a marked reduction in risk in the G-CSF group as noted by the Vogel study (28). The Ziddani study, which had a risk of approximately 20% in the control group, used daily G-CSF rather than pegfilgrastim and showed a similar benefit in risk reduction in non-Hodgkin's lymphoma patients (30). This suggests that the benefit is not unique to pegfilgrastim versus filgrastim, or disease setting, but may be more related to the ability of nearly eliminating moderate neutropenia with myeloid growth factors.

Most importantly, this analysis had the opportunity to look at infection-related mortality and early mortality across these studies. Both endpoints showed statistically significant risk reduction. In terms of infection-related mortality, the relative risk reduction for the G-CSF patients compared to control was 0.552 (0.338–0.902) $p = 0.018$. The relative risk for early mortality in the G-CSF group was 0.599 (0.433–0.832) $p = 0.002$. Thus, these data suggest that the selection of patients for primary prophylaxis with myeloid growth factors impacts not only the risk of febrile neutropenia and consequent morbidity and hospitalization, but also potential mortality.

RECOMMENDATIONS BY PRACTICE GUIDELINE COMMITTEES

Based on the data reviewed above, the NCCN, ASCO, and EORTC (3–5) all have concurred that chemotherapy patients at risk of 20% or greater for febrile neutropenia should be considered for first cycle prophylaxis. To quote the ASCO committee who had previously set a threshold of 40%, "the 2005 update committee agreed unanimously that reduction in febrile neutropenia was an important clinical outcome with justified use of CSFs, regardless of impact and other factors, when the risk of febrile neutropenia (FN) was approximately 20% and no other equally effective that did not require CSFs was available" (3).

The NCCN guidelines panel was the first group to recommend that 20% risk of febrile neutropenia be considered high risk, and warrant first cycle CSF prophylaxis, further qualified their decision analysis by evaluating patients in terms of curative, life prolonging, or palliative approaches (4). Above the risk of 20% first cycle prophylaxis was indicated for all three groups. However, in the intermediate group of 10% to 20%, consideration might be made for myeloid growth factor support, particularly in the curative and adjuvant settings. The EORTC guidelines (6) further tried to define the intermediate risk population based not only on chemotherapy regimen, but on individual patient factors that may influence the risk of febrile neutropenia. The goal is to identify both the high- and low-risk populations so that strategies of chemotherapy dose administration with or without adjunctive myeloid growth factor support can be made to maximize clinical efficacy and resource utilization.

COMPARATIVE CLINICAL ACTIVITY OF G-CSF AND GM-CSF

The evidence presented thus far regarding reduction of chemotherapy-induced neutropenia and its complications was based on randomized clinical trials of G-CSF. The number of trials with GM-CSF is far less and head-to-head trials have been reviewed in a systematic review (31). The conclusions of this study were that the incidence of fever in the GM-CSF arms was higher and the data was lacking on the comparative abilities of these agents to reduce chemotherapy-induced complications. In other settings of mobilization of peripheral blood progenitor cells, G-CSF has either been found to mobilize more peripheral blood progenitor cells than GM-CSF or the two agents have been comparable (3). Based on the limits of the information, the ASCO guidelines have continued to conclude that no guideline recommendation can be made regarding the equivalence of these agents and that further studies continue to be warranted. In the setting of primary prophylaxis for chemotherapy-induced neutropenia, the NCCN guidelines have concluded that G-CSF is the preferred agent due to the large body of level-one evidence (4).

OTHER CLINICAL ISSUES REGARDING MYELOID GROWTH FACTORS

For patients who did not receive primary prophylaxis with a myeloid growth factor, but developed neutropenia or neutropenic complications, the pros and cons of therapeutic use of myeloid growth factors have already been discussed. However, on the subsequent cycle of chemotherapy, patients would be potential candidates for secondary prophylaxis. Both NCCN and ASCO guidelines have proposed appropriate consideration for secondary prophylaxis, with the main criteria being that consideration should be made for myeloid growth factor use if the alternative strategy of reducing dose would compromise disease-free, overall survival or treatment outcome. While secondary prophylaxis was a major strategy when the threshold for primary prophylaxis was set at 40% risk of febrile neutropenia, the change to 20% has substantially altered this process. It is hoped that patient-specific risk factor identification in the future will allow even better targeting of patients who are candidates for first cycle use.

ASCO guidelines also help clarify the distinction between using myeloid growth factors to increase chemotherapy dose intensity versus maintenance of standard dose intensity, versus the use of dose-dense approaches (3). The use of myeloid growth factors to increase chemotherapy dose intensity outside clinical trials is not indicated. The role of CSF to maintain standard dose intensity of therapy warrants further study, but it is an accepted practice where standard full-dose chemotherapy is felt to improve outcomes. Usually included in this category would be chemotherapy in the adjuvant or curative settings. Individual consideration can also be made with chemotherapy in the life prolonging or even palliative setting depending on clinical benefit. In this setting, NCCN recommends consideration of less myelotoxic chemotherapy regimens if they can provide equivalent benefit.

The use of myeloid growth factors can also be considered in dose-dense regimens. By definition these are regimens most commonly given at three-week intervals, but with the use of myeloid growth factors, the same chemotherapy doses can be delivered every two weeks with acceptable toxicity. Trials in adjuvant treatment of breast cancer (32) and advanced-stage lymphoma patients (33) have demonstrated survival benefit with these strategies. ASCO guidelines have suggested that these clinical uses are established in these particular settings, but that further clinical trials are needed in other settings before such dose-dense approaches can be generalized.

Detailed review of the use of myeloid growth factors in other settings are beyond the scope of this chapter and are well reviewed in the ASCO guidelines (3), but will be summarized briefly here. The use of myeloid growth factors in the setting of acute leukemia and myelodysplastic syndromes warrants longer discussion; but in short, the trials done thus far do not demonstrate increased risk of stimulation of leukemic clones. In induction chemotherapy, modest decreases in duration of neutropenia can be achieved with use of CSFs. This benefit appears greater in older patients where the ability to withstand prolonged neutropenia is compromised and, therefore, clinical benefit of CSFs is easier to demonstrate. In consolidation therapy, where the bone marrow progenitor cells have been restored after induction chemotherapy, the impact of reduction in duration of neutropenia with myeloid growth factors is better established. The use of myeloid growth factors in patients with myelodysplastic syndromes can be considered on an individual patient basis in management of neutropenia.

Another commonly asked question is the use of colony-stimulating factors concurrently with chemotherapy or radiation. Studies of pegfilgrastim given on the same day as chemotherapy have shown either no benefit or a reduction in the benefit of the myeloid growth factor compared to 24 hours after chemotherapy, which remains the standard. In the setting of concurrent chemotherapy and radiotherapy the recommendation has been not to administer myeloid growth factors due to early clinical trials that demonstrated an adverse impact on myeloid recovery. This continues to be the recommendation, although preliminary data have suggested that with current radiation techniques, this approach may be safer and warrants further study. A phase II RTOG trial in patients with limited-stage small cell lung cancer is ongoing to address this issue.

SUMMARY

Much has been learned in the last two decades regarding the impact of myeloid growth factors on hematopoiesis and clinical outcomes in the oncology population. Studies over the next several years will continue to focus on refining their use by better identifying patients' specific risk factors, and conducting prospective clinical trials in targeted populations. Through such studies, hopefully both high- and low-risk populations can be identified so that these agents can be used most effectively to prevent febrile neutropenia and infection, as well as maintain standard-dose chemotherapy and/or support dose-dense treatments. The forthcoming clinical trials in these areas will undoubtedly lead to continued updates of the guidelines of ASCO and NCCN, and the reader is encouraged to follow these updates so that we can maximize the benefits of these agents in our own clinical practices.

REFERENCES

1. Bodey G, Buckley M, Sathe Y, et al. Quantitative relationships between circulating leukocytes and infection in patients with acute leukemia. Ann Intern Med 1966; 64:328–340.
2. Lieschke GJ, Burgess AW. Granulocyte colony-stimulating factor. N Engl J Med 1992; 327:28–35, 99–106.
3. Smith TJ, Khatcheressian J, Lyman GH, et al. Update of recommendations for the use of white blood cell growth factors: an evidence-based clinical practice guideline. JCO 2006; 24(19):3187–3205.
4. Myeloid Growth Factors V.1.2007, NCCN Clinical Practice Guidelines in Oncology™
5. Bokemeyer C, Aapro, Courdi A, et al. EORTC guidelines for the use of erythropoietic proteins in anaemic patients with cancer: 2006 update. Eur J Cancer 2007; 43(2):258–270.
6. Metcalf D, Nicola NA. The hematopoietic colony-stimulating factor. From Biology to Clinical Applications. Cambridge: Cambridge University Press, 1995:44–55, 75, 177–184.
7. Crawford J. Pegfilgrastim: the promise of pegylation fulfilled. Ann Oncol 2003; 14:6–7.
8. Armitage J. Emerging applications of recombinant human granulocyte-macrophage colony-stimulating factor. Blood 1988; 92(12):4491–4508.
9. Korzenik J, Dieckgraefe B, Valentine J, et al., for the Sargramostim in Crohn's Disease Study Group. Sargramostim for active Crohn's disease. N Engl J Med 352:21.
10. Clark OAC, Lyman GH, Castro AA, et al. Colony-stimulating factors for chemotherapy-induced febrile neutropenia: a meta-analysis of randomized controlled trials. JCO 2005; 23(18):4198–4214.
11. Klastersky J, Paesmans M, Georgala A, et al. Outpatient oral antibiotcs for febrile neutropenic cancer patients using a score predictive for complications. JCO 2006; 24(25):4129–4134.
12. Klimm B, Reineke T, Haverkamp H, et al. Role of hematotoxicity and sex in patients with Hodgkin's lymphoma: an analysis from the German Hodgkin Study Group. JCO 2005; Nov 1:8003–8011.
13. Di Maio M, Gridelli C, Gallo C, et al. Chemotherapy-induced neutropenia and treatment efficacy in advanced non-small-cell lung cancer: a pooled analysis of three randomised trials. Lancet Oncology 2005; 6(9):669–677.
14. Gafter-Gvili A, Fraser A, Paul, M, et al. Meta-Analysis: Antibiotic prophylaxis reduces mortality in neutropenic patients. Ann Intern Med 2005; 142(12):979–995.
15. Cullen M, Steven N, Billingham L, et al. Simple investigation in neutropenic individuals of the frequency of infection after chemotherapy +/− antibiotic in a number of tumours (SIGNIFICANT) trial group. Antibacterial prophylaxis after chemotherapy for solid tumors and lymphomas. N Engl J Med 2005; 353(10):988–998.

16. Crawford J, Ozer H, Stoller R, et al. Reduction in the incidence of chemotherapy-induced febrile neutropenia in patients with small cell lung cancer by granulocyte colony-stimulating factor (R-metG-CSF). N Engl J Med 1991; 325:164–171.
17. Trillet-Lenoir V, Green J, Manegold C, et al. Recombinant granulocyte colony stimulating factor reduces the infectious complications of cytotoxic chemotherapy. Eur J Cancer 1993; 16A:319–324.
18. Pettengell R, Gurney H, Radford JA, et al. Granulocyte colony-stimulating factor to prevent dose-limiting neutropenia in non-Hodgkin's lymphoma: a randomized controlled trial. Blood 1992; 80(6):1430–1436.
19. Lyman GH, Kuder NM, Green J, et al. The economics of febrile neutropenia: implications for the use of colony-stimulating factors. Eur J Cancer 1998; 34: 1857–1864.
20. Eldar-Lissai A, Cosler L, Culakova E, et al. Economic analysis of prophylactic pegfilgrastim in adult cancer patients receiving chemotherapy. Value in Health, OnlineEarly Articles, Published article online: Jul 21, 2007. doi:10.1111/j.1524-4733.2007.00242.x.
21. Blackwell S, Crawford J. G-CSF in the chemotherapy setting. In: Morstyn, G, ed. Granulocyte Colony Stimulating Factor in the Clinical. New York: Marcel Dekker, 1994:103–116.
22. Timmer-Bonte J, de Boo T, Smit H, et al. Prevention of chemotherapy-induced febrile neutropenia by prophylactic antibiotics plus or minus granulocyte colony-stimulating factor in small-cell lung cancer: a Dutch randomized Phase III study. JCO 2005; Nov 1:7974–7984.
23. Johnston E, Crawford J, Blackwell S, et al. Randomized, dose-escalation study of SD/01 compared with daily filgrastim in patients receiving chemotherapy, JCO 2000; Jul 1:2522–2528.
24. Holmes FA, O'Shaughnessy JA, Vukelja S, et al. Blinded, randomized, multicenter study to evaluate single administration pegfilgrastim once per cycle versus daily filgrastim as an adjunct to chemotherapy in patients with high-risk Stage II or Stage III/IV breast cancer. JCO 2002; 727–731.
25. Green MD, Koelbl H, Baselga J, et al. A randomized double-blind multicenter phase III study of fixed-dose single-administration pegfilgrastim versus daily filgrastim in patients receiving myelosuppressive chemotherapy. Ann Oncol 2003; 14:29–35.
26. Pinto L, Liu Z, Doan Q, et al. Comparison of pegfilgrastim with filgrastim on febrile neutropenia, grade IV neutropenia and bone pain: a meta-analysis of randomized controlled trials. Curr Med Res Opin 2007; 23(9):2283–2295.
27. Mey U, Maier A, Schmidt-Wolf I, et al. Pegfilgrastim as hematopoietic support for dose-dense chemoimmunotherapy with R-CHOP-14 as first-line therapy in elderly patients with diffuse large B cell lymphoma. Support Care Cancer 2007; 15(7):877–884.
28. Vogel C, Wojtukiewicz M, Carroll R, et al. First and subsequent cycle use of pegfilgrastim prevents febrile neutropenia in patients with breast cancer: a multicenter, double-blind, placebo-controlled phase III study. JCO 2005; Feb 20:1178–1184.
29. Kuderer N, Dale D, Crawford J, et al. Impact of primary prophylaxis with granulocyte colony-stimulating factor on febrile neutropenia and mortality in adult cancer patients receiving chemotherapy: a systematic review. JCO 2007; 25(21):3158–3167.
30. Zinzani PL, Pavone E, Storti S, et al. Randomized trial with or without granulocyte colony-stimulating factor as adjunct to induction VNCOP-B treatment of elderly high-grade non-Hodgkin's lymphoma. Blood 1997; 89:3974–3979.

31. Dubois RW, Pinto LA, Bernal M, et al. Benefits of GM-CSF versus placebo or G-CSF in reducing chemotherapy-induced complications: A systematic review of the literature. Support Cancer Ther 2004; 2:34–41.
32. Citron ML, Berry DA, Cirrincione C, et al. Randomized trial of dose-dense versus conventionally scheduled and sequential versus concurrent combination chemotherapy as postoperative adjuvant treatment of node-positive primary breast cancer: first report of Intergroup Trial C9741/Cancer and Leukemia Group B Trial 9741. J Clin Oncol 2003; 21:1431–1439.
33. Pfreundschuh M, Truemper L, Schmits R, et al. 2-weekly or 3-weekly CHOP chemotherapy with or without etoposide for the treatment of young patients with good prognosis (normal LDH) aggressive lymphomas: Results of the NHL-B1 trial of the DSHNHL. Blood 2004; 104:626–633.
34. Barbour S, Crawford J. Hematopoietic growth factors. In: Cancer management: a multidisciplinary approach. 10th Edition. Pazdur R, Coia L, Hoskins W, Wagman L (Eds). 2007; 901–915.

8

Thrombocytopenia and Thrombopoetic Growth Factors

Jennifer Wright
Baylor College of Medicine, Houston, Texas, U.S.A.

Saroj Vadhan-Raj
The University of Texas M.D. Anderson Cancer Center, Houston, Texas, U.S.A.

THROMBOPOIESIS

It is first important to review normal platelet development and regulation in a healthy system. The hematopoietic stem cell gives rise to the early common myeloid progenitor, which then leads to the development of a common megakaryocyte (MK) erythroid progenitor (MEP). The transcription factor GATA-1 plays an important role in the differentiation of the MEP. The MEP can then either lead to the early and late erythroid progenitors (burst-forming unit erythroid (BFU-E)) and CFU-E or to the MK progenitors (BFU-MK or CFU-MK). As MKs mature, they increase their cytoplasmic mass and undergo endoreduplication and the cytoplasm eventually forms proplatelets. Platelets then either bud off the tip of the proplatelets or are released from a pool when the cytoplasm fragments; around 2000 to 5000 platelets from each cell. This process is controlled by various cytokines working in concert together. In a normal state 10^{11} platelets are produced daily, with platelets lasting about eight to nine days in the circulation (1).

The process of megakaryocytopoiesis and platelet production is controlled by a number of cytokines. Stem cell factor (SCF) (c-Kit ligand) and Interleukin-3 (multi-CSF) act at early stages and stimulate proliferation and differentiation of progenitor cells into MK lineage. The multifunctional cytokines such as IL-1, IL-6, and IL-11 have very little, if any, CSF effect alone but act as costimulating factors in concert with early-acting growth factors and have effect at later stages in the development. In contrast, thrombopoietin has a broader activity, stimulating growth and maturation of MK progenitor cells into mature MKs.

Thrombopoietin was initially identified in 1994 (2–4) and has been shown to be the primary regulator of thrombopoiesis. More specifically, its functions include increasing the size and ploidy of MKs and stimulating formation of proplatelet processes. It also stimulates platelet adhesion and promotes aggregation. It is produced primarily in the liver and binds to c-Mpl receptors on platelets and MKs. Thrombopoietin levels are regulated primarily by the amount of c-Mpl receptors available for binding. The TPO-receptor complex is removed from the system, removing the TPO from circulation. It is the unbound TPO that regulates megakaryocytopoiesis. Thrombopoietin levels are high in cases of thrombocytopenia due to decreased production. However, in cases of increased destruction (such as ITP), the thrombopoietin level is not sufficiently elevated, probably due to the high turnover of TPO with the platelets and their c-Mpl receptors (1). Interleukin-6 is probably responsible for the thrombocytosis seen in cases of acute inflammation (1).

THROMBOCYTOPENIA

Thrombocytopenia results when there is an imbalance between the normal production and destruction cycle. Accordingly, the etiology of thrombocytopenia can be classified into defects in production or destruction of platelets. Decreased production of platelets result when the liver fails to produce sufficient thrombopoietin or the bone marrow fails to produce an adequate supply of platelets (Table 1). Situations not uncommonly seen in cancer patients include marrow infiltration from cancer cells or infection, myelosuppression due to chemotherapy, and concomitant liver disease. Increased destruction, due to ITP or DIC, and splenic sequestration are also important causes of thrombocytopenia. The most common etiology in cancer patients is thrombocytopenia induced by myelosuppressive treatment, observed frequently in patients receiving dose-intensive treatment with stem cell support, in patients with hematologic malignancies, in chemosensitive pediatric malignancies, and in patients with solid tumors where it is more of a cumulative problem after multiple cycles. The introduction of several novel therapeutic agents with increased propensity to cause thrombocytopenia and their use in combination may have further increased the incidence.

Thrombocytopenia is an important problem to consider in the oncology patient for a number of reasons. Thrombocytopenia increases the risk for bleeding complications, the need for platelet transfusions, and may result in dose reduction and treatment delays which may compromise the treatment outcome (5,6). In

Table 1 Etiology of Thrombocytopenia

Decreased production
- Marrow infiltration: tumor cells, infections
- Decreased substrates: vitamin B12, folate, or iron deficiency
- Myelosuppression: viruses, drugs, alcohol
- Congenital: May-Hegglin anomaly, Bernard-Soulier syndrome
- Other: Myelodysplastic syndrome, aplastic anemia

Increased destruction
- Autoimmune destruction: ITP, SLE
- Alloimmune destruction: posttransfusion
- Consumption: DIC
- Drugs
- Microangiopathic hemolytic anemias
- Physical destruction: cardiac valves, large aortic aneurysms

Splenic sequestration

addition, it adds significant cost to the care of these patients—both in terms of costs incurred due to treatment of or complications from the low platelets and in terms of less measurable costs to the patient resulting from delayed chemotherapy. In one study, the mean cost of care for patients during chemotherapy cycles with thrombocytopenia was 40% higher than in those without thrombocytopenia. A substantial portion of those costs stem from prophylactic platelet transfusions and treatment of major bleeding (7). While platelet transfusions can provide a temporary solution, it does not address the underlying cause of thrombocytopenia. Furthermore, the transfusions have several potential risks including transfusion reactions, transmission of infectious agents, alloimmunization, and platelet refractoriness resulting in shortage of platelets.

Current practice guidelines for the management of patients with thrombocytopenia due to myelosuppressive therapy are centered on prophylactic or therapeutic platelet transfusions (8). Clearly, there is a need for alternate management strategies. To address these concerns, a number of studies in the past decade have examined and demonstrated the safety of lowering the threshold for platelet transfusions from the gold standard of 20,000/mm^3 to less than 10,000/mm^3, in patients who are otherwise clinically stable. In addition, advances are being made in the pharmacologic management of thrombocytopenia. The clinical experience with these thrombopoietic agents will be briefly reviewed below.

MULTIFUNCTIONAL CYTOKINES WITH THROMBOPOIETIC ACTIVITY

Various cytokines exhibiting a role in MK and platelet development have been identified including IL-1, IL-3, IL-6, IL-11, SCF, and fusion molecules such as PIXY321 and promegapoietin. These cytokines mediate multiple biologic effects and have increased platelet counts in preclinical and clinical studies. Based on their thrombopoietic activity, clinical trials have examined their potential in reducing chemotherapy-induced thrombocytopenia and other conditions with thrombocytopenia.

Interleukin-1 (IL-1) alpha reduced the duration of thrombocytopenia and raised the platelet nadir in a dose-dependent fashion in patients with recurrent ovarian cancer receiving single-agent carboplatin. However, a significant number of patients suffered from adverse effects of the drug. All patients had fever and chills, about 70% had myalgia and fatigue, 86% had nausea and vomiting, 67% had anorexia, and 81% had tachycardia (9).

IL-3 is primarily produced by activated T lymphocytes, monocytes/macrophages, and stoma cells (10–12). It stimulates proliferation and differentiation of multipotent hematopoietic stem cells (10,11). Phase I and II clinical studies have demonstrated the ability of IL-3 to increase the leukocyte and platelet counts in patients with solid tumors receiving chemotherapy (11) but had a lesser impact in a trial with patients receiving an autologous stem cell transplant (SCT) (10). Fever is a common adverse event, occurring in 75% to 80% of patients, with many of them also having headaches and myalgias. Other common side effects include erythema, facial flushing, and pruritus (11,12). These symptoms can sometimes be managed with acetaminophen or other supportive care measures (9), but are a common cause for cessation of therapy with IL-3, with dropout rates as high as 50% (10).

PIXY321, a genetically engineered agent consisting of portions of both GM-CSF and IL-3 was shown in initial studies to reduce neutropenia and thrombocytopenia in patients with solid tumors receiving modestly myelosuppressive chemotherapy (23). However, phase III trials in myeloablative setting failed to demonstrate significant clinical activity. In addition, neutralizing antibodies to PIXY321 were found to develop in some patients receiving the drug (24).

IL-6, found primarily in monocytes/macrophages, is also found in T cells, endothelial cells, and fibroblasts. IL-6 is important in MK maturation (10). Mixed results have been seen in clinical trials with this agent. Improvement in platelet recovery was seen in patients treated for ovarian carcinoma and sarcoma, but other studies evaluating its use in sarcoma or autologous SCT (for breast cancer) showed no significant benefits. Adverse effects included fever, headache, myalgias, and stimulation of acute-phase reactants. The frequency of these symptoms limits its clinical usefulness (10).

SCF, a ligand for c-kit, resulted in improvement in the recovery of neutrophils and platelets after chemotherapy in patients with lung and breast cancer. When used with G-CSF, it also decreased the number of apheresis procedures required to collect adequate cells in breast cancer patients preparing for high-dose chemotherapy; no effect was seen on platelet recovery, however. The side effects (urticaria, cough, dyspnea, and throat tightness) could be reduced by premedication with a histamine receptor antagonists and inhaled B2 agonists (10,24).

IL-11 is derived from mesenchymal cells and plays a role in MK maturation and proliferation of multipotent cells in contrast with other cytokines. In phase II randomized clinical trial, IL-11 decreased the need for platelet transfusions in patients who had experienced thrombocytopenia requiring platelet transfusion in the previous cycle (14,24). The side effects included fatigue, headache, and myalgias. In addition, anemia, which was thought to be due to volume expansion, atrial arrhythmias, and syncope were also seen (14,24). IL-11 is approved by the FDA for the prevention of severe thrombocytopenia in patients with nonmyeloid malignancies receiving nonmyeloablative chemotherapy. However, it is not widely utilized due to its toxicity profile.

In summary, several cytokines have been found to be modestly effective in raising platelet counts in the setting of chemotherapy-induced thrombocytopenia. Their use, however, is fraught with adverse effects, limiting their clinical utility.

Recombinat Human Thrombopoietins

Thrombopoietin is a 332 amino acid glycoprotein with amino terminals and carboxy terminals. Only the amino domain is essential for thrombopoietic activity; the carboxy domain provides a long half life. Based on this observation, two versions, full-length molecule (rhTPO) and truncated, pegylated (rhpegMGDF), have been investigated in clinical trials. Both these agents have been shown to have promising biologic activity in various clinical settings.

Pegylated Recombinant Human Megakaryocyte Growth and Development Factor

Pegylated recombinant human MK growth and development factor (PEG-rHuMGDF) consists of the receptor-binding domain of thrombopoietin bound to a polyethylene glycol moiety (25). It was originally administered subcutaneously. Phase I and II clinical trials showed improvement in the time required for platelet recovery and subsequently decreased the number of platelet transfusions in breast cancer patients undergoing high-dose chemotherapy followed by an autologous SCT. However, the phase III trial failed to show a significant difference in these endpoints between the groups receiving placebo and PEG-rHuMGDF (17).

Phase I and II trials have frequently shown a higher nadir and a shorter duration of thrombocytopenia in advanced cancer patients receiving modestly myelosuppresive chemotherapy (15,16). However, studies in some solid tumors (16) and acute myeloid leukemia, have found no difference in the platelet nadir or time to platelet recovery. There was an increased incidence of recovery thrombocytosis (18,19).

Some of the differences in the results may be related to timing of administration of the drug. Thrombopoietin appears to affect early MK progenitors with little effect on the release of platelets (19). This explains the delay in thrombopoietin effect—a minimum of eight days in vitro (18) and a peak effect at 10 to 14 days in clinical studies (19). PEG-rHuMGDF has been used successfully in cases of cyclic immune thrombocytopenia (26) and ITP (27). In the report of four patients with ITP treated with PEG-rHuMGDF, three had an improvement in the platelet count and the fourth had cessation of bleeding symptoms, in spite of the platelet count remaining low.

PEG-rHuMGDF was well tolerated by most patients. The platelets that resulted from its use were normal morphologically and functionally. Although there were several patients who developed thrombotic events while taking the drug, they were not in a sufficient number to outweigh the expected number of events, considering the known hypercoagulable state present in patients with malignancies (15). Unfortunately, one unexpected adverse effect led to its withdrawal from clinical trials in the United States. Thrombocytopenia developed in 13 of 325 healthy volunteers and 4 of 650 oncology patients receiving as few as two doses of PEG-rHuMGDF. Antibodies against TPO were identified as the cause (28). It was felt that the subcutaneous administration may have facilitated the development of the antibodies due to the processing of PEG-rHuMGDF by dendritic cells (24).

Recombinant Human Thrombopoietin

Recombinant human thrombopoietin is identical to endogenous thrombopoietin (29) and has also been found to increase the platelet counts in a dose-dependent fashion when given to patients with cancer. The increased platelet count was noticed at day 5 after administration and peaked at a median of 12 days (20). In patients with gynecologic malignancies, it decreased the degree and duration of thrombocytopenia and decreased the need for transfusions when given after carboplatin (which causes a late nadir) (22). The optimal timing of the administration of the drug was found to be important when it was evaluated in patients with sarcoma receiving adriamycin and ifosfamide, which cause earlier nadir (Fig. 1). The platelet nadir was higher when rhTPO was given five days prior to chemotherapy and a day after chemotherapy compared to various dosing schedules given after chemotherapy administration. There was also a decreased need for platelet transfusions (21). These studies demonstrated the importance of timing and schedule of administration based on the biology of TPO on platelet production and timing of chemotherapy-induced nadir.

In the setting of highly myelosuppressive chemotherapy or myeloablative treatment, where TPO may not have an impact on nadir. RhTPO can be used to facilitate autologous platelet transfusions. Giving rhTPO prior to platelet pheresis permitted collection of large numbers of platelets (median of 53 units per patient in one to three collections) (Fig. 2). These units were then cryopreserved in ThromboSol and 2% dimethylsulfoxide and transfused when needed after chemotherapy over the following six months. In spite of the loss of 26% of the platelets during the freezing, thawing, and washing process, there were no differences in the corrected count increment after they were transfused compared to

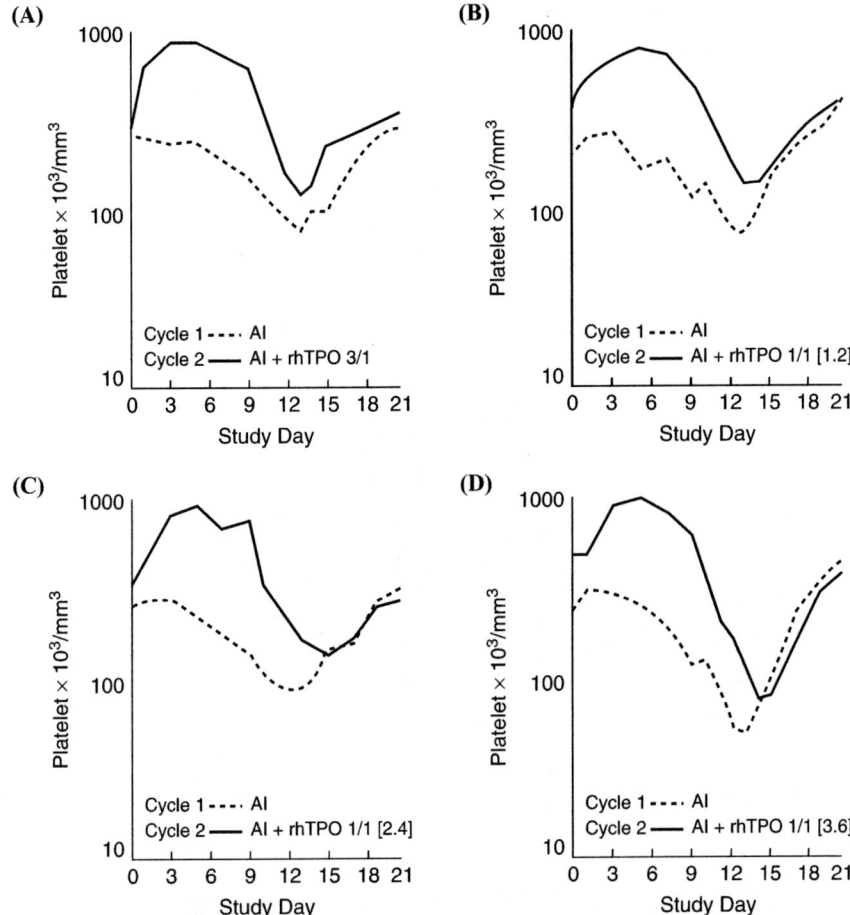

Figure 1 Optimizing predose of recombinant human thrombopoietin (rhTPO). The median platelet counts in cycle 1 (dashed line) and cycle 2 (solid line) in patients who received rhTPO from day 5 as three predoses and one postdose (**A**) or one predose and one postdose (predose rhTPO 1.2 (**B**), 2.4 (**C**), or 3.6 μg/kg (**D**)). *Abbreviation*: AI, doxorubicin and ifosfamide. *Source*: Reprinted from Ref. 21 with permission from the American Society of Clinical Oncology.

transfusion of allogeneic platelets in the same patients. In fact, when the group was analyzed according to whether or not they were responders to platelet transfusions (CCI ≥ 7.5 at one hour), the nonresponders had a significantly higher CCI with the stored autologous platelets compared to the allogeneic platelets (30).

TPO may also play an important role in mobilization of progenitor cells. Initial studies suggested rhTPO was advantageous in the setting of SCT. Although there was no benefit to treating mice with rhTPO after transplant, there was a higher platelet nadir and shorter duration of thrombocytopenia in mice

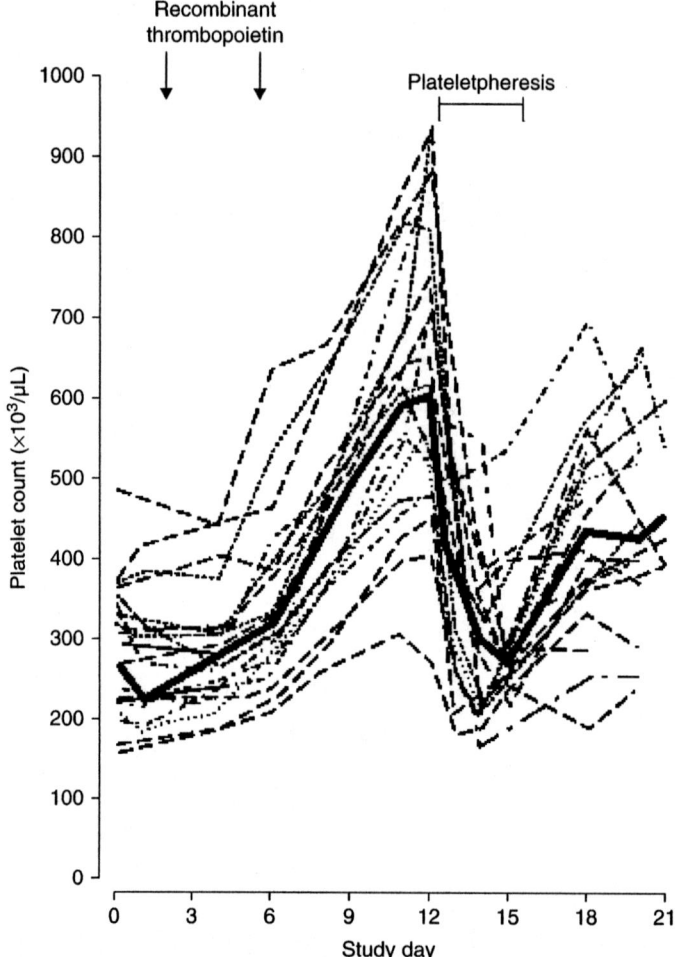

Figure 2 Kinetics of platelet reponse ($n = 21$) after recombinant human thrombopoietin administration (arrows) and plateletpheresis starting from day 12. *Source*: Reprinted from Ref. 30 with permission from Elsevier.

given cells that were obtained from other mice treated with TPO prior to stem cell harvesting (31). Similar findings were seen in studies of humans. In breast cancer patients undergoing high-dose chemotherapy followed by an autologous SCT, those who received rhTPO and G-CSF (as opposed to G-CSF alone) for mobilization had a higher yield of CD34+ cells (61% obtaining the target dose of cells at the first pheresis compared to 10% in the control group). Those patients who received rhTPO also had a quicker granulocyte and platelet recovery and fewer platelet and PRBC transfusions (32).

RhTPO has been well tolerated and no neutralizing antibodies have been identified. One patient developed nonneutralizing antibodies after SQ injection of rhTPO (29). When serial bone marrow biopsies from patients with AML treated with TPO were evaluated, a subset showed hypercellularity, megakaryocytic hyperplasia, and reticulin fibrosis. The megakaryocytic hyperplasia was more pronounced when the biopsy was performed within five days of rhTPO administration. The hyperplasia and fibrosis resolved within three months after rhTPO was stopped (4).

NEWER AGENTS

Due to concerns about the antibodies that developed in patients receiving PEG-rHuMGDF, newer agents have been developed that have the ability to bind to the TPO receptor without having any homology with the endogenous thrombopoietin (33–36). These new agents can be classified TPO peptide mimetics, TPO nonpeptide mimetics, or TPO agonist antibodies.

AMG 531 is a TPO peptide mimetic that has been primarily studied in patients with ITP (Fig. 3). The rationale for the use of TPO agonists in ITP, a condition related to platelet destruction by immune antibody, is based on findings that serum TPO levels are normal or inappropriately low in two-thirds of

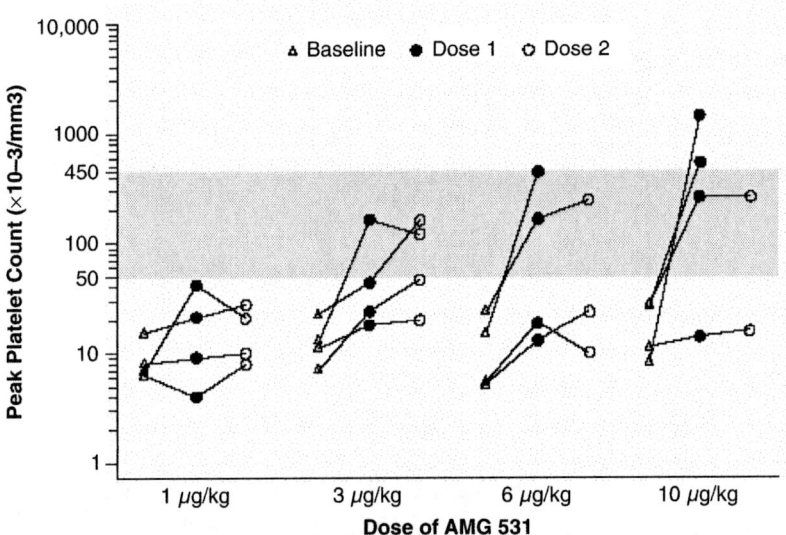

Figure 3 The baseline platelet count and peak platelet count after dose 1 and dose 2 of AMG 531 are shown. There were four patients in each dose cohort. Three patients did not receive a second dose. The shaded area shows the targeted platelet range. Platelet counts associated with the use of rescue medication have been excluded. *Source*: Reprinted from Ref. 36 with permission from the New England Journal of Medicine.

patients, and there may be a defect in platelet production due to apoptosis of the platelet precursor by autoantibody. In a phase I/II trial, 58% of patients achieved a platelet count greater that 50,000/μL, in a median of five to eight days (33). With safety follow-up up to 96 weeks with weekly subcutaneous administrations, the drug continued to be well tolerated. The most common adverse effect was a headache. Four patients were seen to have at least one of the following SAEs reticulin formation in the bone marrow, vaginal hemorrhage, bone pain, and transverse sinus thrombosis. No neutralizing antibodies have been found (34–36). When AMG 531 was discontinued, the platelet count returned to the prior baseline in all patients and a few had transient rebound worsening of the thrombocytopenia (34–36).

Eltrombopag, a TPO nonpeptide mimetic, has been studied in an oral formulation in patients with ITP and HCV patients treated with interferon. In a phase II trial of chronic ITP patients, there was a dose-dependent response noted in the patients who had achieved platelets greater than 50,000/μL. At the higher doses, there was also a trend toward a decrease in the bleeding events when compared to placebo (33). All platelet counts returned to baseline levels when the drug was discontinued (33). In a phase II trial in patients with HCV, at all doses tried, the median platelet count was higher than those patients receiving placebo. Fifty-three to sixty-five percent of those at the 50 or 75 mg dose were able to complete interferon treatment for 12 weeks compared to only 6% of patients taking placebo (35).

Table 2 Multifunctional Cytokines in Treating Thrombocytopenia

Cytokine	Patients studied	Results	Toxicity
IL-1 alpha	Ovarian cancer (9)	Decreased duration of low PLT Increased PLT nadir	Fever 100%; myalgias, fatigue
IL-3	Small cell (11)	Increased leukocyte and PLT	Fever 80%; skin
	Auto SCT (10)	Not effective	50% drop out due to toxicity
IL-6	Ovarian; sarcoma (10)	Improved PLT recovery	Fever, myalgias
	SCT (breast), sarcoma (10)	Not effective	VOD of liver
IL-11	Solid tumors (14)	Decreased severe thrombocytopenia and transfusions	Volume expansion, fatigue, atrial arrhythmias
SCF	Apheresis for auto SCT (10)	Improved mobilization	Toxicity limited by use of histamine blocker and inhaled B2 agonist

Table 3 Clinical Studies of Thrombopoietin

Patients studied	Dosing	Results
PEG-rHuMGDF		
NSCLC (15)	Daily after chemotherapy	Higher PLT nadir, earlier recovery
Solid tumors (16)	Daily after chemotherapy	No change in nadir; earlier recovery
SCT (breast) (17)	After SCT	Higher PLT at recovery, no impact on duration of low PLT
AML (18)	Daily after chemotherapy	Higher peak PLT, no effect on transfusions
AML (19)	Daily after chemotherapy	No effect on time to PLT recovery; no effect on transfusions
RhTPO		
Sarcoma (20)	Single dose, 3 wk prior to chemotherapy	Increased PLT day 4, peak at day 12
Sarcoma (2)	Single dose after chemotherapy	No difference in platelet nadir
Sarcoma (21)	Various dosing schedules	When doses given 5 days prior to chemotherapy and a day after, PLT nadir was higher and fewer transfusions needed
Gynecologic cancer (22)	QOD × 4 doses after chemotherapy	Higher mean PLT nadir and shorter duration of low PLT
Mobilization for autologous SCT (23)	Single dose with G-CSF	Enhanced mobilization, decreased number of apheresis required

SUMMARY AND FUTURE DIRECTIONS

Since the identification of thrombopoietin numerous pharmacologic agents have been developed to combat the thrombocytopenia commonly encountered in oncologic patients. The use of nonspecific cytokines is limited by their side effects (Table 2). The timing of administration of rhTPO in relation to chemotherapy dosing is critical to obtaining optimal responses (Table 3). The newer TPO peptide and nonpeptide mimetics show promise in the management of ITP patients. Further phase III trials in ITP are underway for both AMG 531 (36) and eltrombopag (34). Studies in patients with chemotherapy-induced thrombocytopenia are ongoing. Other TPO peptide mimetics (Fab 59 and Peg-TPOmp), TPO nonpeptide mimetics (AKR-501), and TPO agonist antibodies (TPO minibodies and domain subclass converted TPO agonist antibodies) await further trials in humans to assess their clinical utility.

REFERENCES

1. Deutsch, VR, Tomer, A. Megakaryocyte development and platelet production. BJH 2006; 134:453–466.
2. Vadhan-Raj S. Recombinant human thrombopoietin: clinical experience and in vivo biology. Semin Hematol 1998; 35(3):261–268.
3. Vadhan-Raj S. Clinical experience with recombinant human thrombopoietin in chemotherapy-induced thrombocytopenia. Semin Hematol 2000; 37(2):28–34.
4. Douglas VK, Tallman MS, Cripe LD, et al. Thrombopoietin administered during induction chemotherapy to patients with acute myeloid leukemia induces transient morphologic changes that may resemble chronic myeloproliferative disorders. Am J Clin Pathol 2002; 117:844–850.
5. Hauser CA, Stockler MR, Tattersall MH. Prognostic factors in patients with recently diagnosed incurable cancer: a systematic review. Support Care Cancer 2006; 14(10): 999–1011.
6. Smith, RE. Trends in recommendations for myelosuppressive chemotherapy for the treatment of solid tumors. JNCCN 2006; 4(7):649–658.
7. Elting LS, Cantor SB, Martin CG, et al. Cost of chemotherapy-induced thrombocytopenia among patients with lymphoma or solid tumors. Cancer 2003; 97(6): 1541–1550.
8. Schiffer CA, Anderson KC, Bennett CL, et al. Platelet transfusion for patients with cancer: clinical practice guidelines of the American Society of Clinical Oncology. JCO 2001; 19:1519–1538.
9. Vadhan-Raj S, Kudelka AP, Garrison L, et al. Effects of Interleukin-1alpha on Carboplatin-induced thrombocytopenia in patients with recurrent ovarian cancer. JCO 1994; 12(4):707–714.
10. Maslak P, Nimer SD. The efficacy of IL-3, SCF, IL-6, and IL-11 in treating thrombocytopenia. Semin Hematol 1998; 35(3):253–260.
11. D'Hondt V, Weynants P, Humblet Y, et al. Dose-dependent interleukin-3 stimulation of thrombopoiesis and neutropoiesis in patients with small-cell lung carcinoma before and following chemotherapy: a placebo-controlled randomized phase IB study. JCO 1993; 11(11):2063–2071.
12. Lindemann A, Ganser A, Herrmann F, et al. Biologic effects of recombinant human interleukin 3 in vivo. JCO 1991; 9:2120–2127.
13. Vadhan-Raj S, Papadopoulos NE, Burgess MA, et al. Effects of PIXY321, a granulocyte-macrophage colony stimulating factor/interleukin-3 fusion protein, on chemotherapy-induced multilineage myelosuppression in patients with sarcoma. JOC 1994; 12(4): 715–724.
14. Tepler I, Elias L, Smith JW, et al. A randomized placebo-controlled trial of recombinant human interleukin-11 in cancer patients with severe thrombocytopenia due to chemotherapy. Blood 1996; 87(9):3607–3614.
15. Fanucchi M, Glaspy J, Crawford J, et al. Effects of polyethylene glycol-conjugated recombinant human megakaryocyte growth and development factor on platelet counts after chemotherapy for lung cancer. N Engl J Med 1997; 336:404–409.
16. Basser RL, Rasko JE, Clarke K, et al. Randomized, blinded, placebo-controlled phase I trial of pegylated recombinant human megakaryocyte growth and development factor with filgrastim after dose-intensive chemotherapy in patients with advanced cancer. Blood 1997; 89:3118–3128.

17. Schuster MW, Beveridge R, Frei-Lahr D, et al. The effects of pegylated recombinant human megakaryocyte growth and development factor (PEG-rHuMGDF) on platelet recovery in breast cancer patients undergoing autologous bone marrow transplantation. Exp Hematol 2002; 30:1044–1050.
18. Archimbaud E, Ottmann OG, Yin JA, et al. A randomized, double-blind, placebo-controlled study with pegylated recombinant human megakaryocyte growth and development factor (PEG-rHuMGDF) as an adjunct to chemotherapy for adults with de novo acute myeloid leukemia. Blood 1999; 94:3694–3701.
19. Schiffer CA, Miller K, Larson RA, et al. A double-blind, placebo-controlled trial of pegylated recombinant human megakaryocyte growth and development factor as an adjunct to induction and consolidation therapy for patients with acute myeloid leukemia. Blood 2000; 95:2530–2535.
20. Vadhan-Raj S, Murray LJ, Bueso-Ramos C, et al. Stimulation of megakaryocyte and platelet production by a single dose of recombinant human thrombopoietin in patients with cancer. Ann Int Med 1997; 126:673–681.
21. Vadhan-Raj S, Patel S, Bueso-Ramos C, et al. Importance of predosing of recombinant human thrombopoietin to reduce chemotherapy-induced early thrombocytopenia. JCO 2003; 21(16):3158–3167.
22. Vadhan-Raj S, Verschraegen CF, Bueso-Ramos C, et al. Recombinant human thrombopoietin attenuates carboplatin-induced severe thrombocytopenia and the need for platelet transfusions in patients with gynecologic cancer. Ann Intern Med 2000; 132:364–368.
23. Vadhan-Raj S, Papadopoulos NE, Burgess MA, et al. Effects of PIXY321, a granulocyte-macrophage colony-stimulating factor/interleukin-3 fusion protein, on chemotherapy-induced multilineage myelosuppression in patients with sarcoma. JCO 1994; 12(4):715–724.
24. Demetri GD. Pharmacologic treatment options in patients with thrombocytopenia. Semin Hematol 2000; 37(2 suppl 4):11–18.
25. Begley CG, Basser RL. Biologic and structural differences of thrombopoietic growth factors. Semin Hematol 2000; 37(2 suppl 4):19–27.
26. Rice L, Nichol JL, McMillan R, et al. Cyclic immune thrombocytopenia responsive to thrombopoietic growth factor therapy. Am J Hematol 2001; 68:210–214.
27. Nomura S, Dan K, Hotta T, et al. Effects of pegylated recombinant human megakaryocyte growth and development factor in patients with idiopathic thrombocytopenic purpura. Blood 2002; 100:728–730.
28. Li J, Yang C, Xia Y, et al. Thrombocytopenia caused by the development of antibodies to thrombopoietin. Blood 2001; 98:3241–3248.
29. Kuter DJ, Begley CG. Recombinant human thrombopoietin: basic biology and evaluation of clinical studies. Blood 2002; 100:3457–3469.
30. Vadhan-Raj S, Kavanagh JJ, Freedman RS, et al. Safety and efficacy of transfusions of autologous cryopreserved platelets derived from recombinant human thrombopoietin to support chemotherapy-associated severe thrombocytopenia: a randomized cross-over study. Lancet 2002; 359:2145–2152.
31. Fibbe WE, Heemskerk DP, Laterveer L, et al. Accelerated reconstitution of platelets and erythrocytes after syngeneic transplantation of bone marrow cells derived from thrombopoietin pretreated donor mice. Blood 1995; 86:3308–3313.
32. Somlo G, Sniecinski I, ter Veer A, et al. Recombinant human thrombopoietin in combination with granulocyte colony-stimulating factor enhances mobilization of

peripheral blood progenitor cells, increases peripheral blood platelet concentration and accelerates hematopoietic recovery following high-dose chemotherapy. Blood 1999; 93(9):2798–2806.
33. Bussel J, Cheng G, Saleh M, Kovaleva L, et al. Analysis of bleeding in patients with immune thrombocytopenic purpura (ITP): a randomized, double-blind placebo-controlled trial of eltrombopag, an oral platelet growth factor. Blood 2006; 108: abstract 475.
34. Kutler DJ, Busse J, George JN, et al. Long-term dosing of AMG 531 in thrombocytopenic patients with immune thrombocytopenic purpura: 48 week update. Blood 2006; 108: abstract 476.
35. Kutler, DJ. New thrombopoietic growth factors. Blood 2007; 109:4607–4616.
36. Bussel J, Kuter DJ, George JN, et al. Effect of a thrombopoiesis-stimulating protein (AMG-531) in chronic immune thrombocytopenic purpura. N Engl J Med 2006; 355:1672–1681.
37. Fielder PJ, Gurney AL, Stefanich E, et al. Regulation of thrombopoietin levels by c-mpl-mediated binding to platelets. Blood 1996; 87:2154–2161.
38. Elting LS, Cantor SB, Martin CG. Cost of chemotherapy-induced thrombocytopenia among patients with lymphoma or solid tumors. Cancer 2003; 97(6):1541–15450.
39. Basser RL, Underhill C, Davis I, et al. Enhancement of platelet recovery after myelosuppressive chemotherapy by recombinant human megakaryocyte growth and development factor in patients with advanced cancer. J Clin Oncol 2000; 18: 2852–2861.

9

Venous Thromboembolism and Anticoagulation

Maithili V. Rao, Charles W. Francis, and Alok A. Khorana
*James P. Wilmot Cancer Center and the
Department of Medicine, University of Rochester,
Rochester, New York, U.S.A.*

INTRODUCTION

The association of cancer and thrombosis was first described by Armand Trousseau in 1865 (1). Venous thromboembolism (VTE) manifesting in the forms of deep vein thrombosis (DVT) and pulmonary embolism (PE) are the most common thrombotic events in cancer patients. Arterial events such as stroke or myocardial infarction are also observed, particularly in patients receiving antiangiogenic agents. Epidemiological and population-based studies have established that cancer patients have an increased risk of VTE compared to the general population. Recent evidence indicates that the incidence of cancer-associated thrombosis has been rising since the last decade (2,3). The risk for development of VTE varies between different cancer populations depending on the presence of various risk factors such as the type and stage of underlying cancer and the use of chemotherapy or antiangiogenic drugs. Cancer-associated VTE is a considerable burden on health care resources; it impairs patients' quality of life and may have a negative impact on survival. Cancer patients with VTE have a twofold or greater increase in mortality compared to cancer patients without VTE (4,5). In a prospective observational study of cancer patients receiving chemotherapy, thromboembolism was the second leading cause of death, after cancer itself, accounting for 9% of all deaths (6).

BIOLOGY

Multiple factors contribute to the development of the prothrombotic state commonly observed in cancer patients. There is increased expression of several procoagulant factors in cancer cells and their microenvironment. In particular, TF, the primary initiator of coagulation, is present on neoplastic cells as well as tumor-associated endothelial cells (7). TF expression occurs early in neoplastic transformation, secondary to oncogenic mutations in *KRAS* and *TP53* (8). TF expression is associated with increased angiogenesis, tumor invasiveness, and worsened prognosis in various malignancies (7,9–12). In addition, a recent report suggests that the grade of TF expression by tumor cells is associated with subsequent VTE in pancreatic cancer (13).

Chemotherapy additionally contributes to the prothrombotic state in cancer patients. Several studies have documented changes in markers of thrombin generation, such as thrombin–antithrombin complex, prothrombin F1+2, fibrinopeptide A, and D-dimer, within hours of chemotherapy administration, with effects lasting up to 48 hours (14). The association of antiangiogenic therapy with arterial and venous thrombosis is still under investigation. Interference with platelet and endothelial cell signaling has been suggested as a possible mechanism (15).

EPIDEMIOLOGY

The estimated annual incidence of VTE in the cancer population is 0.5%, compared with 0.1% in the general population (16). Population-based studies report a two- to sevenfold increased risk of VTE in patients with malignancy compared to persons without a malignancy (3,17). In hospitalized cancer patients, retrospective studies have observed an approximate 8% incidence of thrombotic events (2,18). Among ambulatory cancer patients on chemotherapy, one prospective study reported a VTE rate of 0.8% per month (19). More recent studies indicate a rise in VTE incidence beginning in the late 1990s (2,3). It is difficult to ascertain whether this is a "true" increase in incidence, or is related to more aggressive and thrombogenic chemotherapy regimens and newer antiangiogenic agents, or is a result of improved diagnostic techniques and greater awareness of VTE. The incidence of arterial thromboembolism in cancer patients has not been as well studied. In one study of hospitalized neutropenic cancer patients, the risk of an arterial event was 1.72% and increased over the eight-year study period by 124% (2).

RISK FACTORS

Cancer patients comprise a heterogeneous group including patients on active therapy, patients undergoing surgery, hospitalized patients, cancer survivors, and patients with terminal illness. Not only is the risk of VTE different in each of

Table 1 Risk Factors for Cancer-Associated VTE

Patient-related factors
Older age
Race (higher in African Americans, lower in Asians)
Comorbid conditions
    Infection
    Obesity
    Renal disease
    Pulmonary disease
Prothrombotic mutations
    Factor V leiden
    Prothrombin gene mutation
Prior history of VTE or arterial thrombosis
Cancer-related factors
Advanced stage of cancer
Initial period after diagnosis
Site of cancer
    Brain, pancreas, kidney, stomach, lung, bladder, gynecologic, hematologic
Treatment-related factors
Major surgery
Hospitalization
Cancer therapy
    Chemotherapy
    Hormonal therapy
    Antiangiogenic agents (thalidomide, lenalidomide, bevacizumab)
    Recombinant erythropoietins
Central venous catheters
Vena cava filters
Possible risks
Bevacizumab (for VTE)
Myeloid growth factors
Elevated prechemotherapy platelet count
Tissue factor expression by tumor cells

these subgroups, but it also varies over time within each patient, depending on the phase of the disease and the changing constellation of risk factors. A comprehensive list of risk factors for cancer-associated VTE is provided in Table 1.

More VTE events occur in the initial period following a diagnosis of malignancy than at any other time during the natural history of the disease. In a population-based study, the highest odds ratio for VTE development was in the first few months following a diagnosis of cancer (OR 53.5, 95% CI 8.6–334.3) (4,17). This observation may be due, in part, to the high use of anticancer therapies during this period that are associated with a thrombosis risk. Cancer patients with metastastic disease have a 2- to 19-fold increased risk of VTE as compared to patients with localized disease (2,4,17,18,20,21). Several studies have established that particular sites of cancer confer an increased risk of VTE. Cancers of the brain, pancreas, ovary, kidney, stomach, lung, and bladder are consistently associated with the highest rates of VTE (2,3,18,22). Traditionally, hematological malignancies were not thought to be associated with an increased risk of VTE; however, recent evidences, particularly in patients with myeloma and lymphoma, suggest otherwise (2,17,23,24). In one population-based study, patients with hematological malignancies had the highest risk of VTE (OR 28, 95% CI 4.0–200) (17). Hospitalization substantially increases the risk of developing VTE in a cancer patient (2,3,22). A prospective study of cancer patients identified inpatient treatment as an independent predictor for VTE (OR 2.34, 95% CI 1.63–3.36) (25). Cancer patients who undergo surgery have a twofold increased risk of postoperative VTE as compared to non-cancer patients; and this increased risk can persist up to seven weeks after an operation (26,27). Of note, cancer patients who are hospitalized or are undergoing surgery are stratified into the "highest" risk category by the American College of Chest Physicians (ACCP) guidelines for VTE prevention (28).

Anticancer drugs and even supportive therapies increase the risk of VTE in cancer patients. In a population-based study, the presence of cancer alone was associated with a fourfold increased risk of VTE (OR 4.05, 95% CI 1.93–8.52), whereas treatment with chemotherapy increased this risk 6.5-fold (OR 6.5, 95% CI 2.1–20.2) (29). The high rates of VTE reported in clinical trials of breast and lung cancer patients receiving chemotherapy support this association (21,30). In clinical trials tamoxifen therapy in breast cancer patients is associated with an estimated 1.5- to 7.1-fold greater risk of VTE compared to those assigned to placebo or observation (31). This risk is highest in women over the age 60 (32). The combination of chemotherapy and tamoxifen is associated with a much higher incidence of VTE (range, 6.5–13.6%) than when either therapy is given alone (range, 1.8–2.6%) (30,33,34). In contrast, postmenopausal breast cancer patients on adjuvant aromatase inhibitor therapy have a lower likelihood of VTE as compared to similar women treated with tamoxifen; however, rates are still high in comparison to untreated, healthy women. (35). In randomized trials, patients treated with a combination of thalidomide or lenalidomide with dexamethasone have higher VTE rates (8.5–17%) compared to those receiving dexamethasone alone (3–4.5%) (36,37). When thalidomide is combined with doxorubicin-containing chemotherapy, the observed rates of VTE are even higher (28%) (38). Concurrent use of recombinant erythropoietins further increases the risk of VTE (39). Bevacizumab, an antiangiogenic agent, has also been associated with increased risk of thrombosis, particularly arterial thrombosis (40,41). In 2007, the FDA issued safety warnings regarding the increased risk of thromboembolism associated with these agents (42). Cancer patients treated with recombinant erythropoietins such as epoetin and darbepoetin have significantly greater VTE events as compared to untreated controls (RR = 1.67, 95% CI = 1.35–2.06) (43). Myeloid growth factor use may also be a risk factor for VTE in cancer patients, but the meta-analysis was not conclusive (44).

Comorbid conditions, such as obesity, renal disease, pulmonary disease, arterial TE, and the presence of infection, are additional risk factors (2). Other possible risk factors include a prechemotherapy platelet count greater than 350,000/mm^3, central venous access devices, and inherited thrombophilic states, such as factor V leiden and prothrombin gene mutation 20210 (17,19,45,46). Recent studies suggest that tissue factor expression by tumor cells may be predictive of VTE in pancreatic and ovarian cancer patients (13,47).

It becomes apparent from this extensive list of risk factors that cancer-associated thrombosis is multifactorial, and that many risk factors can interact in the same patient. Efforts are ongoing to develop a risk assessment model that stratifies cancer patients into subgroups at low risk or high risk for developing VTE (48). Such a model will help identify the subgroup of cancer patients, particularly in the ambulatory population, who will derive the greatest benefit from thromboprophylaxis strategies.

PREVENTION OF CANCER-ASSOCIATED VTE

Prophylaxis in Surgery

There are only a small number of clinical trials addressing the issue of anticoagulation prophylaxis specifically in cancer patients. Among patients undergoing major abdominal surgery for cancer, the rates of DVT or major bleeding are no different in those randomized to receive in-hospital prophylaxis with subcutaneous low-dose unfractionated heparin (UFH) three times a day or low-molecular-weight heparin (LMWH) once daily (49,50). For cancer patients, postoperative prophylaxis with either UFH 5000 U three times a day or LMWH once daily is considered an acceptable standard (28). Prophylaxis with the factor Xa inhibitor fondaparinux is another alternative. Fondaparinux and the LMWH dalteparin were found to be equally effective in preventing postoperative VTE in patients undergoing abdominal surgery (51). A post hoc analysis for the subpopulation of cancer patients suggested greater protection from VTE in the fondaparinux group. Mechanical methods of prophylaxis, such as graduated compression stockings or intermittent pneumatic compression devices, can reduce rates of VTE and should be used in patients with a serious risk of bleeding. Combining mechanical devices with anticoagulation is suggested for patients at highest risk of VTE. The regimens for postsurgical prophylaxis for VTE in cancer patients are displayed in Table 2.

Two recent randomized trials have suggested that extending the duration of postoperative LMWH prophylaxis for two to four weeks after hospital discharge reduces the incidence of late venographic VTE by 60% in patients undergoing cancer surgery (52,53). Based on this evidence, the 2004 ACCP and 2006 National Comprehensive Cancer Network (NCCN) guidelines recommend extended posthospital discharge prophylaxis for cancer patients (28,54).

Table 2 Selected Regimens for Postsurgical Prophylaxis for Venous Thromboembolism in Cancer Patients

Drug	Regimen	Reference
Enoxaparin	40 mg sc daily	ENOXACAN, 1997 (49)[b]
		ENOXACAN II, 2002 (52)[a,b]
Dalteparin	5000 U sc daily	Rasmussen et al. 2006 (53)[a]
Fondaparinux	2.5 mg sc daily	Agnelli et al. 2005 (51)
Heparin	5000 U sc Q8 hours	2004 ACCP guidelines (28)

[a]Study population comprised of cancer patients only.
[b]Extended anticoagulation prophylaxis after surgery for 4 weeks was superior to 7 day course.

Prophylaxis in Hospitalized Medical Cancer Patients

Most trials investigating prophylaxis for VTE in hospitalized patients are conducted in general medical patients at high-risk of thrombosis secondary to a variety of underlying acute medical illnesses, such as congestive heart failure, respiratory compromise, and infectious diseases. Cancer patients comprise a small subset of this study population. Since it is well established that hospitalized patients with cancer have an extremely high risk of VTE, we can infer that the results from these studies apply to cancer patients.

Three large randomized, double-blinded, placebo-controlled trials have established the benefit of pharmacologic prophylaxis with LMWH in hospitalized medical patients (Table 3). Cancer patients comprised 5% to 15% of the study population in these trials. The primary end point of these studies was the presence of symptomatic or asymptomatic DVT or PE. Most of the patients underwent noninvasive testing at a predetermined time period to screen for the presence of DVT. The Prophylaxis in Medical Patients with Enoxaparin (MEDENOX) study randomized 1102 patients older than 40 years and hospitalized for at least 6 days with an acute illness to receive daily subcutaneous injections of either enoxaparin 40 mg or enoxaparin 20 mg, or placebo for 6 to 14 days (55). There were significantly lower rates of VTE in the enoxaparin 40 mg group, but not the 20-mg group, as compared to placebo (5.5% vs. 14.9%; $p < 0.001$). Similar benefit was reported in a trial of dalteparin, another LMWH. The Prospective Evaluation of Dalteparin Efficacy for Prevention of VTE in Immobilized Patients Trial (PREVENT) randomized 3706 patients, with similar baseline characteristics as the MEDENOX study, to receive dalteparin 5000 IU daily or placebo for 14 days (56). Rates of VTE were reduced from 4.96% in the placebo group to 2.77% in the dalteparin group ($p = 0.002$). The third trial assessed the efficacy of prophylaxis with fondaparinux, a synthetic pentasaccharide that inhibits factor Xa. The Arixtra for Thromboembolism Prevention

Table 3 Selected Recent Trials of Prophylaxis of Venous Thromboembolism in Hospitalized Acutely Ill Medical Patients

Study[a]	Drug	Regimen	Total patients	Cancer patients (%)	% placebo vs. treatment events
MEDENOX (55)	Enoxaparin	40 mg sc daily	579	72 (12.4)	14.9 vs. 5.5 $p < 0.001$ RRR 63%
PREVENT (56)	Dalteparin	5000 U sc daily	3706	190 (5.1)	4.9 vs. 2.7 $p = 0.002$ RRR 44%
ARTEMIS (57)	Fondaparinux	2.5 mg sc daily	849	131 (15.4)	10.5 vs. 5.6 $p = 0.03$ RRR 47%

Abbreviations: sc, subcutaneous; RRR, relative risk reduction.
[a]All are placebo-controlled, randomized trials.

in a Medical Indications Study (ARTEMIS) compared fondaparinux 2.5 mg subcutaneously daily with placebo for 6 to 14 days in 849 hospitalized medical patients (57). There was a significant reduction in the incidence of VTE in patients who received fondaparinux compared to those assigned to placebo (5.6% vs. 10.5%, $p = 0.03$). In both the MEDENOX and the PREVENT studies, the benefits of prophylaxis extended through the three-month follow-up period, with no difference in the rates of mortality or bleeding between the treatment or placebo arms. However, the ARTEMIS study reported lower one-month mortality in the patients receiving fondaparinux as compared to placebo (33% vs. 6%, $p = 0.06$).

UFH 5000 U subcutaneously every 8 hours or every 12 hours is also an acceptable regimen for prophylaxis in the hospitalized general medical patients (58,59). A meta-analysis of eight randomized trials that compared prophylaxis with UFH versus LMWH in hospitalized medical patients concluded that there were no difference in VTE rates between the two treatments, but the rate of major bleeding was lower in patients who received LMWH (RR 0.48, 95% CI 0.23–1.00) (60). Nonpharmacological strategies for VTE prophylaxis such as graduated compression stockings or pneumatic compression devices have proven to be effective in the postoperative period (61,62). However, their effectiveness has not been fully characterized in the hospitalized medical or cancer patient. For patients with obvious contraindications to anticoagulation, including those who are actively bleeding or severely thrombocytopenic, these nonpharmacological measures are safe choices.

Prophylaxis in Ambulatory Cancer Patients

Cancer patients who are ambulatory, particularly those recently diagnosed, having advanced disease or receiving active anticancer therapies, are also at increased risk of thrombosis. Attempts have been made to explore the potential benefits of prophylactic anticoagulation in these patients in small randomized trials. In one study of 311 metastatic breast cancer patients receiving chemotherapy, those assigned to 1 mg of daily warfarin had an 85% relative risk reduction in VTE events (1 event vs. 7 events, $p = 0.031$) without an increased risk of bleeding (63). However, this finding was not confirmed by two other placebo-controlled, randomized trials of prophylactic LMWH in metastatic breast and lung cancer patients receiving chemotherapy (64). The Fragmin Advanced Malignancy Outcome Study (FAMOUS) study randomized 382 patients with advanced cancer to dalteparin 5000 U sc once daily or placebo for 9 months. There were no significant differences between the groups in either the primary end point of survival or the secondary endpoint of symptomatic VTE (65). In summary, there is no compelling evidence to support the implementation of routine thromboprophylaxis in unselected ambulatory cancer patients. Once reliable risk-assessment models are fully developed, they may provide a basis for prospective studies to evaluate the effectiveness of thromboprophylaxis in high-risk ambulatory cancer patients.

One established high-risk group in the ambulatory setting is multiple myeloma patients receiving antiangiogenic therapy. The expert consensus is that all newly diagnosed patients treated with thalidomide-lenalidomide-containing regimens should receive thromboprophylaxis (38). Fixed low-dose warfarin (1 to 2 mg) has been modestly effective at decreasing VTE complications in patients on thalidomide-dexamethasone, but was ineffective for patients treated with thalidomide chemotherapy (38). The use of prophylactic-dose LMWH has been shown to eliminate excess VTE risk resulting from adding thalidomide to doxorubicin-containing chemotherapy regimens (66,67). Recent nonrandomized studies in patients treated with lenalidomide-dexamethasone and thalidomide-chemotherapy suggest that effective VTE risk reduction can be achieved with prophylactic aspirin (80 or 325 mg) (68,69). Since none of these anticoagulation regimens have been compared head-to-head, no one regimen can be specifically recommended. In contrast, patients receiving the antiangiogenic agent bevacizumab have high risk of both major and minor bleeding complications, and primary thromboprophylaxis has therefore not been tested in this setting.

Prophylaxis for Central Venous Catheters

The rate of symptomatic central venous catheters (CVC)-related thrombosis among patients on chemotherapy followed prospectively ranges from 4.3% to 14%, depending primarily on the duration of follow-up (70,71). Several factors influence the rate, including the presence of CVC-related infection, catheter-tip position and placement, more than one insertion attempt, presence of ovarian cancer, and type of anticancer therapy (70,72,73). Prospective, randomized trials in cancer patients have failed to demonstrate a decrease in rate of symptomatic CVC-associated thrombosis with fixed low-dose warfarin, warfarin dose-adjusted to INR of 1.5 to 2.0, or low-dose LMWH compared to placebo or no therapy (74–76). In one study, cancer patients randomized to warfarin dose adjusted to INR of 1.5 to 2.0 had lower rates of symptomatic CVC-associated thrombosis compared to those receiving fixed-dose warfarin, albeit at a cost of increased major bleeding events (76). Patients on warfarin have higher rates of bleeding complications, and even a fixed low-dose regimen (1 mg) may result in marked increases in the INR (76,77). The 2004 ACCP and 2006 NCCN consensus guidelines recommend against the use of routine anticoagulation for prevention of CVC-associated VTE in cancer patients (28,54).

TREATMENT OF VTE IN CANCER PATIENTS

Anticoagulation is the mainstay of therapy for VTE. The initial phase of anticoagulation helps relieve acute symptoms and prevents thrombus extension or embolization. This is followed by a second long-term phase of anticoagulation for 3 to 12 months with a goal of preventing recurrent VTE (78). Traditionally, this was accomplished with the initial use of parenteral UFH, followed by transition to therapeutic dose of oral warfarin to achieve an INR between 2 and 3 (79). However, based on their convenience and strong evidence of efficacy, LMWHs have become the preferred, and in some situations even the standard, agents of choice both for acute and long-term anticoagulation of VTE. There are certain key aspects of treatment for VTE in cancer patients that merit discussion.

INITIAL ANTICOAGULATION

Until the early 1990s, initial therapy with UFH followed by long-term warfarin remained the standard (80). With the availability of LMWHs, which do not require frequent laboratory monitoring, are convenient to use, and are potentially applicable to outpatient use, this traditional approach to initial anticoagulation has been revised. Phase III trials and meta-analyses have demonstrated a lower risk of recurrent VTE and major bleeding and suggest a survival benefit with LMWH compared to UFH (81–83). It is unclear if these results are applicable to patients with cancer who comprise only a minority of the study populations. However, considering the many practical advantages of LMWHs, they remain an attractive and widely used alternative to UFH in the initial treatment of acute VTE in cancer patients.

Recently, fondaparinux has been approved for acute treatment. In a randomized study of 2213 patients with acute symptomatic PE, including 356 (16%) with cancer, those assigned to receive initial anticoagulation with fondaparinux had significantly fewer recurrent VTE events at three months as

Table 4 Regimens for Treatment of Venous Thromboembolism in Cancer Patients

Drug	Regimen	Reference
Initial anticoagulation		
Dalteparin	200 U/kg sc daily	CLOT study (90)
Heparin	80 U/kg IV bolus, then 18 U/kg/hr IV (adjust based on PTT) for 5–7 days	2004 ACCP guidelines (78)
Enoxaparin	1.5 mg/kg sc daily	CANTHANOX and ONCENOX studies (93,94)
Tinzaparin	175 U/kg sc once daily	LITE study (91)
Fondaparinux	<50 kg, 2.5 mg sc daily; 50–100 kg, 5 mg sc daily; >100 kg, 7.5 mg sc daily	MATISSE study (84)
Long-term anticoagulation		
FDA-approved regimen		
Dalteparin	200 U/kg sc once daily for one month, thereafter 150 U/kg sc once daily	CLOT study (90)
Other regimens		
Enoxaparin	1.5 mg/kg sc once daily	CANTHANOX and ONCENOX studies (93,94)
Tinzaparin	175 U/kg sc once daily	LITE study (91)
Warfarin	5–10 mg orally once daily, begin on first day of IV UFH or LMWH. Adjust dose to achieve INR 2–3	2004 ACCP guidelines (78)

Abbreviations: PTT, partial-thromboplastin time; sc, subcutaneously; LMWH, low-molecular-weight heparin; UFH, unfractionated heparin; INR, international normalized ratio.

compared to those who received IV UFH (3.8% vs. 5%, 95% CI 3–0.5) (84). The standard anticoagulation regimens for initial treatment of VTE in cancer patients are listed in Table 4.

Long-Term Anticoagulation

Warfarin has long been the standard anticoagulant used in the long-term treatment of VTE in cancer patients. Despite adequate anticoagulation with warfarin, cancer patients with VTE have an increased risk of recurrent thrombosis. In a prospective cohort of over 800 patients on warfarin, the 12-month cumulative incidence of recurrent VTE was significantly greater in cancer patients (20.7%, 95% CI 15.6–25.8) compared to those without cancer (6.8%, 95% CI 3.9–9.7) (85). In the same study, the rate of major bleeding on warfarin was also higher in cancer patients (12.4% vs. 4.9%). While the bleeding risk in noncancer patients is related to INR levels and appears to plateau after the first month on warfarin, patients with cancer have a elevated risk of bleeding that persists throughout the duration of warfarin therapy and is not only associated with high INR levels (86). In addition to the risk of bleeding and recurrent thrombosis, oral anticoagulation has limitations that complicate the care and reduce quality of life of cancer patients. These include the unpredictability of INR in the face of drug interactions, erratic absorption from GI disturbances, liver dysfunction, and impaired nutritional status, all of which are common problems in cancer patients (87). The need for frequent venipuncture and laboratory visits to monitor INR poses additional burdens on the patient and family. The process of interrupting and reversing anticoagulation during invasive procedures and periods of chemotherapy-induced thrombocytopenia followed by reinstitution of therapeutic INR can be cumbersome.

LMWHs offer several advantages over long-term warfarin therapy, including fewer drug interactions, stable absorption, and no necessity for laboratory monitoring. Drawbacks include the necessity for self-injection, which may be burdensome, the relative contraindication in patients with renal insufficiency, and a small risk of heparin-induced thrombocytopenia. Meta-analyses of several small, randomized trials comparing long-term anticoagulation with LMWH versus warfarin in non-cancer patients suggested a benefit for LMWH in terms of lower rates of recurrent VTE and bleeding complications (88,89). In patients with cancer, the benefits of LMWH become more apparent. The CLOT trial randomized 676 cancer patients with DVT and/or PE to receive either six months of dalteparin or initial anticoagulation with dalteparin followed by six months of warfarin (target INR 2.5) (90). Patients assigned to dalteparin alone were given a dose of 200 IU/kg for the first one month followed by 75% to 80% of this dose for the next five months. Recurrent symptomatic VTE event was noted in 27 of 338 patients in the dalteparin group and in 53 of 338 patients in the warfarin group (HR 0.48, 95% CI 0.30–0.77). This translates into greater than 50% risk reduction for recurrent VTE with LMWH. Figure 1 demonstrates the Kaplan–Meier estimates of the probability of recurrent VTE in the two study groups. There was no difference in bleeding complications or mortality between the two groups. This landmark trial established the superiority of long-term anticoagulation with LMWH over warfarin in the population of cancer patients. In May 2007, the FDA approved dalteparin for long-term treatment of cancer-associated thrombosis. Another LMWH, tinzaparin, has also been studied in this setting. The LITE study randomized patients with VTE to tinzaparin 175 U/kg once daily for three months or initial therapy of IV UFH followed by warfarin (91). There were significantly fewer bleeding complications in the tinzaparin group as compared to the warfarin group (19.8% vs. 13%, $p = 0.01$). Although rates of recurrent VTE were the same in both groups for the entire study

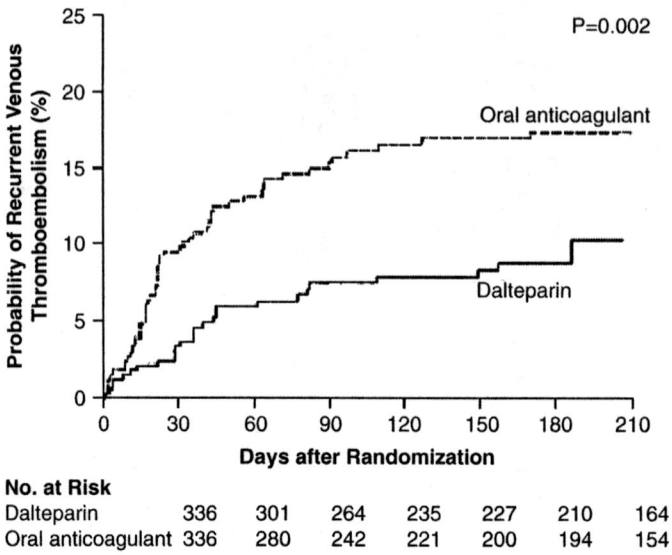

Figure 1 The cumulative risks of recurrent VTE comparing six months of treatment with LMWH dalteparin versus an oral vitamin K antagonist. Hazard ratio 0.48 (95% CI 0.30–0.77). *Source*: Reprinted with permission from Ref. 90.

population, among the subgroup of 200 patients with cancer, the LMWH regimen was more effective in reducing rates of recurrent VTE (16% vs. 7%, $p = 0.44$) (92). Two trials evaluating long-term anticoagulation with the LMWH enoxaparin in cancer patients failed to show a statistically significant reduction in symptomatic VTE as compared to warfarin (93,94). The small sample sizes in these studies may account for the lack of statistical significance. However, in one study, the enoxaparin-treated patients fared better than the warfarin group in the primary end-point measure of combined major bleeding and recurrent VTE events (21.1% vs. 10.5%, RR 2.02, 95% CI 0.88–4.65) (93). In summary, long-term LMWH is associated with a lower rate of symptomatic recurrent VTE in cancer patients without an increased risk of bleeding. Based on this evidence, practice guidelines issued by expert consensus panels, including the ACCP and NCCN, recommend long-term anticoagulation with LMWH for cancer patients with VTE (54,78). Table 4 displays the regimens for long-term anticoagulation in cancer patients.

There are little data, particularly in the cancer patient population, comparing the efficacy of once or twice daily injection regimens of LMWH. For the initial management of acute DVT, one randomized trial compared intravenous UFH versus enoxaparin 1 mg/kg twice daily versus enoxaparin 1.5 mg/kg once daily (95). For the overall patient population, there were no differences in the rates of recurrent VTE or bleeding. However, for the subgroup of patients with cancer, once daily enoxaparin was associated with a twofold, albeit statistically nonsignificant, increase in risk of recurrent VTE compared to the twice-daily regimen. For long-term treatment, only once-daily regimens have been studied.

Duration of Therapy

The optimal duration of anticoagulation in cancer patients with VTE is not known. Since patients with metastatic disease theoretically have a persistent risk factor for thrombosis, the general recommendation is for "indefinite" anticoagulation. For patients without metastasis, extended anticoagulation beyond the standard six months should be considered if they have "active" cancer or are receiving anticancer treatments. Thereafter, the risk-benefit ratio should be weighed periodically and an individualized decision regarding the duration of anticoagulation is recommended (54,78)

Vena Cava Filters

The PREPIC study is the only randomized trial to assess potential late complications of recurrent DVT and/or PE with use of vena cava filters (VCF) (96). In this prospective randomized, controlled trial of 200 patients (including 56 with cancer) on anticoagulation, those who received a VCF had short-term protection from PE, but suffered significantly more recurrent DVT and filter-site thrombosis compared to those who did not have VCF placed (20.8% vs. 11.6%, OR 1.87, 95% CI 1.10–1.38). Retrospective studies have noted a 32% to 40% incidence of recurrent DVT in cancer patients who receive VCF (97,98). It is clear that the risk of thrombosis in cancer patients is not attenuated, but may actually be increased by VCF placement. Filters should be used conservatively and only temporarily in situations where there is serious contraindication to anticoagulation.

SUMMARY

Cancer patients are at high risk for the development of VTE compared to the general population. The risk of VTE varies considerably between cancer patients depending on the course of the disease and presence of specific risk factors. LMWHs are effective and proven superior to warfarin in preventing recurrent VTE events without an increased risk of bleeding complications in the long-term anticoagulation of VTE in cancer patients. Anticoagulation prophylaxis with UFH, LMWH, or fondaparinux is recommended for hospitalized acutely ill and postsurgical cancer patients. There is insufficient evidence to recommend routine thromboprophylaxis in ambulatory cancer patients with the exception of multiple myeloma patients receiving thalidomide- or lenalidomide-containing regimens. The results of ongoing investigations will help identify high-risk subgroups in the ambulatory cancer population that may benefit from anticoagulation prophylaxis strategies.

REFERENCES

1. Khorana AA. Malignancy, thrombosis and trousseau: the case for an eponym. J Thromb Haemost 2003; 1(12):2463–2465.
2. Khorana AA, Francis CW, Culakova E, et al. Thromboembolism in hospitalized neutropenic cancer patients. J Clin Oncol 2006; 24(3):484–490.
3. Stein PD, Beemath A, Meyers FA, et al. Incidence of venous thromboembolism in patients hospitalized with cancer. Am J Med 2006; 119(1):60–68.
4. Chew HK, Wun T, Harvey D, et al. Incidence of venous thromboembolism and its effect on survival among patients with common cancers. Arch Intern Med 2006; 166(4): 458–464.
5. Sorensen HT, Mellemkjaer L, Olsen JH, et al. Prognosis of cancers associated with venous thromboembolism. N Engl J Med 2000; 343(25):1846–1850.
6. Khorana AA, Francis CW, Culakova E, et al. Thromboembolism is a leading cause of death in cancer patients receiving outpatient chemotherapy. J Thromb Haemost 2007; 5(3):632–634.
7. Rickles FR, Patierno S, Fernandez PM. Tissue factor, thrombin, and cancer. Chest 2003; 124(3 suppl):58S–68S.
8. Yu JL, May L, Lhotak V, et al. Oncogenic events regulate tissue factor expression in colorectal cancer cells: implications for tumor progression and angiogenesis. Blood 2005; 105(4):1734–1741.
9. Lopez-Pedrera C, Barbarroja N, Dorado G, et al. Tissue factor as an effector of angiogenesis and tumor progression in hematological malignancies. Leukemia 2006; 20(8):1331–1340.
10. Jiang X, Bailly MA, Panetti TS, et al. Formation of tissue factor-factor VIIa-factor xa complex promotes cellular signaling and migration of human breast cancer cells. J Thromb Haemost 2004; 2(1):93–101.
11. Kakkar AK, Lemoine NR, Scully MF, et al. Tissue factor expression correlates with histological grade in human pancreatic cancer. Br J Surg 1995; 82(8):1101–1104.
12. Nitori N, Ino Y, Nakanishi Y, et al. Prognostic significance of tissue factor in pancreatic ductal adenocarcinoma. Clin Cancer Res 2005; 11(7):2531–2539.
13. Khorana AA, Ahrendt SA, Ryan CK, et al. Tissue factor expression, angiogenesis, and thrombosis in pancreatic cancer. Clin Cancer Res 2007; 13(10):2870–2875.
14. Weitz I, Liebman H, Chemotherapy-induced hemostatic activation and thrombosis in cancer. In: Khorana, AA, Francis, CW (Eds): Cancer-Associated Thrombosis: New Findings in Translational Science, Prevention and Treatment. Informa Healthcare (New York), 2007.
15. Kuenen BC, Levi M, Meijers JC, et al. Potential role of platelets in endothelial damage observed during treatment with cisplatin, gemcitabine, and the angiogenesis inhibitor SU5416. J Clin Oncol 2003; 21(11):2192–2198.
16. Lee AY, Levine MN. Venous thromboembolism and cancer: risks and outcomes. Circulation 2003; 107(23 suppl 1):I17–I21.
17. Blom JW, Doggen CJ, Osanto S, et al. Malignancies, prothrombotic mutations, and the risk of venous thrombosis. JAMA 2005; 293(6):715–722.
18. Sallah S, Wan JY, Nguyen NP. Venous thrombosis in patients with solid tumors: determination of frequency and characteristics. Thromb Haemost 2002; 87(4):575–579.
19. Khorana AA, Francis CW, Culakova E, et al. Risk factors for chemotherapy-associated venous thromboembolism in a prospective observational study. Cancer 2005; 104(12): 2822–2829.

20. Blom JW, Vanderschoot JP, Oostindier MJ, et al. Incidence of venous thrombosis in a large cohort of 66,329 cancer patients: results of a record linkage study. J Thromb Haemost 2006; 4(3):529–535.
21. Blom JW, Osanto S, Rosendaal FR. The risk of a venous thrombotic event in lung cancer patients: higher risk for adenocarcinoma than squamous cell carcinoma. J Thromb Haemost 2004; 2(10):1760–1765.
22. Levitan N, Dowlati A, Remick SC, et al. Rates of initial and recurrent thromboembolic disease among patients with malignancy versus those without malignancy. risk analysis using medicare claims data. Medicine (Baltimore) 1999; 78(5):285–291.
23. Komrokji RS, Uppal NP, Khorana AA, et al. Venous thromboembolism in patients with diffuse large B-cell lymphoma. Leuk Lymphoma 2006; 47(6):1029–1033.
24. Zangari M, Barlogie B, Thertulien R, et al. Thalidomide and deep vein thrombosis in multiple myeloma: risk factors and effect on survival. Clin Lymphoma 2003; 4(1): 32–35.
25. Kroger K, Weiland D, Ose C, et al. Risk factors for venous thromboembolic events in cancer patients. Ann Oncol 2006; 17(2):297–303.
26. Bergqvist D. Venous thromboembolism and cancer: prevention of VTE. Thromb Res 2001; 102(6):V209–V213.
27. Kikura M, Takada T, Sato S. Preexisting morbidity as an independent risk factor for perioperative acute thromboembolism syndrome. Arch Surg 2005; 140(12): 1210–1217; discussion 1218.
28. Geerts WH, Pineo GF, Heit JA, et al. Prevention of venous thromboembolism: the seventh ACCP conference on antithrombotic and thrombolytic therapy. Chest 2004; 126(3 suppl):338S–400S.
29. Heit JA, Silverstein MD, Mohr DN, et al. Risk factors for deep vein thrombosis and pulmonary embolism: a population-based case-control study. Arch Intern Med 2000; 160(6):809–815.
30. Saphner T, Tormey DC, Gray R. Venous and arterial thrombosis in patients who received adjuvant therapy for breast cancer. J Clin Oncol 1991; 9(2):286–294.
31. Deitcher SR, Gomes MP. The risk of venous thromboembolic disease associated with adjuvant hormone therapy for breast carcinoma: a systematic review. Cancer 2004; 101(3):439–449.
32. Fisher B, Dignam J, Bryant J, et al. Five versus more than five years of tamoxifen therapy for breast cancer patients with negative lymph nodes and estrogen receptor-positive tumors. J Natl Cancer Inst 1996; 88(21):1529–1542.
33. Pritchard KI, Paterson AH, Paul NA, et al. Increased thromboembolic complications with concurrent tamoxifen and chemotherapy in a randomized trial of adjuvant therapy for women with breast cancer. National cancer institute of canada clinical trials group breast cancer site group. J Clin Oncol 1996; 14(10):2731–2737.
34. Fisher B, Dignam J, Wolmark N, et al. Tamoxifen and chemotherapy for lymph node-negative, estrogen receptor-positive breast cancer. J Natl Cancer Inst 1997; 89 (22):1673–1682.
35. Howell A, Cuzick J, Baum M, et al. Results of the ATAC (arimidex, tamoxifen, alone or in combination) trial after completion of 5 years' adjuvant treatment for breast cancer. Lancet 2005; 365(9453):60–62.
36. Rajkumar SV, Blood E, Vesole D, et al. Phase III clinical trial of thalidomide plus dexamethasone compared with dexamethasone alone in newly diagnosed multiple

myeloma: a clinical trial coordinated by the Eastern Cooperative Oncology Group. J Clin Oncol 2006; 24(3):431–436.
37. Dimopoulos MA, Spencer A, Attal M, et al. Study of lenalidomide plus dexamethasone versus dexamethasone alone in relapsed or refractory multiple myeloma (MM): results of a phase 3 study (MM-010). ASH Annual Meeting Abstracts 2005; 106(11):6.
38. Zangari M, Elice F, Fink L, et al. Thrombosis in multiple myeloma. Expert Rev Anticancer Ther 2007; 7(3):307–315.
39. Knight R, DeLap RJ, Zeldis JB, et al. Lenalidomide and venous thrombosis in multiple myeloma. N Engl J Med 2006; 354(19):2079–2080.
40. Kabbinavar F, Hurwitz HI, Fehrenbacher L, et al. Phase II, randomized trial comparing bevacizumab plus fluorouracil (FU)/leucovorin (LV) with FU/LV alone in patients with metastatic colorectal cancer. J Clin Oncol 2003; 21(1):60–65.
41. Shah MA, Ilson D, Kelsen DP. Thromboembolic events in gastric cancer: high incidence in patients receiving irinotecan- and bevacizumab-based therapy. J Clin Oncol 2005; 23(11):2574–2576.
42. http://www.fda.gov/Medwatch/Safety/2004/avastin_deardoc_mod.pdf. Accessed Jan.1, 2008
43. Bohlius J, Wilson J, Seidenfeld J, et al. Recombinant human erythropoietins and cancer patients: updated meta-analysis of 57 studies including 9353 patients. J Natl Cancer Inst 2006; 98(10):708–714.
44. Barbui T, Finazzi G, Grassi A, et al. Thrombosis in cancer patients treated with hematopoietic growth factors: a meta-analysis on behalf of the Subcommittee on Haemostasis and Malignancy of the Scientific and Standardization Committee of the ISTH. Thromb Haemost 1996; 75(2):368–371.
45. Kennedy M, Andreescu AC, Greenblatt MS, et al. Factor V leiden, prothrombin 20210A and the risk of venous thrombosis among cancer patients. Br J Haematol 2005; 128(3):386–388.
46. Eroglu A, Kurtman C, Ulu A, et al. Factor V leiden and PT G20210A mutations in cancer patients with and without venous thrombosis. J Thromb Haemost 2005; 3(6):1323–1324.
47. Uno K, Homma S, Satoh T, et al. Tissue factor expression as a possible determinant of thromboembolism in ovarian cancer. Br J Cancer 2007; 96(2):290–295.
48. Khorana AA, Francis CW, Culakova E, et al. Risk factors for chemotherapy-associated venous thromboembolism in a prospective observational study: a proposed predictive model. J Thromb haemost 2005; 3(suppl 1):abstract number OR058.
49. ENOXACAN Study Group. Efficacy and safety of enoxaparin versus unfractionated heparin for prevention of deep vein thrombosis in elective cancer surgery: a double-blind randomized multicentre trial with venographic assessment. Br J Surg 1997; 84(8):1099–1103.
50. McLeod RS, Geerts WH, Sniderman KW, et al. Subcutaneous heparin versus low-molecular-weight heparin as thromboprophylaxis in patients undergoing colorectal surgery: results of the canadian colorectal DVT prophylaxis trial. A randomized, double-blind trial. Ann Surg 2001; 233(3):438–444.
51. Agnelli G, Bergqvist D, Cohen AT, et al. Randomized clinical trial of postoperative fondaparinux versus perioperative dalteparin for prevention of venous thromboembolism in high-risk abdominal surgery. Br J Surg 2005; 92(10):1212–1220.

52. Bergqvist D, Agnelli G, Cohen AT, et al. Duration of prophylaxis against venous thromboembolism with enoxaparin after surgery for cancer. N Engl J Med 2002; 346 (13):975–980.
53. Rasmussen MS, Jorgensen LN, Wille-Jorgensen P, et al. Prolonged prophylaxis with dalteparin to prevent late thromboembolic complications in patients undergoing major abdominal surgery: a multicenter randomized open-label study. J Thromb Haemost 2006; 4(11):2384–2390.
54. Wagman LD, Baird MF, Bennett CL, et al. Venous thromboembolic disease. Clinical practice guidelines in oncology. J Natl Compr Canc Netw 2006; 4(9):838–869.
55. Samama MM, Cohen AT, Darmon JY, et al. A comparison of enoxaparin with placebo for the prevention of venous thromboembolism in acutely ill medical patients. Prophylaxis in medical patients with enoxaparin study group. N Engl J Med 1999; 341(11):793–800.
56. Leizorovicz A, Cohen AT, Turpie AG, et al. Randomized, placebo-controlled trial of dalteparin for the prevention of venous thromboembolism in acutely ill medical patients. Circulation 2004; 110(7):874–879.
57. Cohen AT, Davidson BL, Gallus AS, et al. Efficacy and safety of fondaparinux for the prevention of venous thromboembolism in older acute medical patients: randomized placebo controlled trial. BMJ 2006; 332(7537):325–329.
58. Halkin H, Goldberg J, Modan M, et al. Reduction of mortality in general medical in-patients by low-dose heparin prophylaxis. Ann Intern Med 1982; 96(5):561–565.
59. Gardlund B. Randomised, controlled trial of low-dose heparin for prevention of fatal pulmonary embolism in patients with infectious diseases. The heparin prophylaxis study group. Lancet 1996; 347(9012):1357–1361.
60. Mismetti P, Laporte-Simitsidis S, Tardy B, et al. Prevention of venous thromboembolism in internal medicine with unfractionated or low-molecular-weight heparins: a meta-analysis of randomised clinical trials. Thromb Haemost 2000; 83(1):14–19.
61. Amaragiri SV, Lees TA. Elastic compression stockings for prevention of deep vein thrombosis. Cochrane Database Syst Rev 2000; 3:CD001484.
62. Agu O, Hamilton G, Baker D. Graduated compression stockings in the prevention of venous thromboembolism. Br J Surg 1999; 86(8):992–1004.
63. Levine M, Hirsh J, Gent M, et al. Double-blind randomised trial of a very-low-dose warfarin for prevention of thromboembolism in stage IV breast cancer. Lancet 1994; 343(8902):886–889.
64. Haas SK, Kakkar AK, Kemkes-Matthes B, et al. Prevention of venous thromboembolism with low-molecular-weight heparin in patients with metastatic breast or lung cancer: results of the TOPIC studies. J Thromb Haemost 2005; 3(suppl 1):OR059 (abstr).
65. Kakkar AK, Levine MN, Kadziola Z, et al. Low molecular weight heparin, therapy with dalteparin, and survival in advanced cancer: the fragmin advanced malignancy outcome study (FAMOUS). J Clin Oncol 2004; 22(10):1944–1948.
66. Zangari M, Barlogie B, Anaissie E, et al. Deep vein thrombosis in patients with multiple myeloma treated with thalidomide and chemotherapy: effects of prophylactic and therapeutic anticoagulation. Br J Haematol 2004; 126(5):715–721.
67. Minnema MC, Breitkreutz I, Auwerda JJ, et al. Prevention of venous thromboembolism with low molecular-weight heparin in patients with multiple myeloma treated with thalidomide and chemotherapy. Leukemia 2004; 18(12):2044–2046.
68. Zonder JA. Thrombotic complications of myeloma therapy. Hematol Am Soc Hematol Educ Program 2006; 348–355.

69. Baz R, Li L, Kottke-Marchant K, et al. The role of aspirin in the prevention of thrombotic complications of thalidomide and anthracycline-based chemotherapy for multiple myeloma. Mayo Clin Proc 2005; 80(12):1568–1574.
70. Lee AYY, Levine MN, Butler G, et al. Incidence, risk factors, and outcomes of catheter-related thrombosis in adult patients with cancer. J Clin Oncol 2006; 24(9):1404–1408.
71. Tesselaar MET, Ouwerkerk J, Nooy MA, et al. Risk factors for catheter-related thrombosis in cancer patients. Eur J Cancer 2004; 40(15):2253–2259.
72. Linenberger ML. Catheter-related thrombosis: risks, diagnosis, and management. J Natl Compr Canc Netw 2006; 4(9):889–901.
73. van Rooden CJ, Schippers EF, Barge RMY, et al. Infectious complications of central venous catheters increase the risk of catheter-related thrombosis in hematology patients: a prospective study. J Clin Oncol 2005; 23(12):2655–2660.
74. Couban S, Goodyear M, Burnell M, et al. Randomized placebo-controlled study of low-dose warfarin for the prevention of central venous catheter-associated thrombosis in patients with cancer. J Clin Oncol 2005; 23(18):4063–4069.
75. Verso M, Agnelli G, Bertoglio S, et al. Enoxaparin for the prevention of venous thromboembolism associated with central vein catheter: a double-blind, placebo-controlled, randomized study in cancer patients. J Clin Oncol 2005; 23(18):4057–4062.
76. Young AM, Begum G, Billingham LJ, et al. WARP: a multicentre prospective randomized controlled trial of thrombosis prophylaxis with warfarin in cancer patients with central venous catheters. J Clin Oncol 2005; ASCO Ann Meeting Proc 2005; 23(16S part I, June 1 supplement): 8004 (abstr).
77. Masci G, Magagnoli M, Zucali PA, et al. Minidose warfarin prophylaxis for catheter-associated thrombosis in cancer patients: can it be safely associated with fluorouracil-based chemotherapy? J Clin Oncol 2003; 21(4):736–739.
78. Buller HR, Agnelli G, Hull RD, et al. Antithrombotic therapy for venous thromboembolic disease: the seventh ACCP conference on antithrombotic and thrombolytic therapy. Chest 2004; 126(3 suppl):401S–428S.
79. Ansell J, Hirsh J, Poller L, et al. The pharmacology and management of the vitamin K antagonists: the seventh ACCP conference on antithrombotic and thrombolytic therapy. Chest 2004; 126(3 suppl):204S–233S.
80. Brandjes DP, Heijboer H, Buller HR, et al. Acenocoumarol and heparin compared with acenocoumarol alone in the initial treatment of proximal-vein thrombosis. N Engl J Med 1992; 327(21):1485–1489.
81. Gould MK, Dembitzer AD, Doyle RL, et al. Low-molecular-weight heparins compared with unfractionated heparin for treatment of acute deep venous thrombosis. A meta-analysis of randomized, controlled trials. Ann Intern Med 1999; 130(10): 800–809.
82. van Dongen CJ, van den Belt AG, Prins MH, et al. Fixed dose subcutaneous low molecular weight heparins versus adjusted dose unfractionated heparin for venous thromboembolism. Cochrane Database Syst Rev 2004; 4:CD001100.
83. Dolovich LR, Ginsberg JS, Douketis JD, et al. A meta-analysis comparing low-molecular-weight heparins with unfractionated heparin in the treatment of venous thromboembolism: examining some unanswered questions regarding location of treatment, product type, and dosing frequency. Arch Intern Med 2000; 160(2):181–188.

84. Buller HR, Davidson BL, Decousus H, et al. Subcutaneous fondaparinux versus intravenous unfractionated heparin in the initial treatment of pulmonary embolism. N Engl J Med 2003; 349(18):1695–1702.
85. Prandoni P, Lensing AW, Piccioli A, et al. Recurrent venous thromboembolism and bleeding complications during anticoagulant treatment in patients with cancer and venous thrombosis. Blood 2002; 100(10):3484–3488.
86. Palareti G, Legnani C, Lee A, et al. A comparison of the safety and efficacy of oral anticoagulation for the treatment of venous thromboembolic disease in patients with or without malignancy. Thromb Haemost 2000; 84(5):805–810.
87. Wells PS, Holbrook AM, Crowther NR, et al. Interactions of warfarin with drugs and food. Ann Intern Med 1994; 121(9):676–683.
88. Iorio A, Guercini F, Pini M. Low-molecular-weight heparin for the long-term treatment of symptomatic venous thromboembolism: meta-analysis of the randomized comparisons with oral anticoagulants. J Thromb Haemost 2003; 1(9):1906–1913.
89. van der Heijden JF, Hutten BA, Buller HR, et al. Vitamin K antagonists or low-molecular-weight heparin for the long term treatment of symptomatic venous thromboembolism. Cochrane Database Syst Rev 2002; 1:CD002001.
90. Lee AY, Levine MN, Baker RI, et al. Low-molecular-weight heparin versus a coumarin for the prevention of recurrent venous thromboembolism in patients with cancer. N Engl J Med 2003; 349(2):146–153.
91. Hull RD, Pineo GF, Mah AF, et al. A randomized trial evaluating long-term low-molecular-weight heparin therapy for three months versus intravenous heparin followed by warfarin sodium. Blood 2002; 100:148a (abstr).
92. Hull RD, Pineo GF, Brant RF, et al. Long-term low-molecular-weight heparin versus usual care in proximal-vein thrombosis patients with cancer. Am J Med 2006; 119(12):1062–1072.
93. Meyer G, Marjanovic Z, Valcke J, et al. Comparison of low-molecular-weight heparin and warfarin for the secondary prevention of venous thromboembolism in patients with cancer: a randomized controlled study. Arch Intern Med 2002; 162(15):1729–1735.
94. Deitcher SR, Kessler CM, Merli G, et al. Secondary prevention of venous thromboembolic events in patients with active cancer: enoxaparin alone versus initial enoxaparin followed by warfarin for a 180-day period. Clin Appl Thromb Hemost 2006; 12(4):389–396.
95. Merli G, Spiro TE, Olsson CG, et al. Subcutaneous enoxaparin once or twice daily compared with intravenous unfractionated heparin for treatment of venous thromboembolic disease. Ann Intern Med 2001; 134(3):191–202.
96. Decousus H, Leizorovicz A, Parent F, et al. A clinical trial of vena caval filters in the prevention of pulmonary embolism in patients with proximal deep-vein thrombosis. prevention du risque d'embolie pulmonaire par interruption cave study group. N Engl J Med 1998; 338(7):409–415.
97. Elting LS, Escalante CP, Cooksley C, et al. Outcomes and cost of deep venous thrombosis among patients with cancer. Arch Intern Med 2004; 164(15):1653–1661.
98. Lin J, Proctor MC, Varma M, et al. Factors associated with recurrent venous thromboembolism in patients with malignant disease. J Vasc Surg 2003; 37(5):976–983.

10

Antiemetic Prophylaxis and Treatment of Chemotherapy-Induced Nausea and Vomiting

Karin Jordan, Christoph Sippel, Timo Behlendorf, Hans-Heinrich Wolf, and Hans-Joachim Schmoll
*Department of Internal Medicine IV,
Oncology/Hematology, Martin-Luther-University
Halle-Wittenberg, Halle (Saale), Germany*

INTRODUCTION

The goal of each antiemetic therapy is to abolish nausea and vomiting. Twenty years ago, nausea and vomiting were common adverse events of certain types of chemotherapy and forced up to 20% of patients to postpone or refuse potentially curative treatment (1). Clinical and basic research over the past 25 years has lead to steady improvements in the control of chemotherapy-induced nausea and vomiting (CINV). The development of the 5-HT$_3$-receptor antagonists (5-HT$_3$-RAs) in the early 1990s has been one of the most significant advances in chemotherapy of cancer patients. Corticosteroids are often underestimated although they show when combined with other antiemetic agents good antiemetic efficacy in the prevention of acute and delayed CINV. Another group of antiemetics, the neurokinin-1-receptor antagonists (NK1-RA), has recently been developed, and the first drug in this class, aprepitant, was incorporated in the updated antiemetic guidelines by the American Society of Clinical Oncology (ASCO), Multinational Association of Supportive Care in Cancer (MASCC), and National Comprehensive Cancer Network (NCCN).

Table 1 Three Categories of Chemotherapy-Induced Nausea and Vomiting

Acute nausea and vomiting
- Within the first 24 hr of chemotherapy
- Mainly by serotonin (5 HT) release from the enterochromaffin cells

Delayed nausea and vomiting
- After 24 hr to 5 days of chemotherapy
- Various mechanisms: mainly Substance P mediated, disruption of the blood-brain barrier, disruption of the GI motility, adrenal hormones

Anticipatory nausea and vomiting
- Occurrence is possible after one cycle of chemotherapy
- Involves the element of classic conditioning
- In approximately 30% of patients by the fourth treatment cycle

Classification of CINV: Acute/Delayed/Anticipatory Nausea and Vomiting

CINV may be classified into three categories: acute onset, occurring within 24 hours of initial administration of chemotherapy (mostly serotonin-related); delayed onset, occurring 24 hours to several days after initial treatment (mostly Substance P related); and anticipatory nausea and vomiting, observed in patients whose emetic episodes are triggered by taste, odor sight, thoughts, or anxiety, secondary to a history of poor response to antiemetic agents (Table 1).

EMETOGENICITY OF CHEMOTHERAPEUTIC AGENTS

The emetogenic potential of the chemotherapeutic agents used is the main risk factor for the degree of CINV. With regard to their emetogenic potential, the chemotherapeutic agents are classified into four emetic risk groups: high (90%), moderate (30–90%), low (10–30%), and minimal (<10%) (the figures in parentheses represent the percentage of patients having emetic episode/s when no prophylactic antiemetic protection is provided) (Tables 2 and 3) (2–4). The antiemetic prophylaxis is directed toward the emetogenic potential of the chemotherapy.

Patient-Related Risk Factors

Patient risk factors, including young age, female gender, a history of low alcohol intake, experience of emesis during pregnancy, impaired quality of life, and previous experience of chemotherapy, are known to increase the risk of nausea and vomiting after chemotherapy (2–6). Although less consistent, Osoba et al. also found that low social functioning or high fatigue scores also predicted for a poor outcome (7). They reported that CINV increased almost fourfold in those with any four of the six risk factors they described (female, prechemotherapy nausea, highly emetogenic chemotherapy, lack of maintenance antiemetics, low social functioning, history of low alcohol use). In the assortment of the optimal

Table 2 Emetogenic Risk of Intravenous Chemotherapeutic Agents

High (emesis risk > 90%, without antiemetics)
Carmustine, BCNU	Lomustine
Cisplatin	Mechlorethamine
Cyclophosphamide (>1500 mg/m^2)	Pentostatin
Dacarbazine, DTIC	Streptozotocin
Dactinomycin, actinomycin D	

Moderate (emesis risk 30–90%, without antiemetics)
Altretamine	Ifosfamide
Carboplatin	Irinotecan
Cyclophosphamide (<1500 mg/m^2)	Melphalan i.v.
Cytarabine (>1 g/m^2)	Mitoxantrone (>12 mg/m^2)
Daunorubicin	Oxaliplatin
Doxorubicin	Temozolomide
Epirubicin	Treosulfan
Idarubicin	Trabectedin

Low (emesis risk 10–30%, without antiemetics)
Asparaginase	Mitoxantron (<12 mg/m^2)
Bortezomib	Paclitaxel
Cetuximab	Pegasparaginase
Cytarabine (<1 g/m^2)	Pemetrexed
Docetaxel	Teniposide
Etoposide i.v.	Thiopeta
5-Fluorouracil	Topotecan
Gemcitabine	Trastuzumab
Methotrexat (>100 mg/m^2)	

Minimal (emesis risk <10%, without antiemetics)
Bleomycin	α-, β-, γ-Interferone
Bevacizumab	Melphalan per os
Busulfan	Mercaptopurine
Chlorambucil	Methotrexat (<100 mg/m^2)
Cladribine	Thioguanine
Cytarabin (<100 mg/m^2)	Vinblastine
Fludarabin	Vincristine
Hormone	Vinorelbine
Hydroxyurea	

Source: Adapted from Refs. 2–4.

antiemetic prophylaxis, patient-related risk factors have primarily no influence on the decision. Further research is necessary to verify the usefulness of integrating a patient-related risk factor profile in the primary decision process. This would make sense, considering the wide range of emetogenic potential (30–90%) in the moderate emetogenic setting. However, whether or not such a model would translate into the daily routine praxis is questionable.

Table 3 Emetic Risk of Oral Chemotherapeutic Agents

High (emesis risk >90%, without antiemetics)	
Hexamethylmelamine	Procarbazine
Moderate (emesis risk 30–90%, without antiemetics)	
Cyclophosphamide	Temozolomide
Etoposide	Vinorelbine
Imatinib	
Low (emesis risk 10–30%, without antiemetics)	
Capecitabine	Fludarabine
Minimal (emesis risk <10%, without antiemetics)	
Chlorambucil	Melphalan
Erlotinib	Methotrexate
Gefitinib	Sorafenib
Hydroxyurea	Sunitinib
L-Phenylalanine mustard	6-Thioguanine

Source: Adapted from Refs. 3,4.

Antiemetics

With modern antiemetics, vomiting can completely be prevented in up to 70% to 80% of the patients (8,9). Combination antiemetic regimens have become the standard of care for the control of CINV.

5-HT$_3$ Serotonin Receptor Antagonists

The introduction of 5-HT$_3$-RAs has dramatically improved the management of chemotherapy- and radiotherapy-induced emesis. The wide experience acquired with these drugs in daily clinical practice since the early 1990s has confirmed the remarkable safety profile. 5-HT$_3$-RAs, ondansetron, granisetron, tropisetron, dolasetron, and palonosetron, are currently available in Europe and the United States. The lowest fully effective once-a-day dose for each agent should be used as indicated in Table 4. Oral and intravenous routes are similarly effective.

Mechanism of action: Serotonin is the main neurotransmitter responsible for emesis after chemotherapy. The 5-HT$_3$ receptors are located in three sites: gastrointestinal (GI) tract, chemoreceptor trigger zone (CTZ) located in the area postrema, and nucleus tractus solitarius (NTS) of the vomiting center. The CTZ is a circumventricular organ located at the caudal end of the fourth ventricle. This structure lacks an effective blood–brain barrier, and will detect emetic agents in both the systemic circulation and the cerebrospinal fluid. The vomiting center is located in the brainstem medullary structures. It receives major inputs from the CTZ, and a vagal and symphathetic input from the gut. Following exposure to radiation or cytotoxic drugs, serotonin (5-HT) is released from enterochromaffine cells in the small intestinal mucosa, which are adjacent to the vagal afferent neurones on which 5-HT$_3$ receptors are located (10). The released

Table 4 Dose of Antiemetics

	Route	Recommended dose (once daily)
5-HT$_3$-receptor antagonist		
Ondansetron	p.o.	24 mg (high), 16 mg^a (moderate)
	i.v.	8 mg (0.15 mg/kg)
Granisetron	p.o.	2 mg
	i.v.	1 mg (0.01 mg/kg)
Tropisetron	p.o.	5 mg
	i.v.	
Dolasetron	p.o.	100 mg
	i.v.	100 mg (1.8 mg/kg)
Palonosetron	i.v.	0.25 mg
Steroids		
Dexamethasone	p.o.	12 mg (high emetogenic with aprepitant), 20 mg w/o aprepitant
	i.v.	8 mg (moderate emetogenic), 8 mg (high/moderate) days 2, 3
NK1-receptorantagonist		
Aprepitant	p.o.	125 mg (day 1), 80 mg (days 2+3)

Source: Adapted from Refs. 2–4
^{a}Eight milligram twice daily is recommended,

serotonin activates vagal afferent neurones via the 5-HT$_3$ receptors, which lead ultimately to a severe emetic response mediated via the CTZ within the area postrema (11).

Dose recommendation: When administering 5-HT$_3$-RAs, several points should be taken into consideration (12–14).

1. The lowest fully effective dose for each agent should be used (Table 4); higher doses do not enhance any aspect of activity because of the receptor saturation.
2. Oral and intravenous route are equally effective.
3. No schedule is better than a single dose daily given before chemotherapy.

Dolasetron: A dose of 100 mg or 1.8 mg/kg intravenous and 100 mg oral is recommended.

Granisetron: All guidelines recommend granisetron 1 mg or 0.01 mg/kg intravenous and 2 mg oral (MASCC and ASCO) or 1 to 2 mg oral (NCCN).

Ondansetron: Different statements are given by the NCCN in comparison to MACC and ASCO regarding the ondansetron dose. As such, the NCCN guidelines recommend ondansetron 16 to 24 mg oral and 8 to 12 mg (maximum 32 mg) intravenous, whereas the MASCC and ASCO guidelines recommend ondansetron 24 mg oral (MASCC 16 mg oral for moderate emetogenic chemotherapy) and 8 mg or 0.15 mg/kg intravenous. In a recently published meta-analysis comparing low-dose ondansetron (8 mg) with high-dose ondansetron (24 or 32 mg) in a subanalysis in cisplatin-based chemotherapy, high-dose ondansetron appear to be more effective ($p = 0.012$) (15).

Palonosetron: A dose of 0.25 mg intravenous is the recommended dose. Oral palonosetron is not available yet. Palonosetron has a significantly longer half-life and a higher binding activity in comparison to the other 5-HT$_3$-RAs. The actual role of palonosetron in comparison to the other available 5-HT$_3$-RAs is discussed controversially in the guidelines. However, all three guidelines did not designate a preferred 5-HT$_3$-RA, although palonosetron outperformed in a study ondansetron and dolasetron in some secondary endpoints (16). In a recently published meta-analysis, palonosetron was not included because only two studies were fully published by that time (15,17).

Tropisetron: A dose of 5 mg oral or intravenous is recommended by the guidelines.

Side effects: The adverse effects of 5-HT$_3$-RAs are generally mild, with headache, constipation, diarrhea, and asthenia mainly described (18). Small, transient, reversible changes in electrocardiographic parameters have been shown to occur with all available 5-HT$_3$-RAs. However, after more than 13 years of commercial use, clinically relevant cardiovascular effects have not been reported (19).

Steroids, Dexamethasone

When used in combination with other antiemetics, they appear to exert a booster effect in raising the emetic threshold. Theoretical concerns that steroids may interfere with the antitumor effects of chemotherapy through immunosuppressive mechanisms have not been confirmed in clinical trials. The use of dexamethasone is recommended for the acute prevention of highly, moderately, and low emetogenic chemotherapy. For the prevention of delayed emesis, dexamethasone is recommended *in combination* with aprepitant in high emetogenic chemotherapy, but not in moderate emetogenic chemotherapy.

Mechanism of action: The mechanisms by which steroids exert their antiemetic activity are not fully understood, but they may affect prostaglandin activity in the brain, modify the blood-cerebrospinal fluid barrier, and inhibit cortical input to the vomiting center (20). Further, the anti-inflammatory effect of steroids may act as an antiemetic by either preventing the release of serotonin in the gut or by interfering with the activation of 5-HT$_3$ receptors in the GI tract (21).

Dose recommendation: For prevention of acute CINV, 20 mg (12 mg when coadministered with aprepitant) in highly emetogenic chemotherapy and a single dose of 8 mg dexamethasone in moderately emetogenic chemotherapy should be the dose of choice (22,23), and has been recommended by the MASCC and ASCO guidelines (Table 4) (2,12,24). These dose recommendations are largely driven by the studies from the Italian Group for Antiemetic Research (22,23).

Side effects: Steroids are considered to be safe antiemetics. Side effects are usually dependent on dose and duration of therapy. In a recently published study in patients receiving dexamethasone in the prophylaxis of delayed CINV, patients reported moderate to severe problems with insomnia (45%), indigestion/epigastric discomfort (27%), agitation (27%), increased appetite (19%), weight gain (16%), and acne (15%) in the week following chemotherapy (25). Concerns that steroids may interfere with the antitumor effects of chemotherapy through immunosuppressive mechanisms have not been confirmed in clinical trials (26).

Neurokinin-1 Receptor Antagonist, Aprepitant

Aprepitant is the first representative of this new group and blocks the NK1 receptor in the brainstem emetic center and GI tract (8). The use of aprepitant is unanimously suggested by all three antiemetic guidelines for high emetogenic chemotherapy and in parts for moderate emetogenic chemotherapy. One study in the moderate emetogenic setting is published so far, which formed the basis for recommendation of aprepitant for anthracycline/cyclophosphamide-based emetogenic chemotherapy (27). Because only patients receiving an anthracycline/cyclophosphamide-based regimen were included in this study, the MASCC and ASCO guidelines restrict the recommendation of the triple combination in the moderate emetogenic setting to this "high-risk" chemotherapeutic regimen. The NCCN guidelines however recommended aprepitant in the moderate emetogenic setting in selected patients based on the emetogenic potential of the chemotherapy. Altogether the addition of aprepitant to the standard antiemetic regimen (5-HT$_3$ receptor-antagonist and dexamethasone) significantly improves the protection against vomiting in the acute as well as delayed phase in highly and moderately emetogenic chemotherapies.

Mechanism of action: The antiemetic mechanism of action of aprepitant is believed to be mainly centrally mediated. Substance P, a neuropeptide (mammalian tachykinin), mediates its action through neurokinin-1 (NK1) receptors. The NK1 receptors are abundant in the CTZ, NTS, and GI tract (28). Animal and human studies using Positron Emission Tomography (PET) have shown that Substance P crosses the blood–brain barrier and occupies brain NK1 receptors (29).

Dose recommendation: A randomized study established the most favorable risk profile of aprepitant at doses of 125 mg per os on day 1 and 80 mg per os on days 2 and 3 (Table 4) (30). It is important to acknowledge that aprepitant has to be taken before the start of the chemotherapy. Since Substance P is released and binds to the NK1-receptors the receptor antagonism of aprepitant is alleviated. Aprepitant is a moderate inhibitor of CYP 3A4, therefore the dexamethasone dose has to be reduced. Theoretical concerns that aprepitant might interact with chemotherapeutic agents could not be demonstrated in preclinical and clinical studies so far (31,32).

Side effects: Adverse effects observed during clinical trials with aprepitant have included headache, abdominal pain, dizziness, anorexia, hiccups, and mild transaminase elevation (30,33,34). In general, the incidence of adverse events is similar in patients treated with aprepitant plus a 5-HT$_3$-RA and dexamethasone, and those treated with just 5-HT$_3$-RA and dexamethasone (8,9).

Metoclopramide

Before the introduction of 5-HT$_3$-RAs, metoclopramide (MCP), usually at high doses and in combination with a steroid, played a primary role in the management of acute CINV. MCP was part of the former antiemetic guidelines especially for the prevention of delayed emesis (13,35). Although MCP has to be proven as effective as 5-HT$_3$-Ras, when combined with steroids in the prevention of delayed CINV (36,37), MCP was not recommended again in the new guidelines in this setting. MCP should be reserved for special circumstances, including known intolerance to 5-HT$_3$-RAs or steroids.

Mechanism of action: MCP is a D2-antagonist and is active peripherally in the gut and centrally in the CTZ. Today, it is recognised that the effect of high-dose MCP in patients receiving cisplatin is due to antagonism at 5-HT$_3$ receptors (38,39).

Dose recommendation: MCP has antiemetic properties both in low doses as a dopamine antagonist and in high doses a serotonin antagonist. The usual recommended doses are 20–40 mg p.o. q 4 to 6 hours (conventional dose) or 2–3 mg/kg (high dose) as suggested by Gralla et al. (38).

Side effects: The side effects commonly associated with MCP include mild sedation, dystonic reactions (age related) especially in higher doses, akathisia, diarrhoea, and orthostatic hypotension (38). Dystonic reactions can be dealt with biperiden.

Metopimazine

Metopimazine is a phenothiazine derivate with antidopaminergic activity (40). It exerts its antiemetic effects via the CTZ. The addition of metopimazine to ondansetron or ondansetron plus prednisolone generally significantly increased the efficacy of the regimens in preventing CINV in patients receiving moderately or highly emetogenic chemotherapy. The percentage of patients experiencing no acute emesis with metopimazine plus ondansetron was 63% to 78% as compared with 47% to 50% for ondansetron monotherapy (41–43). Metopimazine combined with prednisolone was significantly less effective than granisetron in the acute setting (44).

Adverse effects occasionally reported with metopimazine include sedation, orthostatic hypotension, and anticholinergic effects. Extrapyramidal symptoms, including dyskinesias, are very uncommon (40).

Cannabinoids

The combination of weak antiemetic efficacy with potentially beneficial side effects (sedation, euphoria) makes cannabinoids a useful adjunct to modern antiemetic therapy in selected patients. However, the associated side effects of dizziness and dysphoria should not be underestimated. The use of cannabinoids is advised in patients intolerant or refractory to 5-HT$_3$-RAs or steroids, and aprepitant. Interestingly, in a systematic review of the efficacy of oral cannabinoids in the prevention of nausea and vomiting, it was found that cannabinoids were slightly better than conventional antiemetics (e.g., MCP, phenothiazines, haloperidol). However, their usefulness was generally limited by the high incidence of toxic effects, such as dizziness, dysphoria, and hallucinations.

Accordingly, dronabinol is recommended for consideration in the treatment of breakthrough or refractory emesis. Doses in the range of 5 to 10 mg/m^2, every three to four hours, orally appear to be among the most useful (45,46). Usually 1 or 2 mg of nabilone twice a day is recommended (47).

Benzodiazepines

Benzodiazepines can be a useful addition to antiemetic regimens in certain circumstances. Trials with lorazepam have shown a high degree of patient acceptance. As such, they serve to reduce anxiety and the risk of anticipatory nausea. Lorazepam may add a small degree of objective antiemetic efficacy, although the effect is limited, and the use of lorazepam as a single-agent antiemetic is not recommended (48). A double-blind randomised study showed that its known antianxiety effects can be quite prominent in the chemotherapy administration setting when added to effective antiemetic combination (10,49).

Midazolam is a short-acting benzodiazepine, which is used for example in patients with prolonged postoperative emesis resistant to usual treatment (50). In a published small phase II study, midazolam was added to granisetron and dexamethasone in patients with refractory acute CINV in previous cycles of highly emetogenic chemotherapy (51). Midazolam was given as a continuous infusion of 0.04 mg/kg during the administration of chemotherapy. With the introduction of midazolam, 73% of the patients had a reduction of at least one grade of nausea and vomiting in comparison to the previous cycle of chemotherapy. No details of potential side effects, such as sedation, were described.

Atypical Neuroleptics

Olanzapine, an atypical antipsychotic drug, has potential antiemetic properties because of its action at multiple receptor sites implicated in the control of nausea and vomiting (52). The latest phase II study shows a high complete response rate over the whole study period (d1–5) when palonosetron and dexamethasone were combined with olanzapine in patients receiving highly or moderately emetogenic chemotherapy (53). Olanzapine showed an acceptable toxicity profile in a dose of 5 mg daily two days prior to chemotherapy and 10 mg daily from start of chemotherapy until seven days after finishing chemotherapy. Mean side effect was a depressed level of consciousness and fatigue (54).

Antihistamines

Although often administered, studies with diphenhydramine or hydroxyzine in the prevention of CINV have not shown any antiemetic activity (2).

Herbs as Antiemetics

Herbs are used by at least 80% of the world's population and are increasingly popular. Some studies showed a potential benefit of ginger and peppermint in postoperative nausea and vomiting as well as in the management of nausea and vomiting in pregnancy.

Ginger (Zingiber officinale Roscoe): The detailed mechanism of action is unknown; although ginger is known to exert its antiemetic effect at the gut and not at the central nervous system level (55). Ginger is consumed via oral ingestion of powdered extract capsules in doses of 500 mg taken up to three times daily. The results of studies done with ginger in patients receiving chemotherapy are controversial and do not demonstrate convincing efficacy (56,57). There is some evidence, however, that ginger might be beneficial as an adjunctive therapy for intractable nausea.

Peppermint (Mentha X piperita Lamiaceae): Peppermint acts as an internal calcium channel-blocking agent, producing intestinal smooth muscle relaxation. Peppermint has supportive evidence for use in patients with dyspepsia, irritable bowel syndrome, and as an intraluminal spasmolytic agent during barium enemas endoscopy (58). Up to now, there is no published study using peppermint as an adjunctive therapy for patients receiving chemotherapy. Peppermint seems to lessen this symptom in the treatment of postoperative nausea (59).

PREVENTION OF CINV

High Emetogenic Chemotherapy

Acute CINV: A combination of $5-HT_3$-RA, dexamethasone, and aprepitant within the first 24 hours is recommended (Tables 5 and 6).

Delayed CINV: An appropriate prophylaxis for delayed CINV is indispensable. All three guidelines suggested the combination of dexamethasone and aprepitant.

Moderate Emetogenic Chemotherapy

Acute CINV: The combination of a $5-HT_3$-RA and dexamethasone with or without aprepitant is recommended. However, the key question in this setting is whether aprepitant should be part of the antiemetic prophylaxis. The ASCO and MASCC guidelines recommend the triple combination ($5-HT_3$-RA, dexamethasone, and aprepitant) when patients receiving the combination of an anthracycline- and cyclophosphamide-based regimen. The NCCN guidelines, however, broaden the spectrum of the use of aprepitant in this setting and advised usage in selected patients receiving other chemotherapies of moderate emetogenic risk (e.g., carboplatin, epirubicin, ifosfamide, irinotecan).

Delayed CINV: Dexamethasone is the preferred agent to use for delayed CINV. Nonetheless, when aprepitant was used for the prevention of acute CINV,

Table 5 Suggested Antiemetic Prophylaxis

Emetogenic potential	Acute phase	Delayed phase
High	5 HT_3 receptor antagonist (5 HT_3-RA): Dolasetron; 200 mg p.o./100 mg i.v. Granisetron; 2 mg p.o. /1mg i.v. Ondansetron; 16–24 mg p.o./8 mg i.v. Palonosetron; 0.25 mg i.v. Tropisetron; 5 mg p.o. /i.v. + **Steroid** Dexamethasone; 12 mg p.o /i.v. + **Neurokinin-1 receptor antagonist** Aprepitant; 125 mg p.o.	**Steroid** Dexamethasone; 8 mg p.o/i.v. for 3 days + **Neurokinin₁ receptor antagonist** Aprepitant; 80 mg p.o. for 2 days
Moderate	*1. anthrazycline/ cyclophosphamide (AC)-based chemotherapy:* same as in high emetogenic chemotherapy *2. other chemotherapies:* **5 HT_3 receptor antagonist** + **Steroid** Dexamethasone; 8 mg p.o/ i.v.	*1. anthrazycline/ cyclophosphamide (AC)-based chemotherapy:* **Neurokinin-1 receptor antagonist** Aprepitant, 80 mg p.o. for 2 days *2. other chemotherapies:* **Steroid** Dexamethasone, 8 mg p.o /i.v. for 2 days or alternatively 5 HT_3 receptor antagonist
Low	**Steroid** Dexamethasone; 8 mg p.o/i.v.	No routine prophylaxis
Minimal	No routine prophylaxis	No routine prophylaxis

then aprepitant should also be used for the prophylaxis of delayed CINV as a monotherapy as stated in the MASCC and ASCO guidelines. As discussed before, the NCCN guidelines suggest aprepitant ± dexamethasone in this situation. A 5-HT_3-RA can be used as an alternative, although the therapeutical role in the

Table 6 Antiemetic Prevention Based on the Emesis Risk Category (MASCC, ASCO, NCCN)

	Recommendation							
	High		Moderate		Low		Minimal	
Group	Acute CINV	Delayed CINV	Acute CINV	Delayed CINV	Acute CINV	Delayed CINV[a]	Acute CINV[a]	Delayed CINV[a]
MASCC	5-HT$_3$-RA + Dexamethasone + Aprepitant	Dexamethasone + Aprepitant	1. Anthracycline/cyclophosphamide 5-HT$_3$-RA + Dexamethasone + Aprepitant 2. Other than anthracycline/cyclophosphamide 5-HT$_3$-RA + Dexamethasone	Aprepitant or Dexamethasone Dexamethasone 5-HT$_3$-RA may be used as an alternative	Dexamethasone	—	—	—
ASCO	5-HT$_3$-RA + Dexamethasone + Aprepitant	Dexamethasone + Aprepitant	1. Anthracycline/cyclophosphamide 5-HT$_3$-RA + Dexamethasone + Aprepitant 2. Other than anthracycline/cyclophosphamide 5-HT$_3$-RA + Dexamethasone	Aprepitant Dexamethasone or a 5-HT$_3$-RA	Dexamethasone	—	—	—

	High	Moderate	Low	Minimal
NCCN	5-HT$_3$-RA + Dexamethasone + Aprepitant ± Lorazepam	Dexamethasone + Aprepitant ± Lorazepam 1. Anthracycline/cyclophosphamide or in selected patients 5-HT$_3$-RA + Dexamethasone + Aprepitant ± Lorazepam 2. Other than anthracycline/cyclophosphamide 5-HT$_3$-RA + Dexamethasone ± Lorazepam or Dexamethasone or 5-HT$_3$-RA both ± Lorazepam	Dexamethasone ± Lorazepam or Prochlorperazine ± Lorazepam or Metoclopramide ± Lorazepam or	—

Source: Adapted from Refs. 2–4.
Abbreviations: CINV, chemotherapy-induced nausea and vomiting; 5-HT$_3$-RA, 5-HT$_3$-receptor antagonist.
[a]No routine prophylaxis.

delayed phase is rather limited (60). In contrast to all three previous published guidelines, MCP is not reflected in the new guidelines as an alternative option.

Low Emetogenic Chemotherapy

The MASCC and ASCO guidelines recommend the use of a steroid alone in the first 24 hours and no prophylaxis beyond 24 hours. The NCCN guidelines recommended as alternative drugs to dexamethasone as well prochlorperazine or MCP.

Minimal Emetogenic Chemotherapy

No antiemetic drug should be routinely administered before chemotherapy.

Management of Breakthrough and Refractory CINV

"Breakthrough CINV" is defined as an event that happens in spite of optimal preventative treatment. "Refractory CINV" recurs in subsequent cycles of therapy when all previous preventive and rescue treatments failed. If optimal treatment has been given as prophylaxis, repeated dosing of the same agents is unlikely to be successful; an addition of dopamine receptor antagonists (MCP) might be useful or adding other agents such as benzodiazepines or neuroleptics. Olanzapine, an atypical neuroleptic could also be considered as suggested by the MASCC and NCCN guidelines. The role of palonosetron, a new 5-HT$_3$-RA, in this setting has not been defined yet (3).

Multiple-Day Chemotherapy

The expert panel creating the MASCC guidelines recommended for multiple-day cisplatin the use of a 5-HT$_3$-RA in combination with dexamethasone for acute CINV, and dexamethasone alone for delayed CINV. The use of NK1-RA remains to be defined as stated by the MASCC. However, the NCCN guidelines advised the application of aprepitant at least the first three days in analogy to high emetogenic chemotherapy. Furthermore, the NCCN guidelines explicitly mentioned palonosetron in this setting.

REFERENCES

1. Herrstedt J. Nausea and emesis: still an unsolved problem in cancer patients? Support Care Cancer 2002; 10:85–87.
2. Kris MG, Hesketh PJ, Somerfield MR, et al. American Society of Clinical Oncology guideline for antiemetics in oncology: update 2006. J Clin Oncol 2006; 24:2932–2947.
3. Roila F, Hesketh PJ, Herrstedt J. Prevention of chemotherapy- and radiotherapy-induced emesis: results of the 2004 Perugia International Antiemetic Consensus Conference. Ann Oncol 2006; 17:20–28.

4. NCCN. National Comprehensive Cancer Network: Antiemesis, Clinical Practice Guidelines in Oncology, 2007 edition; v.1.
5. Grunberg SM, Osoba D, Hesketh PJ, et al. Evaluation of new antiemetic agents and definition of antineoplastic agent emetogenicity: an update. Support Care Cancer 2005; 13:80–84.
6. Jordan K, Grothey A, Kegel T, et al. Antiemetic efficacy of an oral suspension of granisetron plus dexamethasone and influence of quality of life on risk for nausea and vomiting. Onkologie 2005; 28:88–92.
7. Osoba D, Zee B, Pater J, et al. Determinants of postchemotherapy nausea and vomiting in patients with cancer. Quality of Life and Symptom Control Committees of the National Cancer Institute of Canada Clinical Trials Group. J Clin Oncol 1997; 15:116–123.
8. Hesketh PJ, Grunberg SM, Gralla RJ, et al. The oral neurokinin-1 antagonist aprepitant for the prevention of chemotherapy-induced nausea and vomiting: a multinational, randomized, double-blind, placebo-controlled trial in patients receiving high-dose cisplatin—the Aprepitant Protocol 052 Study Group. J Clin Oncol 2003; 21:4112–4119.
9. Poli-Bigelli S, Rodrigues-Pereira J, Carides AD, et al. Addition of the neurokinin 1 receptor antagonist aprepitant to standard antiemetic therapy improves control of chemotherapy-induced nausea and vomiting. Results from a randomized, double-blind, placebo-controlled trial in Latin America. Cancer 2003; 97:3090–3098.
10. Morrow GR, Roscoe JA. Anticipatory nausea and vomiting: models, mechanisms and management. In: Dicato MA, ed. Medical Management of Cancer Treatment Induced Emesis, Edition London1998:149–166.
11. Leslie RA. Comparative aspects of the area postrema: fine-structural considerations help to determine its function. Cell Mol Neurobiol 1986; 6:95–120.
12. Kris MG, Hesketh PJ, Herrstedt J, et al. Consensus proposals for the prevention of acute and delayed vomiting and nausea following high-emetic-risk chemotherapy. Support Care Cancer 2005; 13:85–96.
13. Gralla RJ, Osoba D, Kris MG, et al. Recommendations for the use of antiemetics: evidence-based, clinical practice guidelines. Am Soc Clin Oncol J Clin Oncol 1999; 17:2971–2994.
14. Ettinger DS, Dwight D, Kris M. National Comprehensive Cancer Network: Antiemesis, Clinical Practice Guidelines in Oncology. In Edition 1. Jenkintown: NCCN 2005.
15. Jordan K, Hinke A, Grothey A, et al. A meta-analysis comparing the efficacy of four 5-HT3-receptor antagonists for acute chemotherapy-induced emesis. Support Care Cancer 2007; 15:1023–1033.
16. Eisenberg P, Figueroa-Vadillo J, Zamora R, et al. Improved prevention of moderately emetogenic chemotherapy-induced nausea and vomiting with palonosetron, a pharmacologically novel 5-HT3 receptor antagonist: results of a phase III, single-dose trial versus dolasetron. Cancer 2003; 98:2473–2482.
17. Gralla R, Lichinitser M, Van Der Vegt S, et al. Palonosetron improves prevention of chemotherapy-induced nausea and vomiting following moderately emetogenic chemotherapy: results of a double-blind randomized phase III trial comparing single doses of palonosetron with ondansetron. Ann Oncol 2003; 14:1570–1577.
18. Goodin S, Cunningham R. 5-HT(3)-receptor antagonists for the treatment of nausea and vomiting: a reappraisal of their side-effect profile. Oncologist 2002; 7:424–436.

19. Navari RM, Koeller JM. Electrocardiographic and cardiovascular effects of the 5-hydroxytryptamine3 receptor antagonists. Ann Pharmacother 2003; 37:1276–1286.
20. Hursti TJ, Fredrikson M, Steineck G, et al. Endogenous cortisol exerts antiemetic effect similar to that of exogenous corticosteroids. Br J Cancer 1993; 68:112–114.
21. Scott SM, Rogers C, Backstrom C. Dexamethasone therapy is associated with a rise in urinary epidermal growth factor concentrations in the preterm infant. Eur J Endocrinol 1995; 132:326–330.
22. Italian Group for Antiemetic Research. Double-blind, dose-finding study of four intravenous doses of dexamethasone in the prevention of cisplatin-induced acute emesis. J Clin Oncol 1998; 16:2937–2942.
23. Italian Group for Antiemetic Research. Randomized, double-blind, dose-finding study of dexamethasone in preventing acute emesis induced by anthracyclines, carboplatin, or cyclophosphamide. J Clin Oncol 2004; 22:725–729.
24. Herrstedt J, Koeller JM, Roila F, et al. Acute emesis: moderately emetogenic chemotherapy. Support Care Cancer 2005; 13:97–103.
25. Vardy J, Chiew KS, Galica J, et al. Side effects associated with the use of dexamethasone for prophylaxis of delayed emesis after moderately emetogenic chemotherapy. Br J Cancer 2006; 94:1011–1015.
26. Herr I, Ucur E, Herzer K, et al. Glucocorticoid cotreatment induces apoptosis resistance toward cancer therapy in carcinomas. Cancer Res 2003; 63:3112–3120.
27. Warr DG, Hesketh PJ, Gralla RJ, et al. Efficacy and tolerability of aprepitant for the prevention of chemotherapy-induced nausea and vomiting in patients with breast cancer after moderately emetogenic chemotherapy. J Clin Oncol 2005; 23:2822–2830.
28. Diemunsch P, Grelot L. Potential of substance P antagonists as antiemetics. Drugs 2000; 60:533–546.
29. Hargreaves R. Imaging substance P receptors (NK1) in the living human brain using positron emission tomography. J Clin Psychiatr 2002; 63(suppl 11):18–24.
30. Chawla SP, Grunberg SM, Gralla RJ, et al. Establishing the dose of the oral NK1 antagonist aprepitant for the prevention of chemotherapy-induced nausea and vomiting. Cancer 2003; 97:2290–2300.
31. Nygren P, Hande K, Petty KJ, et al. Lack of effect of aprepitant on the pharmacokinetics of docetaxel in cancer patients. Cancer Chemother Pharmacol 2005; 55:609–616.
32. Loos WJ, de Wit R, Freedman SJ, et al. Aprepitant when added to a standard antiemetic regimen consisting of ondansetron and dexamethasone does not affect vinorelbine pharmacokinetics in cancer patients. Cancer Chemother Pharmacol 2007; 59:407–412.
33. Van Belle S, Lichinitser MR, Navari RM, et al. Prevention of cisplatin-induced acute and delayed emesis by the selective neurokinin-1 antagonists, L-758,298 and MK-869. Cancer 2002; 94:3032–3041.
34. Merck&Co. Emend [package literature]. In Edition Merck& Co., 2003.
35. Antiemetic Subcommittee of the Multinational Association of Supportive Care in Cancer (MASCC). Prevention of chemotherapy- and radiotherapy-induced emesis: results of Perugia Consensus Conference. Ann Oncol 1998; 9:811–819.
36. Moreno I, Rosell R, Abad A, et al. Comparison of three protracted antiemetic regimens for the control of delayed emesis in cisplatin-treated patients. Eur J Cancer 1992; 28A:1344–1347.

37. Kris MG, Gralla RJ, Tyson LB, et al. Controlling delayed vomiting: double-blind, randomized trial comparing placebo, dexamethasone alone, and metoclopramide plus dexamethasone in patients receiving cisplatin. J Clin Oncol 1989; 7:108–114.
38. Gralla RJ, Itri LM, Pisko SE, et al. Antiemetic efficacy of high-dose metoclopramide: randomized trials with placebo and prochlorperazine in patients with chemotherapy-induced nausea and vomiting. NEJM 1981; 305:905–909.
39. Gralla RJ, Tyson LB, Bordin LA, et al. Antiemetic therapy: a review of recent studies and a report of a random assignment trial comparing metoclopramide with delta-9-tetrahydrocannabinol. Cancer Treat Rep 1984; 68:163–172.
40. Herrstedt J. Chemotherapy-induced nausea and vomiting with special emphasis on metopimazine. Dan Med Bull 1998; 45:412–422.
41. Sigsgaard T, Herrstedt J, Handberg J, et al. Ondansetron plus metopimazine compared with ondansetron plus metopimazine plus prednisolone as antiemetic prophylaxis in patients receiving multiple cycles of moderately emetogenic chemotherapy. J Clin Oncol 2001; 19:2091–2097.
42. Herrstedt J, Sigsgaard T, Handberg J, et al. Randomized, double-blind comparison of ondansetron versus ondansetron plus metopimazine as antiemetic prophylaxis during platinum-based chemotherapy in patients with cancer. J Clin Oncol 1997; 15:1690–1696.
43. Herrstedt J, Sigsgaard T, Boesgaard M, et al. Ondansetron plus metopimazine compared with ondansetron alone in patients receiving moderately emetogenic chemotherapy. NEJM 1993; 328:1076–1080.
44. Sigsgaard T, Herrstedt J, Andersen LJ, et al. Granisetron compared with prednisolone plus metopimazine as anti-emetic prophylaxis during multiple cycles of moderately emetogenic chemotherapy. Br J Cancer 1999; 80:412–418.
45. Kwiatkowska M, Parker LA, Burton P, et al. A comparative analysis of the potential of cannabinoids and ondansetron to suppress cisplatin-induced emesis in the Suncus murinus (house musk shrew). Psychopharmacology (Berl) 2004; 174:254–259.
46. Radbruch L, Nauck F. Review of cannabinoids in the treatment of nausea and vomiting. Schmerz 2004; 18:306–310.
47. Williams PI, Higgs A. Effect of nabilone on nausea and vomiting. Br J Anaesth 1995; 74:111; author reply 111–112.
48. Kris MG, Hesketh PJ, Somerfield MR, et al. American Society of Clinical Oncology Guideline for Antiemetics in Oncology: Update 2006. J Clin Oncol 2006; 24:2932–2947.
49. Aapro MS, Molassiotis A, Olver I. Anticipatory nausea and vomiting. Support Care Cancer 2005; 13:117–121.
50. Watts JC, Brierly A. Midazolam for treatment of postoperative nausea. Anaesthesia 2001; 56:1129.
51. Mandala M, Cremonesi M, Rocca A, et al. Midazolam for acute emesis refractory to dexamethasone and granisetron after highly emetogenic chemotherapy: a phase II study. Support Care Cancer 2005; 13:375–380.
52. Bymaster FP, Calligaro DO, Falcone JF, et al. Radioreceptor binding profile of the atypical antipsychotic olanzapine. Neuropsychopharmacology 1996; 14:87–96.
53. Navari RM, Einhorn LH, Loehrer Sr., PJ, et al. A phase II trial of olanzapine, dexamethasone, and palonosetron for the prevention of chemotherapy-induced nausea and vomiting: a Hoosier oncology group study. Support Care Cancer 2007; 15:1285–1291.
54. Passik SD, Navari RM, Jung SH, et al. A phase I trial of olanzapine (Zyprexa) for the prevention of delayed emesis in cancer patients: a Hoosier Oncology Group study. Cancer Invest 2004; 22:383–388.

55. Sharma SS, Gupta YK. Reversal of cisplatin-induced delay in gastric emptying in rats by ginger (*Zingiber officinale*). J Ethnopharmacol 1998; 62:49–55.
56. Dupuis LL, Nathan PC. Options for the prevention and management of acute chemotherapy-induced nausea and vomiting in children. Paediatr Drugs 2003; 5:597–613.
57. Manusirivithaya S, Sripramote M, Tangjitgamol S, et al. Antiemetic effect of ginger in gynecologic oncology patients receiving cisplatin. Int J Gynecol Cancer 2004; 14:1063–1069.
58. Koretz RL, Rotblatt M. Complementary and alternative medicine in gastroenterology: the good, the bad, and the ugly. Clin Gastroenterol Hepatol 2004; 2:957–967.
59. Tate S. Peppermint oil: a treatment for postoperative nausea. J Adv Nurs 1997; 26:543–549.
60. Grunberg SM, Deuson RR, Mavros P, et al. Incidence of chemotherapy-induced nausea and emesis after modern antiemetics. Cancer 2004; 100:2261–2268.

11

Mucositis in Patients Receiving High-Dose Cancer Therapy

Douglas E. Peterson and Rajesh V. Lalla
Section of Oral Medicine, Department of Oral Health and Diagnostic Sciences and Head & Neck/ Oral Oncology Program, Neag Comprehensive Cancer Center, University of Connecticut Health Center, Farmington, Connecticut, U.S.A.

INTRODUCTION

There have been multiple strategic advances associated with mucositis research and management in the past 10 years. Mucositis is no longer an orphan toxicity to be inevitably tolerated as a consequence of high-dose cancer therapy. Based on the collective advances, including those described below, it may become possible in the coming years to customize the delivery of molecularly targeted drugs to prevent and treat the toxicity.

The trajectory of mucositis research and its clinical applications has been robust over the past 15 years, following the National Institutes of Health (NIH) 1989 Consensus Development Conference titled "Oral Complications of Cancer Therapies: Diagnosis, Prevention and Treatment" (1). Oral mucositis was specifically highlighted at the conference as a toxicity for which further research and novel therapeutic models were needed. A new pathobiologic model for oral mucositis was established in 1998 (2). An additional NIH conference in 2000 highlighted research strategies based on models of healthy and diseased oral and gastrointestinal (GI) mucosa in the cancer patient (3). This modeling was then framed in the concept of alimentary tract mucositis (4).

The clinical translation of this paradigm has been noteworthy as well, in recent years. The first molecularly targeted drug, palifermin (keratinocyte growth factor-1) was approved by the U.S. Food and Drug Administration (FDA) in 2004; other drugs continue in pipeline development. An international panel of clinicians and researchers with experience in the toxicity has produced evidence-based guidelines for oral and GI mucositis (5,6). In 1996, "mucositis" was added to the United States Library of Medicine MeSH library of search terms, and can thus be utilized for cataloguing of articles identified via MEDLINE/PubMed as related to mucosal injury associated with cancer therapies.

In sum, this collective evolution of the mucositis paradigm, including identification in gaps in knowledge, new molecular models for pathogenesis, development of molecularly targeted drugs, and contemporary guidelines for clinical practice, represent key advances over the past several years.

This chapter will address the clinical and economic significance, pathobiology, clinical features, and management of mucositis. It will also highlight current research directions that may lead to safe and effective strategies for prevention and treatment in the future. Much of this chapter will focus on oral mucositis, since a large part of the basic and clinical research on this toxicity has been on the upper aerodigestive tract.

ORAL MUCOSITIS

Oral mucositis refers to inflammation of the oral mucosa caused by cytotoxic cancer therapy including high-dose chemotherapy or ionizing head/neck radiation. The lesion typically manifests as erythematous and ulcerative lesions of the oral mucosa. The condition may be exacerbated by trauma, infection, poor oral hygiene, and other local factors.

As described below, pain is a prominent component of oral mucositis and accounts for a considerable number of the supportive care interventions required to manage the patient when moderate to severe mucosal toxicity develops. Complications include impairment of oral hygiene and nutritional intake, need for opioid narcotic management, and overall compromised quality of life. The patients with severe oral mucositis often require hospitalization in order to manage the collective range of toxicities. In some cases, oral mucositis can be a dose-limiting complication of cancer therapy.

Morbidity of Mucositis

Incidence and severity of oral mucositis in cancer patients varies, depending upon the cancer treatment regimens being utilized. For example, virtually all head and neck cancer patients receiving approximately 6,000 to 7,000 cGy over six to seven weeks develop severe oral mucositis. Oral mucositis incidence and severity is especially elevated in patients with primary tumors involving the oral cavity, oropharynx or nasopharynx, as well as patients who receive higher total doses and hyperfractionated radiation schedules (7,8). The majority of patients receiving radiation therapy for head and neck cancer are unable to continue eating by mouth due to mucositis pain and the need to receive nutrition via a gastrostomy tube or intravenous line. Patients with oral mucositis are significantly more likely to have severe pain and a weight loss of $\geq 5\%$ (8). Ulcerations of radiation therapy–induced oral mucositis may also become secondarily infected and lead to systemic infection, especially in patients who are immunosuppressed due to concomitant chemotherapy. In one study, approximately 16% of patients receiving radiation therapy for head and neck cancer were hospitalized due to mucositis (9). Further, 11% of the patients receiving radiation therapy for head and neck cancer had unplanned breaks in radiation therapy due to severe mucositis (9). Oral mucositis can thus be a major dose-limiting toxicity of radiation therapy to the head and neck region.

Oral mucositis is also a significant problem in patients undergoing chemotherapeutic management for solid tumors. In one study, it was reported that 303 of 599 patients receiving chemotherapy for solid tumors or lymphoma developed oral and/or GI mucositis. Oral mucositis developed in 22% of 1236 cycles of chemotherapy, GI mucositis in 7% of cycles, and both oral and GI mucositis in 8% of cycles (10). Importantly, a reduction in the next dose of chemotherapy was twice as common after cycles with mucositis than after cycles without mucositis (10). Thus, mucositis can be a dose-limiting toxicity of cancer chemotherapy with direct effects on patient survival. Single protocol chemotherapeutic drugs that frequently cause oral mucositis include methotrexate, doxorubicin, 5-fluorouracil (5-FU), busulfan, and bleomycin. Multidrug regimens can cause increased risk for clinically significant mucositis as compared to single agent regimens. For example, 5-FU, with or without leucovorin, is associated with a 22% incidence of oral mucositis only, 8% incidence of GI mucositis only, and a 16% incidence of both oral and GI mucositis (10). Most anthracycline-based regimens are associated with an approximately 10% risk of clinically significant oral mucositis, except when the regimen includes 5-FU. Thus, the combination of docetaxel with 5-FU is associated with a much higher risk of clinically significant oral mucositis, in the range of 58 to 74% (11).

Oral mucositis is also a frequent, serious toxicity of conditioning chemotherapy prior to hematopoietic cell transplant (HCT). Approximately 80% of patients who receive high-dose chemotherapy or chemoradiotherapy as conditioning prior to HCT develop clinically significant oral mucositis (12). Oral mucositis can be very painful and can significantly affect nutritional intake, mouth care, oral function, and quality of life (13). For patients receiving intensive myeloablative conditioning regimes prior to HCT, oral mucositis has been reported to be the single most debilitating complication (14). In patients with hematologic malignancies receiving allogeneic HCT, severity of oral mucositis was found to be significantly associated with the number of days of total parenteral nutrition and parenteral narcotic therapy, number of days with fever, incidence of significant infection, time in hospital, and total inpatient charges (12). In addition, oral mucositis may contribute to an overall constellation of symptom burden in cancer patients, analogous to modeling reported in cohorts such as those receiving autologous HCT (15).

Economic Impact of Mucositis

Chemotherapy patients who have significant oral mucositis typically require several supportive care measures such as use of total parenteral nutrition, fluid replacement, and prophylaxis against infections. These can add substantially to the total cost of care. For example, in patients receiving chemotherapy for solid tumors or lymphoma, the estimated cost of hospitalization was $3893 per chemotherapy cycle without mucositis, $6277 per cycle with oral mucositis and $9132 per cycle with both oral and GI mucositis (10). A single point increase in peak mucositis scores in HCT patients is associated with one additional day of fever, a 2.1-fold increase in risk of significant infection, 2.7 additional days of total parenteral nutrition, 2.6 additional days of injectable narcotic therapy, 2.6 additional days in hospital and a 3.9-fold increase in 100-day mortality risk, collectively contributing to over $25,000 in additional hospital charges (16). Radiation-induced oral mucositis also has a significant economic impact due to costs associated with pain management, liquid diet supplements, gastrostomy tube placement or total parenteral nutrition, management of secondary infections and hospitalizations. In one study of patients receiving radiation therapy for head and neck cancer, oral mucositis was associated with an increase in costs ranging from $1700 to $6000 per patient, depending on the grade of oral mucositis (8).

Pathogenesis

The oral mucosa is a complex physical and chemical barrier that, when functioning normally, provides critical defense against pathogens and other challenges. Recent studies have indicated that the fundamental mechanisms involved in mucositis pathogenesis are much more complex than direct damage to epithelium alone (17). The current pathobiologic model of oral mucositis incorporates five stages (11,18) (Fig. 1). While these steps are presented in a linear fashion, it is important to recognize that the damage actually occurs with both simultaneous and sequential patterns of damage. Furthermore, the whole process will be repeated with each successive administration of chemotherapy.

1. *Initiation of tissue injury*: Radiation and/or chemotherapy cause cellular damage resulting in clonogenic cell death of the basal epithelial cells. Generation of reactive oxygen species by radiation or chemotherapy is also believed to exert a role in the initiation of mucosal injury.

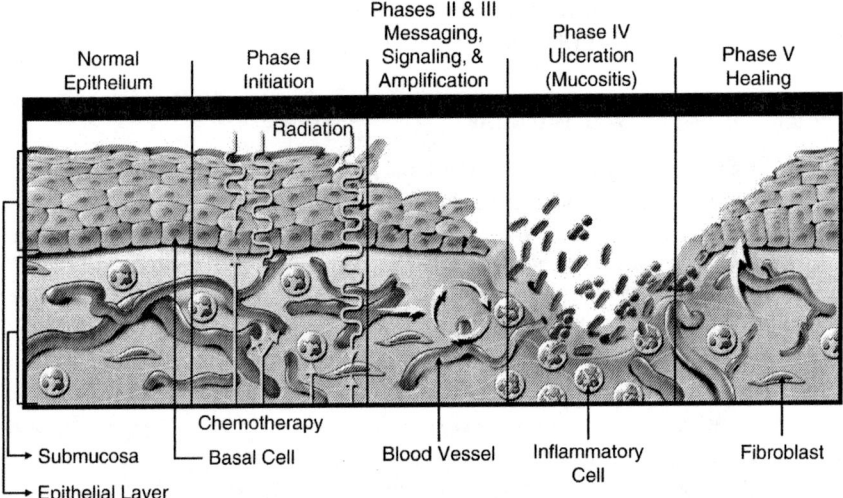

Figure 1 Five-phase model for the pathogenesis of oral mucositis. *Source*: From Ref. 49.

2. *Upregulation via generation of messenger signals*: In addition to causing direct cell death, radiation or chemotherapy may also induce activation of second messengers such as ceramide. Activation of these second messengers can lead to upregulation in production of proinflammatory cytokines as well as tissue injury and cell death.
3. *Signaling and amplification*: Upregulation of proinflammatory cytokines such as tumor necrosis factor-alpha (TNF-α causes injury to mucosal cells, and also activates molecular pathways that amplify mucosal injury.
4. *Ulceration and inflammation*: There is a significant inflammatory cell infiltrate associated with the mucosal ulcerations, theorized to be based in part on metabolic byproducts of colonizing microflora. Production of proinflammatory cytokines is also further upregulated (19).
5. *Healing*: Renewal of epithelial proliferation as well as cellular and tissue differentiation are hallmarks of this phase (20). It is important to note, however, that the appearance of the clinically normal mucosa, particularly in the early weeks post-resolution, does not necessarily indicate normalcy of subclinical cellular and tissue function.

The collective interactions of these parameters, coupled with underlying genetic governance, are thus postulated to govern risk, clinical trajectory and severity of mucosal injury secondary to cancer therapy (18). Enhanced understanding of this paradigm may identify novel strategies for mucositis prevention and treatment. For example, recent studies have indicated that pathways associated with COX-2, NF-κB, toll-like receptor, P13k/Akt, IL-6, and p38 MAPK are upregulated in oral mucositis. These genes and/or their gene products may thus represent potential therapeutic targets (21,22).

Clinical Course of Oral Mucositis

Oral mucositis typically presents as erythema of the oral mucosa, with progression to erosion and ulceration over the next 7 to 10 days depending on the intensity of the cancer therapy. The ulcerations may be covered by a white pseudomembrane. Oral mucositis lesions are usually limited to nonkeratinized areas of the mouth such as the lateral and ventral tongue, buccal mucosa, and soft palate. Histologic changes associated with these clinical findings most commonly include vascular inflammation, collagen degeneration, and epithelial atrophy.

Selected agents such as antimetabolites and alkylating agents cause a higher incidence and severity of oral mucositis (23). Patients who experience oral mucositis during one course of chemotherapy often experience mucositis of similar extent and location during subsequent courses of the same regimen. Mucositis will generally peak between 6 and 12 days after the last dose of chemotherapy and will typically resolve between 10 and 18 days after cessation of chemotherapy. Resolution of oral toxicity, including mucositis and infection, usually coincides with neutrophil recovery. However, this relationship may be temporally but not causally related. Hypothetically, neutrophil recovery could promote control of oral microflora invading into ulcerated tissues, mitigate damage that the microflora induce, and thus enhance mucosal healing. This concept is supported by studies examining the effect of granulocyte macrophage colony-stimulating factor on oral mucositis where the hematopoietic growth factor did not affect severity of mucositis, but appeared to promote more rapid healing. This and related theoretic relationships warrant further investigation (24).

Similar but not identical modeling exists relative to oral mucositis in HCT patients. The first three weeks following HCT are the most risky period for development of clinically significant oral mucositis. During the neutropenic phase, oral complications arise primarily from direct and indirect stomatotoxic toxicities associated with high-dose chemotherapy or chemoradiotherapy and their sequel. Mucositis, xerostomia, and those lesions related to myelosuppression, thrombocytopenia, and anemia predominate. This phase is typically the period of high prevalence and severity of oral complications. Oral mucositis usually begins 7 to 10 days after initiation of cytotoxic therapy, and remains present for approximately two to three weeks after stem cell infusion. Viral, fungal, and bacterial infections may arise, with incidence depending on use of prophylactic regimens, oral status prior to chemotherapy, and duration/severity of neutropenia. The frequency of infection declines upon resolution of mucositis and increasing neutrophil engraftment. However, the patient may remain at risk for infection depending on the status of overall immune reconstitution.

In radiation-induced oral mucositis, lesions are limited to the tissues in the field of radiation, with nonkeratinized tissues affected more often. Lesions are

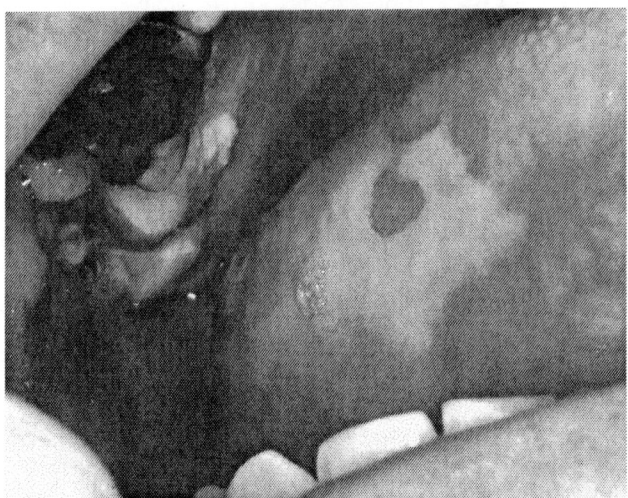

Figure 2 Extensive mucositis ulcer involving the right lateral and ventral tongue. This patient had received 5200 cGy of a total planned regimen of 7200 cGy radiation therapy with concurrent chemotherapy for treatment of a squamous cell carcinoma of the right tongue. The patient was not able to ingest any food by mouth, and was being fed through a gastrostomy tube. He was receiving topical lidocaine mouthrinse as well as systemic opioid analgesics. The oral mucositis also affected the patient's ability to perform mouth care, as evidenced by plaque accumulation on the maxillary molars adjacent to the lesion.

similar in appearance to those caused by chemotherapy (Fig. 2). The clinical severity is directly proportional to the dose of radiation administered. Most patients who have received more than 50 Gy to the oral mucosa will develop severe ulcerative oral mucositis (25). Ulcerations may not completely resolve clinically until several weeks after high-dose radiation therapy has ended.

Measurement of Oral Mucositis

A wide variety of scales have been used to record the extent and severity of oral mucositis in clinical practice and research. The World Health Organization (WHO) scale is a simple, user-friendly scale suitable for daily use in clinical practice. This scale combines both subjective and objective measures of oral mucositis (Table 1). The National Cancer Institute (NCI) Common Terminology Criteria for Adverse Events (CTCAE) version 3.0 includes separate subjective and objective scales for mucositis (Table 2). The Oral Mucositis Assessment Scale (OMAS) is an objective scale that measures erythema and ulceration at nine different sites in the oral cavity. This scale was validated in a multicenter trial with high inter-observer reproducibility and strong correlation of objective mucositis scores with patient symptoms (26).

Table 1 World Health Organization (WHO) Scale for Oral Mucositis

Grade 0 = no oral mucositis
Grade 1 = erythema and soreness
Grade 2 = ulcers, able to eat solids
Grade 3 = ulcers, requires liquid diet (due to mucositis)
Grade 4 = ulcers, alimentation not possible (due to mucositis)

Source: http://www.fda.gov/cder/cancer/toxicityframe.htm

Table 2 National Cancer Institute (NCI) Common Terminology Criteria for Adverse Events (CTCAE) Version 3.0

Oral mucositis (clinical exam)
  Grade 1 = Erythema of the mucosa
  Grade 2 = Patchy ulcerations or pseudomembranes
  Grade 3 = Confluent ulcerations or pseudomembranes; bleeding with minor trauma
  Grade 4 = Tissue necrosis; significant spontaneous bleeding; life-threatening consequences
  Grade 5 = Death
Oral mucositis (functional/symptomatic)
  Grade 1 = Minimal symptoms, normal diet
  Grade 2 = Symptomatic but can eat and swallow modified diet
  Grade 3 = Symptomatic and unable to adequately aliment or hydrate orally
  Grade 4 = Symptoms associated with life-threatening consequences
  Grade 5 = Death

Source: http://www.fda.gov/cder/cancer/toxicityframe.htm

Clinical Management of Oral Mucositis

Pain Management

Pain is a significant component of moderate to severe oral mucositis, and typically results in clinically significant sequel that increase the cost of patient care (27). Given the prominence of this pain, most oral mucositis regimens incorporate a combination of different agents and treatments that can be applied with escalating intensity of pain relief. Basic oral hygiene is the foundation of mucositis management. Bland rinses, often containing sodium bicarbonate, are also initiated to help moisturize oral tissues, rinse away debris, and to provide symptomatic relief for mild mucositis. As mucosal breakdown and pain increase, topical anesthetics can be added. A wide variety of topical agents are available, ranging from antihistamines (e.g., diphenhydramine), anesthetics (e.g., lidocaine, benzocaine), and analgesics (e.g., benzydamine, doxepin). Topical, directed application of anesthetic agents allows the patient to concentrate the anesthetic effect to the most symptomatic oral sites. The most common complication associated with topical anesthetic use is inadvertent mucosal damage due to trauma and irritation when trying to eat or perform oral hygiene when mouth is numb. Generalized oral rinsing/gargling with anesthetics also carries the risk of impairing the gag reflex due to oropharyngeal anesthesia, which can result in aspiration and pneumonia. Therefore, local application to areas of ulceration may be more appropriate than extensive oral rinsing.

Many centers empirically utilize oral rinses that are compounded by combining a number of agents. These rinses will often include topical anesthetic agents (lidocaine, diphenhydramine, etc.), a coating agent (e.g., antacid or kaolin solution) and an antifungal (nystatin solution). Before prescribing these combinations, it is reasonable to consider (1) the degree to which the patient will benefit from the multiple agents compounded in the rinse, (2) tolerability of the product by the patient (e.g., taste, texture, physical appearance), and (3) cost effectiveness of the multiagent compounded rinse in relation to a single agent (e.g., viscous lidocaine).

Systemic pain medications represent the highest step of mucositis pain management; these drugs can be utilized either with or without bland rinses and topical anesthetics. Systemic pain medications, especially opioids, are indicated when bland rinses and topical anesthetic fail to produce sufficient pain relief. Opiates including hydromorphone, meperidine, and time-release oral or intravenous morphine and fentanyl (intravenous, transdermal patches, and oral transmucosal) can be used. Morphine has generally been the most frequently utilized agent for inpatients and has been found to be extremely effective when administered with patient-controlled analgesia. A detailed discussion of these specific pain management strategies may be found in the Chapter 17.

Nutritional Support

Nutrition in the cancer patient with oral mucositis is also an important concern. Nutritional intake can be severely compromised by the pain associated with severe oral mucositis. In addition, taste changes can also occur secondary to chemotherapy and/or radiation therapy (28,29). It is very important that the patient's nutritional intake and weight be monitored by a dietician or other professional working together with family caregivers. Soft diet and/or liquid diet supplements are more easily tolerated during mucositis. In patients expected to develop severe mucositis, a gastrostomy tube is sometimes placed prophylactically.

The following guidelines can be used to mitigate difficulties with nutritional intake:

1. Eat a bland diet, avoiding spiced, acidic, or salted foods.
2. Avoid foods with coarse texture, using blenderized foods if necessary.
3. Avoid extremely hot or cold foods.
4. Supply added calories and nutrients by drinking shakes prepared with nutritional supplements or ice cream.
5. Chew sugar-free gum or sugar-free hard candy to stimulate saliva if xerostomia is a problem.

6. Use nasogastric or nasoduodenal tube feedings, or total parenteral nutrition if necessary.
7. Use antiemetics as indicated.

Therapeutic Interventions

Establishment of a pathophysiologic model has contributed to significant research devoted to development of agents that extend beyond symptom management, and target molecular pathways associated with causation (30). The advances in molecularly based pharmacologic approaches have been complemented by development of evidence-based guidelines by the Mucositis Study Group of the Multinational Association for Supportive Care in Cancer and the International Society of Oral Oncology (MASCC/ISOO) (5). These guidelines are based on extensive, evidence-based reviews utilizing American Society of Clinical Oncology criteria. The guidelines are referenced below as applicable, and are summarized in Table 3.

Mouth Care. Maintenance of effective oral hygiene has been reported to result in both reduced incidence and severity of oral mucositis (31–33). Multiple studies have demonstrated that good oral hygiene plays an important role in the management of oral mucositis (31–33). Therefore, a mouth care protocol should be incorporated into management strategies for oral mucositis. The MASCC/ISOO guidelines recommend as good clinical practice the use of a standardized oral care protocol including brushing with a soft toothbrush, flossing, and the use of nonmedicated rinses (e.g., saline, sodium bicarbonate rinse). It is important that patients, staff, and caregivers be educated about the importance of good oral hygiene (34).

Cryotherapy. Multiple studies have indicated that the use of cryotherapy in patients receiving bolus doses of chemotherapeutic agents with short half-lives reduces the severity of oral mucositis. It has been hypothesized that topical administration of ice chips to the oral cavity during administration of chemotherapy results in decreased delivery of the chemotherapeutic agent to the oral mucosa. This effect may be mediated through local vasoconstriction and reduced blood flow. Several studies have demonstrated that cryotherapy reduces the severity of oral mucositis in patients receiving bolus doses of chemotherapeutic agents. For example, 5-FU has a short plasma half-life (5–20 min); thus oral cryotherapy is well suited to reduce the risk of mucositis secondary to bolus administration regimens of this agent. The MASCC/ISOO guidelines recommend use of cryotherapy to reduce oral mucositis in patients receiving bolus doses of 5-fluorouracil, melphalan, and edatrexate (35). Ice chips are placed in the mouth, beginning 5 minutes before administration of chemotherapy and replenished as needed, usually for up to 30 minutes.

Table 3 Summary of Evidence-based MASCC/ISOO Clinical Practice Guidelines for Care of Patients with Oral and/or Gastrointestinal Mucositis

I. Oral Mucositis
Basic oral care and good clinical practices
1. The panel suggests the following
    Oral care protocols which include patient and staff education should be used to attempt to reduce the severity of oral mucositis from chemotherapy and/or radiation therapy.
    Protocol development should be multidisciplinary and that the impact of the oral care and educational protocols should be evaluated.
    The oral care protocol should include use of a soft toothbrush that is replaced on a regular basis. Elements of good clinical practice should include the regular assessment, using validated tools, of oral pain, and oral cavity health status. Inclusion of dental professionals is vital throughout the treatment and follow-up phases.
2. The panel recommends patient-controlled analgesia with morphine as the treatment of choice for oral mucositis pain in patients undergoing HCT. Regular oral pain assessment using validated instruments for self-report is essential.

Radiotherapy: prevention
3. To reduce mucosal injury, the panel recommends the use of midline radiation blocks and three-dimensional radiation treatment.
4. The panel recommends benzydamine for prevention of radiation-induced mucositis in patients with head and neck cancer receiving moderate-dose radiation therapy.
5. The panel recommends that chlorhexidine *not* be used to prevent oral mucositis in patients with solid tumors of the head and neck who are undergoing radiotherapy.
6. It is recommended that antimicrobial lozenges *not* be used for the prevention of radiation-induced oral mucositis.

Radiotherapy: treatment
7. It is recommended that sucralfate not be used for the treatment of radiation-induced oral mucositis

Standard-dose chemotherapy: prevention
8. The panel recommends that patients receiving bolus 5-FU chemotherapy undergo 30 min of oral cryotherapy to prevent oral mucositis.
9. The panel suggests that 20–30 min of oral cryotherapy be used to attempt to decrease mucositis in patients treated with bolus doses of edatrexate.
10. The panel recommends that acyclovir and its analogues *not be used* routinely to prevent mucositis.

Standard-dose chemotherapy: treatment
11. The panel recommends that chlorhexidine not be used to treat established oral mucositis.

High-dose chemotherapy with or without total body irradiation plus HCT: prevention
12. In patients with hematological malignancies receiving high-dose chemotherapy and total body irradiation with autologous HCT, the panel recommends the use of

(*Continued*)

Table 3 Summary of Evidence-based MASCC/ISOO Clinical Practice Guidelines for Care of Patients with Oral and/or Gastrointestinal Mucositis (*Continued*)

keratinocyte growth factor-1 (Palifermin) in a dose of 60 μg/kg/day for 3 days prior to conditioning treatment and for 3 days post-transplant for the prevention of oral mucositis.

13. The panel suggests the use of cryotherapy to prevent oral mucositis in patients receiving high-dose melphalan.
14. The panel does not recommend the use of pentoxifylline to prevent mucositis in patients undergoing HCT.
15. The panel suggests that GM-CSF mouthwashes *not be used* for the prevention of oral mucositis in patients undergoing HCT.
16. Low-level laser therapy (LLLT) requires expensive equipment and specialized training. Because of interoperator variability, clinical trials are difficult to conduct, and their results are difficult to compare; nevertheless, the panel is encouraged by the accumulating evidence in support of LLLT. The panel suggests that, for centers able to support the necessary technology and training, LLLT be used to attempt to reduce the incidence of oral mucositis and its associated pain in patients receiving high-dose chemotherapy or chemoradiotherapy before HCT.

II. Gastrointestinal mucositis
Basic bowel care and good clinical practices
17. The panel suggests that basic bowel care should include the maintenance of adequate hydration, and that consideration should be given to the potential for transient lactose intolerance, and the presence of bacterial pathogens.

Radiotherapy: prevention
18. The panel suggests the use of 500 mg sulfasalazine orally twice daily to help reduce the incidence and severity of radiation-induced enteropathy in patients receiving external beam radiotherapy to the pelvis.
19. The panel suggests that amifostine in a dose of at least 340 mg/kg may prevent radiation proctitis in those receiving standard-dose radiotherapy for rectal cancer.
20. The panel recommends that oral sucralfate *not be used* to reduce related side effects of radiotherapy; it does not prevent acute diarrhea in patients with pelvic malignancies undergoing external beam radiotherapy, and compared with placebo it is associated with more gastrointestinal side effects, including rectal bleeding.
21. The panel recommends that 5-amino salicylic acid and its related compounds mesalazine and olsalazine *not be used* to prevent GI mucositis.

Radiotherapy: treatment
22. The panel suggests the use of sucralfate enemas to help manage chronic radiation-induced proctitis in patients who have rectal bleeding.

Standard-dose and high-dose chemotherapy: prevention
23. The panel recommends either ranitidine or omeprazole for the prevention of epigastric pain following treatment with cyclophosphamide, methotrexate, and 5-FU or treatment with 5-FU with or without folinic acid chemotherapy.
24. The panel recommends that systemic glutamine *not be used* for the prevention of GI mucositis.

(*Continued*)

Standard-dose and high-dose chemotherapy: treatment
25. When loperamide fails to control diarrhea induced by standard-dose or high-dose chemotherapy associated with HCT, the panel recommends octreotide at a dose of at least 100 μg subcutaneously, twice daily.

Combined chemotherapy and radiotherapy: prevention
26. The panel suggests the use of amifostine to reduce esophagitis induced by concomitant chemotherapy and radiotherapy in patients with non–small-cell lung cancer.

Abbreviations: MASCC/ISOO, Multinational Association for Supportive Care in Cancer/International Society of Oral Oncology; HCT, hematopoietic cell transplant; 5-FU, 5-fluorouracil; GM-CSF, granulocyte macrophage colony-stimulating factor.
Source: From Ref. 5 with permission from John Wiley & Sons, Inc.

Growth factors. A number of growth factors have been studied for the management of oral mucositis, since damage to the proliferative capacity of oral epithelial cells is thought to play a role in the pathogenesis of mucositis. An important advance in mucositis management was achieved in 2004 with the FDA's approval of intravenous recombinant human keratinocyte growth factor-1 (palifermin) as the first-ever agent approved for mucositis. This approval was based on a clinically and statistically significant reduction in oral mucositis in patients undergoing autologous HCT transplant for hematologic malignancies and who received palifermin prior to and immediately after conditioning chemotherapy (36). The MASCC/ISOO guidelines recommend use of palifermin in patients with hematologic malignancies receiving high-dose chemotherapy and total body irradiation before autologous HCT (37).

Interestingly, a related compound, human keratinocyte growth factor-2 (Repifermin, Human Genome Sciences Rockville, MD), was found to be ineffective in reducing the percentage of subjects who experienced severe mucositis (38). Intravenous human fibroblast growth factor-20 (Velafermin, CuraGen Corp. Branford, CT) was in clinical development for mucositis secondary to high-dose chemotherapy in autologous HCT patients (39). However, the company has discontinued further development of Velafermin effective October 2007, based on Phase II results. The safety of this class of growth factors has not been established in patients with nonhematologic malignancies. There is theoretical concern that these growth factors may promote growth of tumor cells, which may have receptors for the respective growth factor. However, one recent study found no significant difference in survival between subjects with colorectal cancer receiving palifermin or placebo at a median follow-up duration of 14.5 months (40). Further studies are warranted to confirm the safety of epithelial growth factors in the solid tumor setting.

Promoters of healing. While use of oral glutamine or the addition of glutamine to intravenous nutritional supplements has been shown to decrease the severity and duration of oral mucositis in some clinical trials, other studies have been unable to show promising results. However, a recent phase III study of L-glutamine administered orally via a proprietary drug-delivery system demonstrated efficacy in reducing incidence and severity of ≥ Grade 2 WHO oral mucositis in breast cancer patients receiving anthracycline-based chemotherapeutic regimens (41). The drug product, Saforis™ (MGI Pharma, Bloomington, MN), is a proprietary oral suspension of L-glutamine that enhances the uptake of this amino acid into epithelial cells. Further study of oral administration of L-glutamine delivered via drug delivery enhancing technology is needed. By comparison, the MASCC/ISOO guidelines recommend that systemically administered glutamine not be used for the prevention of GI mucositis (42).

Antiinflammatory agents. Since evidence supports a role for proinflammatory cytokines in oral mucositis, a wide variety of antiinflammatory agents have been tested. Benzydamine hydrochloride is a nonsteroidal antiinflammatory drug that inhibits proinflammatory cytokines including TNF-α. In one phase III trial, benzydamine hydrochloride mouthrinse reduced severity of mucositis in head and neck cancer patients up to cumulative doses of 50 Gy radiation therapy (43). Based on this and previous studies, the MASCC/ISOO guidelines recommended use of this agent in patients receiving moderate-dose radiation therapy (44). However, this agent has not received approval from the FDA; furthermore, most head and neck cancer patients receive over 50 Gy radiation doses, often with concomitant chemotherapy. A more recent phase III trial of this agent in radiation-induced oral mucositis in head and neck cancer patients was halted on the basis of negative results of an interim analysis.

Antioxidants. Amifostine (Ethyol™, MedImmune, Gaithersburg, MD) is thought to act as a scavenger for harmful reactive oxygen species. Amifostine is a pro-drug that is dephosphorylated in tissues to a free thiol metabolite that can act as a scavenger for reactive oxygen species. Despite numerous studies, results have been inconsistent and there was insufficient evidence of benefit to establish a MASCC/ISOO guideline for oral mucositis in chemotherapy or radiation therapy patients. The use of amifostine was recommended for the prevention of esophagitis in patients receiving chemoradiation for non–small cell lung cancer (45).

EN3285 (Endo Pharmaceuticals, Chadds Ford, PA) consists of the antioxidant *N*-acetylcysteine in a proprietary matrix for topical application in the oral cavity. In a phase II trial in head and neck cancer patients, this agent reduced incidence of severe oral mucositis at 50 Gy radiation therapy (46).

Antimicrobial agents. It has been hypothesized that microbial colonization of oral mucositis lesions exacerbates the severity of oral mucositis. However, clinical trials with antimicrobial agents have generally yielded negative results. The MASCC/ISOO guidelines recommend against the routine use of antimicrobial lozenges or of acyclovir and its analogues to prevent oral mucositis. However, drugs such as acyclovir have a well-established role in prophylaxis and treatment of lesions caused by the herpes viruses. The guidelines also recommend against the use of chlorhexidine mouthrinse to prevent or treat oral mucositis (42).

Topical coating agents. A number of studies have evaluated topical sucralfate for its ability to benefit patients with oral mucositis by topically coating the oral mucosa. Due to inadequate evidence for a beneficial effect in chemotherapy patients, no MASCC/ISOO guideline was possible for this agent. In radiation-induced oral mucositis, adequate evidence was available to develop a guideline against the use of sucralfate. While some oral bioadhesive gels have been approved by the FDA as safe medical devices for use in patients with oral mucositis, there was insufficient evidence of efficacy to develop a MASCC/ISOO guideline for these agents (42).

Laser therapy. The efficacy of intraoral low-level laser therapy to reduce the severity of oral mucositis has been reported by several clinical trials; however, the mechanism by which laser therapy influences mucositis is unknown. Further, clinical trials are generally difficult to compare due to different laser and treatment variables (wavelength, energy density, and administration schedules). Nevertheless, due to the promising data to date the MASCC/ISOO guidelines for chemotherapy patients suggest the use of laser therapy at centers able to support the necessary technology and training (35).

GASTROINTESTINAL MUCOSITIS

Multiple symptoms, including diarrhea as well as nausea and emesis, can be considered as components of the constellation of symptoms associated with GI mucositis. Interestingly and unlike oral mucositis, GI pain is usually not a prominent symptom associated with high-dose chemotherapy. Although there are unique molecular pathways that contribute to each of the GI complications, there is increasing evidence that both global and tissue-specific factors account for mucositis expression (47). In this modeling, gender, race, and underlying systemic disease are examples of global factors, while epithelial histology and tissue architecture, the intrinsic endocrine system, mucosal cellular and tissue function, and local microbial environment represent selected local factors. Recent evidence also highlights the likely central role that gene expression changes over time exert relative to governance of clinical expression of GI mucositis (48). In addition to these novel research directions, there are important current clinical issues that confront the patient and health professional. Specific information relative to these issues is presented in Chapters 10 and 12.

FUTURE DIRECTIONS IN MUCOSITIS RESEARCH

With the advent of a current pathobiologic model, drug development directed to molecular pathways has escalated strategically in the past five years. As described previously in this chapter, palifermin is the first such approved drug; numerous other drugs are in the developmental pipeline.

There is a strategic need to continue research directed to etiopathogenesis as well as to drug development to prevent or reduce the toxicity across a broader cohort of at risk patients. Important basic and clinical research efforts are underway to identify agents capable of reducing or eliminating the oral mucosal injury that characterizes mucositis. The role of biological response modifiers, including epithelial cell mitogens, continues to be under intense investigation, as do other classes of drugs including antiinflammatories. In addition to the active agents themselves, additional research directed to oral drug-delivery technology may lead to strategic improvement of targeting the bioactive agent to the specific tissue compartments at risk.

Based on this collective research, it may become possible to utilize combinations of agents in order to achieve optimal outcomes. For example it may prove useful to (1) initially administer an epithelial growth factor to increase mucosal thickness prior to chemotherapy followed by (2) administration of an inhibitor of epithelial cell cycling to reduce cytotoxicity during chemotherapy along with an antiinflammatory agent to minimize mucosal damage and, then (3) additional administration of an epithelial growth factor following chemotherapy to enhance recovery of normal mucosal thickness. Prevention of ulcerative mucositis using this strategy might in turn ultimately provide the setting for escalating the intensity of cancer therapy, leading to more durable remissions and increased patient survival.

REFERENCES

1. National Institutes of Health Consensus Development Conference on Oral Complications of Cancer Therapies: Diagnosis, prevention, and treatment. Bethesda, Maryland, April 17–19, 1989. NCI Monogr 1990(9):1–184.
2. Sonis ST. Mucositis as a biological process: a new hypothesis for the development of chemotherapy-induced stomatotoxicity. Oral Oncol 1998; 34(1):39–43.
3. Peterson DE, Sonis ST. Future research directions. J Natl Cancer Inst Monogr 2001 (29):3–5.
4. Keefe DM. Gastrointestinal mucositis: a new biological model. Support Care Cancer 2004; 12(1):6–9.
5. Keefe DM, Schubert MM, Elting LS, et al. Updated clinical practice guidelines for the prevention and treatment of mucositis. Cancer 2007; 109(5):820–831.
6. Rubenstein EB, Peterson DE, Schubert M, et al. Clinical practice guidelines for the prevention and treatment of cancer therapy-induced oral and gastrointestinal mucositis. Cancer 2004; 100(9 suppl):2026–2046.
7. Vera-Llonch M, Oster G, Hagiwara M, et al. Oral mucositis in patients undergoing radiation treatment for head and neck carcinoma. Cancer 2006; 106(2):329–336.
8. Elting LS, Cooksley CD, Chambers MS, et al. Risk, outcomes, and costs of radiation-induced oral mucositis among patients with head-and-neck malignancies. Int J Radiat Oncol Biol Phys 2007.
9. Trotti A, Bellm LA, Epstein JB, et al. Mucositis incidence, severity and associated outcomes in patients with head and neck cancer receiving radiotherapy with

or without chemotherapy: a systematic literature review. Radiother Oncol 2003; 66(3):253–262.
10. Elting LS, Cooksley C, Chambers M, et al. The burdens of cancer therapy. Clinical and economic outcomes of chemotherapy-induced mucositis. Cancer 2003; 98(7): 1531–1539.
11. Sonis ST, Elting LS, Keefe D, et al. Perspectives on cancer therapy-induced mucosal injury: pathogenesis, measurement, epidemiology, and consequences for patients. Cancer 2004; 100(S9):1995–2025.
12. Vera-Llonch M, Oster G, Ford CM, et al. Oral mucositis and outcomes of allogeneic hematopoietic stem-cell transplantation in patients with hematologic malignancies. Support Care Cancer 2007; 15(5):491–496.
13. Lalla RV, Sonis ST, Peterson DE. Management of oral mucositis in patients who have cancer. Woo S-B, Treister NS (eds.). Management of the Oncologic Patient. Dent Clin N Am. 2008; 52:61–77.
14. Bellm LA, Epstein JB, Rose-Ped A, et al. Patient reports of complications of bone marrow transplantation. Support Care Cancer 2000; 8(1):33–39.
15. Anderson KO, Giralt SA, Mendoza TR, et al. Symptom burden in patients undergoing autologous stem-cell transplantation. Bone Marrow Transplant 2007; 39(12): 759–766.
16. Sonis ST, Oster G, Fuchs H, et al. Oral mucositis and the clinical and economic outcomes of hematopoietic stem-cell transplantation. J Clin Oncol 2001; 19(8): 2201–2205.
17. Treister N, Sonis S. Mucositis: biology and management. Curr Opin Otolaryngol Head Neck Surg 2007; 15(2):123–129.
18. Anthony L, Bowen J, Garden A, et al. New thoughts on the pathobiology of regimen-related mucosal injury. Support Care Cancer 2006; 14(6):516–518.
19. Sonis ST, Peterson RL, Edwards LJ, et al. Defining mechanisms of action of interleukin-11 on the progression of radiation-induced oral mucositis in hamsters. Oral Oncol 2000; 36(4):373–381.
20. Dorr W, Emmendorfer H, Haide E, et al. Proliferation equivalent of 'accelerated repopulation' in mouse oral mucosa. Int J Radiat Biol 1994; 66(2):157–167.
21. Sonis S, Haddad R, Posner M, et al. Gene expression changes in peripheral blood cells provide insight into the biological mechanisms associated with regimen-related toxicities in patients being treated for head and neck cancers. Oral Oncol 2007; 43(3):289–300.
22. Logan RM, Gibson RJ, Sonis ST, et al. Nuclear factor-kappaB (NF-kappaB) and cyclooxygenase-2 (COX-2) expression in the oral mucosa following cancer chemotherapy. Oral Oncol 2007; 43(4):395–401.
23. Barasch A, Peterson DE. Risk factors for ulcerative oral mucositis in cancer patients: unanswered questions. Oral Oncol 2003; 39(2):91–100.
24. Johnston EM, Crawford J. Hematopoietic growth factors in the reduction of chemotherapeutic toxicity. Semin Oncol 1998; 25(5):552–561.
25. Epstein JB, Gorsky M, Guglietta A, et al. The correlation between epidermal growth factor levels in saliva and the severity of oral mucositis during oropharyngeal radiation therapy. Cancer 2000; 89(11):2258–2265.
26. Sonis ST, Eilers JP, Epstein JB, et al. Validation of a new scoring system for the assessment of clinical trial research of oral mucositis induced by radiation or chemotherapy. Mucositis Study Group. Cancer 1999; 85(10):2103–113.

27. Epstein JB, Elad S, Eliav E, et al. Orofacial pain in cancer: part II—clinical perspectives and management. Journal of dental research 2007; 86(6):506–518.
28. Oral complications of chemotherapy and head/neck radiation. National Cancer Institute, Accessed 10 May, 2007 (http://www.nci.nih.gov/cancerinfo/pdq/supportivecare/oralcomplications/healthprofessional/)
29. Raber-Durlacher J, Barasch A, Peterson DE, et al. Oral Complications and management considerations in patients treated with high-dose cancer chemotherapy. supportive cancer therapy 2004; 1(4):219–229.
30. Lalla RV, Peterson DE. Treatment of mucositis, including new medications. Cancer J 2006; 12(5):348–354.
31. Cheng KK, Molassiotis A, Chang AM, et al. Evaluation of an oral care protocol intervention in the prevention of chemotherapy-induced oral mucositis in paediatric cancer patients. Eur J Cancer 2001; 37(16):2056–2063.
32. Levy-Polack MP, Sebelli P, Polack NL. Incidence of oral complications and application of a preventive protocol in children with acute leukemia. Spec Care Dentist 1998; 18(5):189–193.
33. Borowski B, Benhamou E, Pico JL, et al. Prevention of oral mucositis in patients treated with high-dose chemotherapy and bone marrow transplantation: a randomised controlled trial comparing two protocols of dental care. Eur J Cancer B Oral Oncol 1994; 30B(2):93–97.
34. McGuire DB, Correa ME, Johnson J, et al. The role of basic oral care and good clinical practice principles in the management of oral mucositis. Support Care Cancer 2006; 14(6):541–547.
35. Migliorati CA, Oberle-Edwards L, Schubert M. The role of alternative and natural agents, cryotherapy, and/or laser for management of alimentary mucositis. Support Care Cancer 2006; 14(6):533–540.
36. Spielberger R, Stiff P, Bensinger W, et al. Palifermin for oral mucositis after intensive therapy for hematologic cancers. NEJM 2004; 351(25):2590–2598.
37. von Bultzingslowen I, Brennan MT, Spijkervet FK, et al. Growth factors and cytokines in the prevention and treatment of oral and gastrointestinal mucositis. Support Care Cancer 2006; 14(6):519–527.
38. Human Genome Sciences reports, results of phase 2 clinical trial of Repifermin in patients with cancer therapy-induced mucositis (press release, 2 February, 2004). Rockville, MD, Human Genome Sciences; 2004.
39. Lalla RV. Velafermin (CuraGen). Curr Opin Investig Drugs 2005; 6(11):1179–1185.
40. Rosen LS, Abdi E, Davis ID, et al. Palifermin reduces the incidence of oral mucositis in patients with metastatic colorectal cancer treated with fluorouracil-based chemotherapy. J Clin Oncol 2006; 24(33):5194–5200.
41. Peterson DE, Jones JB, Petit II, RG. Randomized, placebo-controlled trial of Saforis for prevention and treatment of oral mucositis in breast cancer patients receiving anthracycline-based chemotherapy. Cancer 2007; 109(2):322–331.
42. Barasch A, Elad S, Altman A, et al. Antimicrobials, mucosal coating agents, anesthetics, analgesics, and nutritional supplements for alimentary tract mucositis. Support Care Cancer 2006; 14(6):528–532.
43. Epstein JB, Silverman Jr., S, Paggiarino DA, et al. Benzydamine HCl for prophylaxis of radiation-induced oral mucositis: results from a multicenter, randomized, double-blind, placebo- controlled clinical trial. Cancer 2001; 92(4):875–885.

44. Lalla RV, Schubert MM, Bensadoun RJ, et al. Anti-inflammatory agents in the management of alimentary mucositis. Support Care Cancer 2006; 14(6):558–565.
45. Bensadoun RJ, Schubert MM, Lalla RV, et al. Amifostine in the management of radiation-induced and chemo-induced mucositis. Support Care Cancer 2006; 14(6): 566–572.
46. RxKinetix completes its end of phase 2 meeting with the FDA for RK-0202 in oral mucositis and is now moving into phase 3 (press release, March 1, 2006). Boulder, CO: RxKinetix, Inc.; 2006.
47. Keefe DM. Intestinal mucositis: mechanisms and management. Current opinion in oncology 2007; 19(4):323–327.
48. Bowen JM, Gibson RJ, Tsykin A, et al. Gene expression analysis of multiple gastrointestinal regions reveals activation of common cell regulatory pathways following cytotoxic chemotherapy. Int J Cancer 2007; 121(8):1847–1856.
49. Sonis ST. A biological approach to mucositis. J Support Oncol 2004; 2(1):21–32.

12

Diarrhea and Constipation

Joyson Karakunnel and Apurva A. Modi
*National Institutes of Health, Bethesda,
Maryland, U.S.A.*

CONSTIPATION

Introduction

Constipation is an extremely common symptom in the U.S. population as a whole, with the prevalence in advanced cancer patients and in those receiving cancer treatments as high as 55% and 50%, respectively (1). It is associated with a considerable amount of distress in oncology patients, which in turn leads to frequent and recurrent hospital visits. To avoid prolonged and costly hospital admissions, appropriate prevention and treatment guidelines are imperative to improve quality of life in a cost-effective manner.

Definition

Constipation can be defined by the presence of two or more criteria (Rome II criteria) listed below (2). The criteria should be present for at least 12 weeks within the last year, but do not have to be consecutive. There should also be an absence of loose stools and insufficient criteria for diagnosing irritable bowel syndrome (IBS).

1. Straining in at least 25% of defecations
2. Feeling of incomplete evacuation in at least 25% of defecations

3. Hard or lumpy stools in at least 25% of defecations
4. Sensation of anorectal obstruction/blockade in at least 25% of defecations
5. Use of manual maneuvers (e.g., digital evacuation) in at least 25% of defecations
6. Frequency of stools of less than three per week

Etiology

Constipation can be classified as primary, secondary, or iatrogenic.

Primary Causes

Primary constipation results from inadequate fluid intake due to chronic debilitating illnesses, nausea, weakness, or depression. Consumption of diets low in fiber can also exacerbate the problem. The lack of activity resulting from surgery, dramatic weight loss, or lethargy is another primary cause of constipation.

Secondary Causes

The secondary causes can be broadly classified into obstructive lesions of the gastrointestinal tract (strictures, colon cancer, postsurgical lesions), neurogenic (autonomic neuropathy, diabetes, spinal cord injury), metabolic (hypercalcemia, uremia, hypokalemia), and endocrine abnormalities (hypothyroidism, panhypopituitariam).

Iatrogenic Causes

Iatrogenic constipation results from the use of pharmacological agents, chemotherapeutic drugs, and medical intervention. This probably is the most common cause of constipation in individuals with cancer. The drugs commonly involved are non-steroidal alkaloids, antidiarrheals, opiates, anticholinergics, and vinca alkaloids.

Pathophysiology

Constipation can be classified into normal transit constipation, pelvic floor dysfunction, and slow transit constipation. In the largest series of 1000 patients with intractable constipation, 59% had normal colonic transit, 28% had pelvic floor dysfunction, and 13% had slow colonic transit (3).

Normal transit constipation is defined as normal rate of stool movement through the colon with normal frequency. Patients may have increased stress, and hence, perceive problems with constipation (4). Symptoms usually respond to treatment with dietary fiber and/or osmotic laxatives (5).

Pelvic floor dysfunction, also known as anismus, outlet obstruction, obstructed defecation, pelvic floor dyssynergia, dyschezia, and paradoxical pelvic floor contraction, is defined as normal or slightly slowed colonic transit with extended periods of stool storage in the rectum (3,6). The inability to evacuate contents from the rectum may be secondary to the loss of coordination between the abdominal, rectoanal, and pelvic floor muscles during defecation (7). Other mechanisms proposed are incomplete relaxation or paradoxical contraction of the pelvic floor muscles and external anal sphincter during defecation (6). Symptoms include feeling of anal blockage, severe straining, prolonged defecation, and manual disimpaction.

Slow transit constipation is defined as slow rate of stool transit through the colon and the rectum. In patients with minimal delay, dietary and cultural factors may play a role, and this can be reversed with a high-fiber diet. In patients with more severe slow transit constipation, two subtypes have been identified:

1. Colonic inertia: No increase in motor activity is observed after meals or after the administration of bisacodyl (8), cholinergic agents, or anticholinesterases (9). This is related to the dysfunction and alterations in the enteric nerve plexus neurons expressing the excitatory neurotransmitter substance P (10) as well as a decrease in the number of interstitial cells of Cajal (11), which regulate gastrointestinal motility.
2. Uncoordinated motor activity: This happens in the distal colon and acts as a functional barrier to normal transit (12).

Clinical Evaluation

A diagnostic algorithm for the evaluation of a patient with constipation is illustrated in Figure 1. The first step includes a thorough history and physical examination. The history should comprise,

1. Detailed drug history with emphasis on the use of opiods, anticholinergics, and calcium channel blockers
2. Family history significant for inflammatory bowel disease or colon cancer; weight loss, anorexia, malaise, and blood in stools could suggest a malignant process such as colon cancer
3. Questions about symptoms associated with systemic diseases that cause constipation
4. Frequency, consistency of stools, and amount of straining associated with defecation; excessive and prolonged straining along with the need for perineal or vaginal pressure or digital evacuation could suggest slow transit constipation

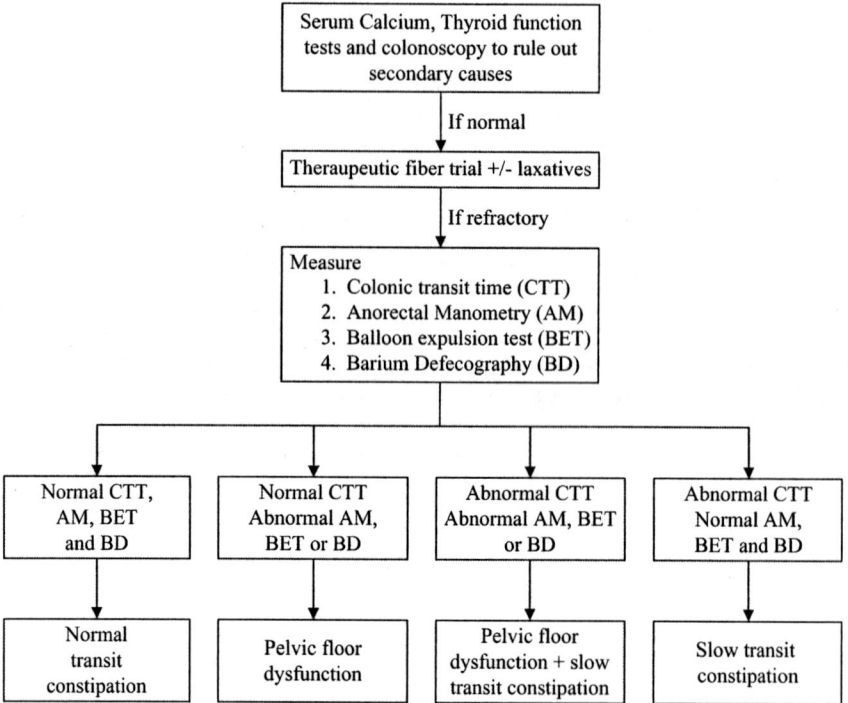

Figure 1 Work up for Constipation. *Source*: Adapted from Ref. 37.

5. Symptoms of alternating diarrhea and constipation with abdominal pain, bloating, and malaise that occurs between bowel movements could suggest IBS (13)
6. Frequency, dosage, and type of laxatives, suppositories, or enemas used to relieve constipation

Physical Examination

1. Inspect the perianal region for tumors, external hemorrhoids, scars, fistulas, fissures, or fecal soiling. The anal reflex can be tested by a scratch test.
2. Observe the descent of the perineum by asking the patient to bear down. Reduced descent (normal is between 1.0 and 3.5 cm) may indicate pelvic floor dysfunction and increased descent may indicate laxity of the perineal muscles (e.g., after multiple pregnancies), which may lead to incomplete evacuation (14).
3. Observe for prolapse of anorectal mucosa during the act of straining.

Diarrhea and Constipation

4. Digital rectal examination:
   a. Examine for tumors, strictures, internal hemorrhoids, or fecal impaction
   b. Evaluate the anal sphincter tone. A patulous opening may raise the suspicion for a neurologic disorder or trauma as the cause of constipation.
   c. Palpate the posterior border of the rectum formed by the puborectalis muscle. Tenderness along this border suggests puborectalis spasm syndrome.
   d. Ask the patient to simulate the act of defecation with the examiner's finger in place, to test coordination of pelvic muscles responsible for defecation.
   e. Test a sample of the stool for occult blood.
5. Examine for rectocele and consider a gynecologic consultation.

Diagnostic Tests

Initial diagnosis of a patient with constipation should include tests to rule out secondary causes. The laboratory tests to be performed are serum electrolytes and calcium, blood glucose, thyroid function tests, complete blood count, endoscopy, and barium studies. Colonoscopy is useful to detect lesions, which occlude the bowel-like polyps, strictures, or tumors. Barium enema is useful for detecting obstructive lesions of the colon, diagnosing megacolon and megarectum, as well as demonstrating proximal dilatation of the aganglionic colonic segment in Hirschsprung's disease. Once the secondary causes have been ruled out, further tests to determine the cause of constipation can be performed. The tests performed are as follows:

1. *Colonic transit time testing* is performed by making the patient swallow radio-opaque markers in a gelatin capsule, followed by abdominal radiographs 120 hours later (15). Prolonged transit is indicated by the retention of 20% or more of the markers (normal colonic transit time is 72 hr).
2. *Defecography* is performed by introducing thickened barium into the patient's rectum. Evacuation of the barium is observed by radiographic films or videos taken during fluoroscopy with the patient sitting on a specially constructed radiolucent commode (16). It helps to detect the anorectal angle during defecation, the degree of pelvic floor descent, and anatomic abnormalities, such as rectocele, solitary rectal ulcers, anal mucosal prolapse, or intussusception (17).
3. *Balloon expulsion test* is performed by inserting a latex balloon into the patient's rectum and then filling it up with 50 cc of water or air. It helps to quantify the ability of a patient to expel the balloon. Failure to do so within two minutes suggests a defecation dysfunction. This test is usually combined with anorectal manometry.

4. *Anorectal manometry* provides measurements of external and internal anal sphincteric pressure. Increased resting external anal sphincteric pressure suggests the presence of anal fissures, whereas increased resting internal anal sphincteric pressure suggests obstructed constipation (18).

Treatment

The first step in treatment of constipation is an increase in fluid intake and physical activity. This should be followed by increasing fiber intake to 20 to 25 g per day for a few weeks, either by incorporating into the diet or with commercial fiber supplements. Patients who do not respond to fiber therapy should begin treatment with a saline osmotic laxative such as milk of magnesia. More expensive agents, such as lactulose and polyethylene glycol, should be reserved for patients who are refractory to fiber or osmotic laxatives.

Laxatives

Laxatives can be grouped into two major categories—oral and rectal laxatives. The classification of oral laxatives according to their mode of action is illustrated in Table 1. Rectal laxatives include suppositories, clysmas, and enemas that act by inhibiting the reabsorption of fluid and sodium from the bowel lumen or as stool softeners (Table 1).

Medications

1. *Prokinetic agents*: Tegaserod improves stool consistency and frequency in patients with constipation as the predominant feature of IBS (19). Recently, Tegaserod has been noted to be associated with increased cardiovascular ischemic complications resulting in suspension of its marketing and sales (20).
2. *Prostaglandin analogs*: Misoprostol causes diarrhea as a major side effect and hence, could be used to treat constipation. However, its high cost limits its use (21).
3. *Colchicine*: Colchicine increases the frequency of bowel movements and accelerates colonic transit. Hence, It can be used in patients with constipation refractory to other medications (22).
4. *Opioid antagonists*: Methylnaltrexone reverses opioid-induced constipation by acting on the peripheral opioid receptors. It does not cross the blood-brain barrier, and hence, does not interfere with analgesia.

Biofeedback Therapy

Biofeedback therapy encompasses visual and auditory feedback on functioning of a patient's anal sphincter and pelvic floor muscles. Patients can be trained to relax the pelvic floor muscles along with appropriate coordination of the

Table 1 Medications Commonly Used for Treatment of Constipation

Medication	Trade Name	Dose	Onset of Action	Mechanism of Action	Side Effects
Standard Laxatives					
Bulk Laxatives				Increases stool bulk; Decreases colonic tranist time.	
Psyllium	Metamucil, Perdiem	1 tsp up to tid	12–72 h		Bloating, flatulence, fluid overlaod
Methylcellulose	Citrucel	1 tsp up to tid	12–72 h		Lesser bloating, flatulence, fluid overload
Polycarbophil	Fibercon, Equalactin	2 to 4 tabs qd	24–48 h		Bloating, flatulence, fluid overload
Bran		1 cup qd			Bloating, flatulence, iron and calcium malabsorption
Osmotic laxatives				Fluid osmotically drawn into the intestines.	
Saline Laxatives					
Magnesium hydroxide	Milk of magnesia	15–30 ml qd or bid	1–3 h		Hypermagnesemia, dehydration abdominal cramps
Sodium phosphate	Fleet Phospho-Soda	10–25 ml			Hyperphosphatemia

(*Continued*)

Table 1 Medications Commonly Used for Treatment of Constipation (*Continued*)

Medication	Trade Name	Dose	Onset of Action	Mechanism of Action	Side Effects
Sugar Laxatives					
Polyethylene glycol (PEG)	Golytely, Miralax	17–36 g qd or bid	0.5–1 h	Retains water and electrolytes by osmotic effect.	Lesser bloating and flatulence
Surfactant					
Docusate sodium	Colace	100 mg bid	12–72 h	Lowers surface tension of stool, allowing water to enter stool.	Skin rash
Stimulant Laxatives					
Anthraquinones					
Senna	Senokot	2–4 tab qd	6–12 h	Increases motility by stimulating myentric plexus.	Malabsorption, Melanosis coli
Diphenyl-methanes					
Bisacodyl	Dulcolax	10–30 mg PO qd 10 mg suppository qhs	6–10 h 15–60 min	Stimulates secretion and increases motility of small intestine and colon	Hyperkalemia, abdominal cramps

Sodium picosulfate	Lubrilax	5–15 mg qhs	Stimulates secretion and motility only of colon	
Lubricant				
Mineral oil	Fleet Mineral Oil	5–15 ml qhs	6–8 h	Lubricates stool	Dehydration, malabsorption of fat soluble vitamins, lipid pnuemonia
Enemas			Initiates evacuation by softening hard stools and distending the rectum.	
Mineral oil retention enema	Fleet mineral oil enema	100 ml qd	6–8 h		Incontinence, mechanical trauma
Phosphate enema	Fleet enema	120 ml qd	5–15 min		Hyperphosphatemia, mechanical trauma
Tap water enema		500 ml qd	5–15 min		Mechanical trauma

Source: Adapted from Ref. 37.

abdominal muscles during the act of defecation. The training can be achieved with the aid of "Fecom"—a silicon-filled artificial stool (23). Patient and therapist motivation along with the development of a rapport are key to successful therapy.

Surgery

Surgery should only be considered in patients with severe constipation who have failed all medical therapies. Total colectomy with ileorectal anastomosis is the preferred treatment for patients with slow transit constipation (3). Rectal surgery should be considered in patients with rectocele-induced constipation (24).

DIARRHEA

Introduction

Chemotherapeutic agents have been utilized in the fight against cancer for several years. These therapeutics have several side effects associated with them. Diarrhea is a severe side effect that can have increased risk of mortality with different regimens (25). In addition, as higher doses of chemotherapy are utilized, there can be a limitation on the oncologist to give the most optimal dose to the patient. The definition of diarrhea is dependent upon three criteria—frequency greater then three bowel movements a day, consistency of the stool, and increased fecal weight (26).

Diarrhea is not only limited to chemotherapeutics, but is present in adjunct therapies that an oncology patient may undergo. Radiation therapy is currently in use for several different cancers, and damage to the mucosa leads to profuse amounts of diarrhea. In addition, bone marrow transplant patients not only undergo high doses of chemotherapy, but are also prone to infections and graft versus host disease. The fragile condition of these patients can cause even minor episodes of diarrhea to be deadly.

Pathology

Several chemotherapeutic agents can lead to severe mucosal damage to the intestinal mucosa. Histopathologic studies of the intestinal mucosa have demonstrated several abnormalities related to chemotherapeutics. Specifically, 5FU and CPT-11 were evaluated, which showed acute mucosal damage, secretion of prostaglandins, leukotrines, cytokines, as well as free radicals, loss of brush border enzymes, mitotic arrest, and initiation of apoptosis (27,28). These pathologic findings are for chemotherapeutic agents, but with several other causes that can lead to slowing of peristalsis or infectious damage to the intestines. The etiology should be established before further work-up is initiated.

Etiology

Diarrhea can occur in several different situations in the oncology patient. Some etiologies consist of radiation therapy, chemotherapeutic agents, decreased physical performance, graft versus host disease, and infections. Careful analysis of the causative agent can lead to more accurate management and early intervention can help in preventing severe complications that may be irreversible.

Evaluation

The initial evaluation of the patient is extremely crucial. It is during the history and physical examination that a health care provider is able to assess the severity of the situation so that the appropriate therapy can be started. During the history, such questions about the duration, frequency, and quantity can provide valuable information to judge the severity of the problem. Physical examination can add to the source of the diarrhea. It is important to evaluate antibiotics the patient has taken in the past and the volume status of the patient. Laboratory evaluation can help to confirm the volume status of the patient as well as if electrolytes need to be repleted. In addition, consultation may help to confirm or exclude a diagnosis of graft versus host disease in transplant patients. Also, infectious etiology (viral, bacterial, or fungal) has to be excluded and the appropriate tests should be sent for culture.

In addition, part of the history should include the medications that the patient is currently taking. Many herbal remedies and over-the-counter medication may be causing diarrhea, and so should be inquired about. Dietary regimen can also lead to diarrhea when there are interactions with medication. Specifically, chemotherapeutic medication can lead to destruction of the gastric mucosa. Therefore, patients may not be able to absorb foods that were previously not leading to diarrhea. A thorough dietary history should be taken, and if necessary a dietician should be consulted for recommendations.

Several oncology patients are neutropenic and need urgent treatment of severe diarrhea as it can be fatal. In addition, patients with colostomy bags are also at risk for diarrhea and should be monitored closely. The severity of diarrhea can be graded by the NCI Common Criteria Toxicity (29). This allows for a common nomenclature so that health care practitioners are able to have a unified method of describing diarrhea.

Initial evaluation can help to divide diarrhea into several different types, which can help to narrow the differential. The types of diarrhea are fatty, motility disorders, watery, and inflammatory (30). A diagnostic analysis of the stool, urine, and blood should be carried out. The stool should be evaluated for pH, electrolytes, minerals, WBCs, and fat. In addition, fecal culture should be sent for infectious etiology. Occult blood should be sent for tumors or infectious etiology, but this can be of questionable importance and should be followed up with further testing. The urine should be tested for vanillylmandelic acid (VMA),

5-hydroxyindole acid, and laxatives. The blood should be tested for vasoactive intestinal peptide, electrolytes, vitamin B12, and pancreatic enzymes.

Management

In some chemotherapeutic regimens, there is life-threatening diarrhea; there are several ways that such diarrhea can be treated (Table 2) (32). The appropriate treatment of this diarrhea can not only allow for better outcomes as patients will be able to tolerate the regimen better, but also help improve the quality of life of the individuals. Nutritional therapy may also benefit some patients who present with acute diarrhea (30,31). Some beneficial therapy consists of clear liquids with electrolytes and minerals, small meals, soluble fiber, protein-rich foods, and eating slowly. Some guidelines for items to avoid include spicy food, alcohol, diary products, and high-osmolar, sugar and fat foods.

After initial evaluation, patients may need fluid restoration and/or admission to the hospital. Health care practitioners should keep in mind that the only goal is not to stop the diarrhea, but to discover if there is an underlying etiology that can be treated. In particular, infectious etiology may need to be treated before stopping the diarrhea. Also, the practitioner should pay special attention to determine if an obstruction is the reason for the diarrhea. Caution should be used when dealing

Table 2 Approach to Chemotherapy-Induced Diarrhea

Evaluation of the patient
- History and physical
- Diet
- Medications
    1. Does the patient have complications or is hemodynamically unstable? If yes, then consideration Inpatient admission and consider
        - Octreotide
        - Tincture of opium
        - Fluid resuscitation
        - Check electrolytes and replete
        - Stop medication that may be felt to be causative agent

       If no, then continue with outpatient management
        - Consider dietary changes

       If ineffective, then
        - Consider pharmacologic therapy

       If no benefit with pharmacologic therapy and **NO** complications, then treat as outpatient
        - Check electrolytes
        - Replace fluids
        - Infectious etiology

       If no benefit and **complications**, patient should be seen as inpatient (see above)

with refractory diarrhea as a complete diagnosis consisting of gastroenterology consult maybe necessary to determine if cancer is the cause of the diarrhea, i.e., colon cancer or a carcinoid syndrome. If these factors have been excluded and it is appropriate after a through examination, then pharmacologic therapy can be started to limit the frequency and quantity of the diarrhea.

It should be noted that opioids are extremely helpful medication in mild to moderate diarrhea management, but are many a times overlooked. Specifically, tincture of opium and morphine may be more useful then codeine. In patients who may have excess bile acid secretions of bismuth, medicinal fiber and cholestyramine may be of use. There are also several ways that the stool consistency may be changed by providing absorbents, such as clays, activated charcoal, or psyllium. The other option is that of steroids such as budesonide, which has a low systemic absorption because of firs- pass mechanism in the liver and used in Crohn's disease (30). It should be kept in mind that using medications that are anticholinergics can be used as a last resort, but their toxicity at higher doses should be taken into consideration.

The pharmacologic armament for diarrhea can be divided into several different categories. Antibiotics is one group that consists of metronidazole, amoxicillin, and neomycin. Bile acid agents are bismuth, medicinal fiber, and cholestyramine. The absorbents consist of clay, activated charcoal, and psyllium. In addition, the opiates are excellent agents in the termination of diarrhea. Some other agents include anticholinergics, octreotide, loperamide, and budenoside.

Two popular medications for the treatment of chemotherapy-induced diarrhea will be emphasized. Loperamide is an antidiarrheal that inhibits peristalsis and prolongs transit time by acting on the intestinal mucosa while enhancing fluid and electrolyte movement through the intestinal mucosa. The current indication is for mild to moderate uncomplicated diarrhea. Initially, the patient should be started on 4 mg orally, then 2 mg after each stool. If the diarrhea persists past 24 hours, then an increase in dose is appropriate. If refractory to initial dose, then begin with 2 mg every 2 hours until the patient is free of diarrhea for 12 hours (25). Side effects that may be experienced are increase in paralytic ileus, distension, cramping, bloating, drowsiness, fatigue, and dizziness. The second drug of importance is octreotide, which is a synthetic somatostatin analog that acts on somatostatin receptors. The indication is for moderate to severe diarrhea. Initially, the sarting dose is 100 to 150 µg SC thrice a day or IV (25–50 µg/hr). If worsening symptoms are observed, increase the dose to 500 µg until the diarrhea is controlled (31). Some side effects that may be experienced include bloating, flatulence, and cramping. Glucose should be monitored at higher doses as hyperglycemia may occur, and patients with cardiac history should be monitored for bradycardia. In addition, further studies have compared the 100 µg dose to the 500 µg dose and found increased efficacy in eliminating diarrhea without a greater number of side effects (33). In a trial of patients that received 5-FU or a modified 5-FU regimen, dose escalation up to 2500 µg thrice a day was beneficial in stopping diarrhea (34).

Many of these experimental medications have explored prevention as well as therapy for specific chemotherapy-induced diarrhea. For example, oral glutamine, thalidomide, and oral neomycin/bacitracin are currently being investigated in irinotecan-induced therapy. There are also several substances that show promising results in animal studies. Keratinocyte growth factor has helped in proliferation and differentiation of epithelial cells. This has been shown to be useful in animal models in the prevention of diarrhea (35). Also, IL-15 has shown promise in reducing chemotherapy-induced diarrhea in animal models (36).

REFERENCES

1. Oi-Ling K, Man-Wah DTSE, Kam-Hung DNG. Symptoms as rated by advanced care patients, care givers and physicians in the last week of life. Pall Med 2005; 19: 228–233.
2. Thompson WG, Creed F, Drossman DA, et al. Functional bowel disorders and functional abdominal pain. Gut 1999; 45:1143–1147.
3. Nyam DC, Pemberton JH, Ilstrup DM, et al. Long-term results of surgery for chronic constipation. Dis Colon Rectum 1997; 40:273–279.
4. Ashraf W, Park F, Lof J, et al. An examination of the reliability of reported stool frequency in the diagnosis of idiopathic constipation. Am J Gastroenterol 1996; 91: 26–32.
5. Voderholzer WA, Schatke W, Muhldorfer BE, et al. Clinical response to dietary fiber treatment of chronic constipation. Am J Gastroenterol 1997; 92:95–98.
6. Preston DM, Lennard-Jones JE. Anismus in chronic constipation. Dig Dis Sci 1985; 30:413–418.
7. Camilleri M, Thompson WG, Fleshman JW, et al. Clinical management of intractable constipation. Ann Intern Med 1994; 121:520–528.
8. Preston DM, Lennard-Jones JE. Pelvic motility and response to intraluminal bisacodyl in slow-transit constipation. Dig Dis Sci 1985; 30:289.
9. Bassotti G, Chiarioni G, Imbimbo BP, et al. Impaired colonic motor response to cholinergic stimulation in patients with severe chronic idiopathic (slow transit type) constipation. Dig Dis Sci 1993; 38:1040–1045.
10. Tzavella K, Riepl RL, Klauser AG, et al. Decreased substance P levels in rectal biopsies from patients with slow transit constipation. Eur J Gastroenterol Hepatol 1996; 8:1207–1211.
11. He CL, Burgart L, Wang L, et al. Decreased interstitial cell of Cajal volume in patients with slow transit constipation. Gastroenterology 2000; 118:14–21.
12. Snape WJJR. Role of colonic motility in guiding therapy in patients with constipation. Dig Dis Sci 1997; 15:104–111.
13. Mertz H, Naliboff B, Mayer E. Physiology of refractory chronic constipation. Am J Gastroenterol 1999; 94:609–615.
14. Harewood GC, Coulie B, Camilleri M, et al. Descending perineum syndrome: audit of clinical and laboratory features and outcome of pelvic floor retaining. Am J Gastroenterol 1999; 94:126–130.

15. Hinton JM, Lennard-Jones JE, Young AC. A new method for studying gut transit times using radioopaque markers. Gut 1969; 10:842–847.
16. Wald A, Caruana BJ, Freimanis MG, et al. Contributions of evacuation proctography and anorectal manometry to the evaluation of adults with constipation and defecatory difficulty. Dig Dis Sci 1990; 35:481.
17. Schweiger M, Alexander-Williams J. Solitary rectal ulcer syndrome of the rectum: its association with occult rectal prolapse. Lancet 1977; 1:1970–1971.
18. Diamant NE, Kamm MA, Wald A, Whitehead WE. AGA technical review on anorectal testing techniques. Gastroenterology 1999; 116:735–760.
19. Muller-Lissner SA, Fumagalli I, Bardhan KD, et al. Tegaserod, a 5-HT (4) receptor partial agonist, relieves symptoms in irritable bowel syndrome patients with abdominal pain, bloating and constipation. Aliment Pharmacol Ther 2001; 15:1655–1666.
20. Novartis Pharmaceuticals Corporation, June 11, 2007 (http://www.zelnorm.com:80/Zelnrom_PR_US_330_Final_12_1007.pdf)
21. Soffer EE, Metcalf A, Launspach J. Misoprostol is effective treatment for patients with severe constipation. Dig Dis Sci 1994; 39:929–933.
22. Verne GN, Davis RH, Robinson ME, et al. Treatment of chronic constipation with colchicine: Randomized, double-blind, placebo-controlled, crossover trial. Am J Gastroeneterol 2003; 98:1112–1116.
23. Pelsang RE, Rao SS, Welcher K. FECOM: a new artificial stool for evaluating defecation. Am J Gastroenterol 1999; 94:183–186.
24. Sarles JC, Arnaud A, Selezneff I, et al. Endo-rectal repair of rectocele. Int J Colorectal Dis 1989; 4:167–171.
25. Rothenberg ML, Meropol NJ, Poplin EA, et al. Mortality associated with irinotecan plus bolus fluorouracil/leucovorin: summary findings of an independent panel. J Clin Oncol 2001; 19:3801–3807.
26. Wenzl HH, Fine KD, Schiller LR, et al. Determinants of decreased fecal consistency in patients with diarrhea. Gastroenterology 1995; 108:1729–1738.
27. Dosik GM, Luna M, Valdivieso M, et al. Necrotizing colitis in patients with cancer. Am J Med 1979; 67:646–656.
28. de Roy van Zuidewijn DB, Schillings PH, Wobbes T, et al. Morphometric analysis of the effects of antineoplastic drugs on mucosa of normal ileum and ileal anastomoses in rats. Exp Mol Pathol 1992; 56:96–107.
29. Cancer Therapy Evaluation Program. Common Terminology Criteria for Adverse Events Version 3.0. 2003, NIH publication No. 03-5410.
30. Mercandante S. Diarrhea, malabsorption and constipation. In: Berger A, ed. Principles and Practices of Supportive Oncology, 2002.
31. Lamberts SW, van der Lely AJ, de Herder WW, et al. Octreotide. NEJM 1996; 334:246–254.
32. Benson III AB, Ajani JA, Catalano RB, et al. Recommended guidelines for the treatment of cancer treatment-induced diarrhea. J Clin Oncol 2004; 22:2918–2926.
33. Goumas P, Naxakis S, Christopoulou A, et al. Octreotide acetate in the treatment of fluorouracil-induced diarrhea. Oncologist 1998; 3:50–53.
34. Wadler S, Haynes H, Wiernik PH. Phase I trial of the somatostatin analog octreotide acetate in the treatment of fluoropyrimidine-induced diarrhea. J Clin Oncol 1995; 13:222–226.

35. Farrell CL, Bready JV, Rex KL, et al. Keratinocyte growth factor protects mice from chemotherapy and radiation-induced gastrointestinal injury and mortality. Cancer Res 1998; 58:933–939.
36. Cao S, Troutt AB, Rustum YM. Interleukin 15 protects against toxicity and potentiates antitumor activity of 5-fluorouracil alone and in combination with leucovorin in rats bearing colorectal cancer. Cancer Res 1998; 58:1695–1699.
37. Locke GR 3rd, Pemberton GH, Phillips SF. AGA technical review on constipation. American Gastroenterology Association. Gastroenterology 2000; 119(6):1766–1778.

13

Skeletal Complications: Bone Metabolism and Novel Targeted Agents

Alissa Huston
James P. Wilmot Cancer Center, University of Rochester, Rochester, New York, U.S.A.

INTRODUCTION

Bone represents the most common site of metastases for many solid tumors. Metastases to bone develop in nearly 70% of patients with either breast or prostate cancer, and in approximately 15% to 30% of patients with other solid tumors (lung, colon, thyroid, renal cell, bladder, uterine, or rectal) (1,2). Significant complications result from bone metastasis including hypercalcemia, pathologic fractures, spinal cord compression, and severe bone pain, representing a significant source of morbidity and mortality for patients (2,3). While any form of cancer metastases is associated with a shortened survival, those with metastases to bones only (particularly with breast and prostate cancer) live, on average, years longer than those with visceral metastasis (1,4). Median survival of patients with cancer metastases to bone is on an average 19 to 25 months (5). A mainstay of treatment for bone metastases for the past several years has consisted of bisphosphonate therapy; however, recent advances have identified newer targets and agents, many of which are currently in clinical trial development.

NORMAL BONE HOMEOSTASIS

There are four phases that comprise normal bone remodeling, which include resorption, reversal, formation, and resting. Osteoclasts and osteoblasts play a critical role in maintaining this balance. Bone resorption occurs through the action of osteoclasts, cells derived from the monocyte-macrophage lineage (6). During the resorption phase, osteoclasts form erosion cavities by breaking down bone mineral and matrix (7). Following resorption, there is the reversal phase, characterized by cessation of osteoclast-mediated bone resorption and new bone formation. During this time, material rich in proteoglycans, glycoproteins, and acid phosphatase, but not collagen, is deposited along the resorption pit to prepare the surface for new bone formation (7). Next, coupling takes place in which osteoblasts are recruited and they begin laying down new bone, which under normal circumstances is equal to the amount of bone resorbed (7). Finally, this is followed by a quiescent or resting phase, which lasts until resorption begins again. This tightly balanced process is important for the maintenance of normal bone homeostasis (7).

Several factors, including hormones and cytokines, are involved in this process. Estrogen is a key mediator in regulating osteoclast activation and lifespan (8). The effects of estrogen upon osteoblasts are less characterized, although there are suggestions that it may be involved in mediating osteoblast function and formation (8). Loss of estrogen, either through pharmacological means (as in breast cancer therapy) or through menopause, results in an imbalance between the tightly regulated process of bone remodeling and bone resorption, resulting in larger resorption pits that cannot be effectively filled by osteoblasts (8). The role that androgens play in normal bone homeostasis is less well characterized and currently under investigation (9).

Osteoclast activation in normal bone remodeling is controlled by the molecular factor receptor activator of nuclear factor-κB ligand (RANKL) and its soluble decoy receptor osteoprotegerin (OPG) (2,10). In addition, 1,25-dihydroxyvitamin D_3 ($1,25D_3$), prostaglandin E2 (PGE_2), parathyroid hormone (PTH)/parathyroid hormone-related protein (PTHrP), and various interleukins have also been shown to play a role through increasing the expression of RANKL on neighboring bone marrow stromal cells and osteoblasts (2,11,12). RANKL, a member of the tumor necrosis factor (TNF) family is expressed on the surface of osteoblasts and bone marrow stromal cells and is also expressed by T-lymphocytes (2,13). Binding of RANKL to its receptor RANK located on osteoclast precursor cells leads to osteoclast formation (10). Knock-out models of RANKL or the RANK gene have resulted in severe osteopetrosis due to a lack of osteoclasts (2,14,15). OPG, also a member of the TNF family, is a soluble decoy receptor for RANKL and inhibits osteoclast activation and formation (14). A ratio exists between RANKL and OPG, which regulates the activity of osteoclasts (2). Over- or underproduction of OPG in animal models results in osteopetrosis and osteopenia, respectively (16,17).

Osteoblasts are derived from mesenchymal stem cells that have the ability to differentiate into bone forming cells (osteoblasts), adipocytes, or muscle cells (18). Differentiation into osteoblasts is controlled through the Runx-2 or core binding factor alpha 1 (Cbfa1) transcription factor (19). Knock-out models of Cbfa1 in mice have demonstrated a lack of bone development (20,21). Other factors that are thought to be involved in the differentiation of osteoblasts include platelet-derived growth factor (PDGF), fibroblast growth factor, and transforming growth factor-β (TGF-β) (2,22).

MECHANISMS OF BONE METASTASES

Bone metastases are characterized on the basis of the predominant type of bone involvement present. While the majority of metastases are distinguished based on whether they are osteolytic or osteoblastic, in reality a continuum exists, with both types of bone involvement often being observed. There are a variety of factors involved in the development and propagation of bone metastases, including interactions between tumor cells and bone, tumor cells and the microenvironment, and bone and the microenvironment. Tumor cells migrate to the bone marrow through the CXC chemokine receptor 4 (CXCR4) stromal-derived-factor-1 (SDF-1) or CXCL12 gradient. The CXCR4 chemokine receptor is expressed on many tumor cells and migrates towards its specific ligand (SDF-1 or CXCL12), which is found at high concentrations within the stroma in bone (23). Once migrated to bone, tumor cells develop adhesive interactions within the bone marrow microenvironment that furthers both bone destruction and growth of the tumor cells (24).

Osteolytic

Osteolytic bone metastases are characterized by significant bone destruction without associated new bone formation (3). The most common types of solid tumors associated with osteolytic metastases include renal, breast, and lung (25). On plain X-rays, the hallmark is the classic lytic appearance of the bone lesion. The mechanism behind osteolytic metastases resides with the osteoclasts. When tumor cells spread to bone, there is an association between the tumor cells and neighboring osteoclasts, resulting in an upregulation of osteoclast activity leading to significant bone destruction (3). The most common and widely studied example is the microenvironmental interactions between tumor cells and bone leading to osteolytic bone metastases in solid tumors is breast cancer.

The development of bone metastases is a frequent consequence in patients with advanced breast cancer occurring in approximately 70% of patients, and representing the commonest site of distant relapse (1). Bone metastases occur more frequently in patients with estrogen-receptor and progesterone-receptor positive tumors, and are predominantly osteolytic. The interaction of breast cancer cells and those within the bone marrow lead to an upregulation of osteolytic factors including interlukin (IL)-11, IL-8, IL-6, PGE_2, macrophage colony stimulating factor, and

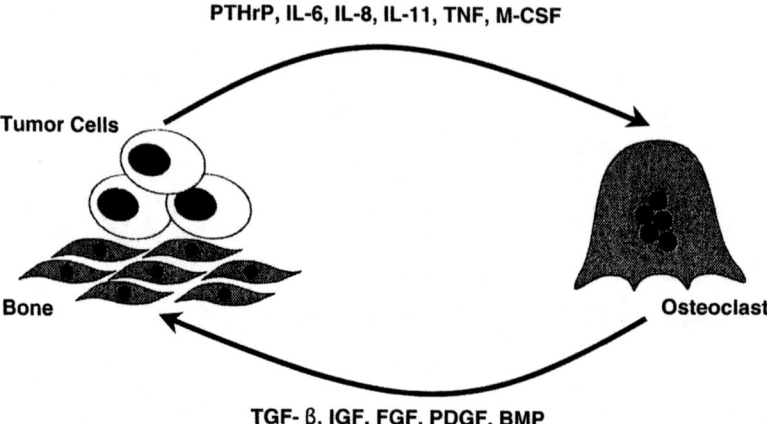

Figure 1 Osteolytic bone metastases.

TNF, leading to increased RANKL expression and subsequent osteoclast activation (Fig. 1) (2,3). There is also data to suggest that IL-8 may stimulate osteoclasts through a RANKL-independent mechanism leading to enhanced bone metastases (26). Factors, including TGF-β, PTHrP, bone morphogenetic proteins, insulin-like growth factors, and fibroblast growth factor, are released from bone during the process of bone resorption (2,3,27,28). The mobilization of these factors leads to subsequent stimulation of breast cancer cell growth. PTHrP, produced by breast cancer cells and other solid tumor cells, leads to osteoclast activation through the induction of RANKL expression within the bone marrow microenvironment, and also leads to the release of TGF-β (27). Expression of TGF-β subsequently results in further PTHrP production by local breast cancer cells and the development of what has been termed a "viscious cycle" leading to enhanced bone destruction and greater tumor burden (2,29). The resulting bone destruction leads to elevated calcium levels, which fuel tumor growth and PTHrP production, further propagating the cycle (30).

Osteoblastic

Osteoblastic bone metastases are characterized by an increase in subsequent bone formation adjacent to areas of tumor involvement. The hallmark on plain X-ray is a sclerotic appearance to the bone. The classic tumor type to result in osteoblastic bone metastases is prostate cancer, although a small proportion of patients with breast cancer (15–20%) develop purely osteoblastic metastases (25,31). Osteoblast activity and bone formation have been shown to be stimulated through endothelin-1 (ET-1) in both breast and prostate cancer (32,33). In patients with prostate cancer, elevated levels have been observed in those with osteoblastic metastases (34).

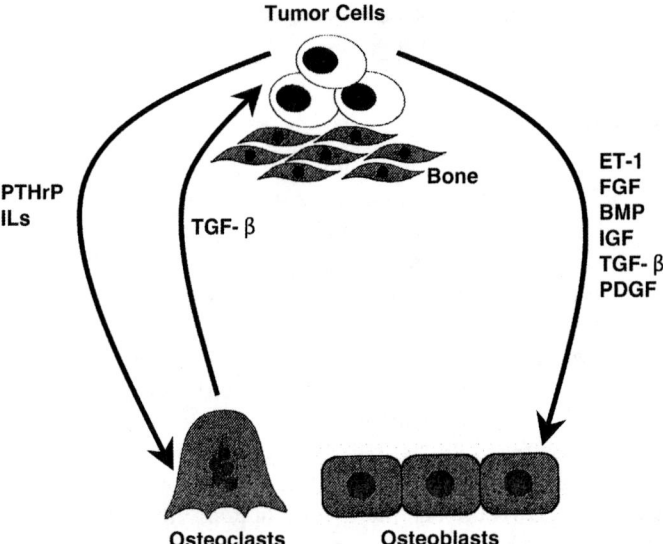

Figure 2 Osteoblastic bone metastases.

Animal models of prostate cancer bone metastases demonstrate a decrease in both metastases and tumor burden following treatment of the animals with an endothelin-A receptor antagonist (2,32). Other factors identified include PTHrP, IL-6, TGF-β, and bone morphogenetic proteins, which are released from tumor cells (Fig. 2) (5), leading to osteoclast activation and formation. Additional data have also suggested roles for platelet-derived growth factor (produced by osteoblasts), urokinase, or prostate-specific antigen (2,35–38). As with breast cancer and osteolytic bone involvement, the most common and widely recognized and studied example of osteoblastic bone metastases is in prostate cancer.

Prostate cancer cells have been demonstrated to release prostate-specific antigen (PSA), a kallikrein serine protease, and urokinase-type plasminogen activator (uPA). In an animal model of prostate cancer, uPA has been shown to enhance osteoblast growth, and increased levels have resulted in an increase in bone metastases (36). PSA has the ability to regulate the activity of PTHrP through cleavage of the protein, and it has also been shown to have a potential role in activating other microenvironmental factors responsible for osteoblast activation and growth including insulin-like growth factors 1 and 2 and TGF-β (38). Interestingly, while metastases from prostate cancer are predominantly osteoblastic, there is evidence of increased markers of bone turnover without corresponding increases in osteoclasts at the pathological level (39). Markers of bone turnover have also been suggested as a more accurate way to follow patients with evidence of bone involvement, as compared to PSA (39). While bisphosphonates are used in prostate cancer, their use appears to be more in prevention of further progression of bone metastases, but not in the inhibition of the development of bone metastases (40–42).

TREATMENT-RELATED BONE LOSS

Many of the therapies currently used in the adjuvant treatment of solid tumors also have detrimental effects upon bone health. These side effects most often stem from the hormonal modulations that result from the initiation of therapy. In the treatment of postmenopausal breast cancer, aromatase inhibition results in a near 99% reduction in the amount of circulating estrogen (43). Aromatase inhibitors [letrozole (Femara®), exemestane (Aromasin®), and anastrozole (Arimidex®)] are considered the standard of care for treating postmenopausal breast cancer. In the ATAC (Arimidex®, Tamoxifen Alone or in Combination) trial, a significant increase in fracture rates was observed following a year of treatment with anastrozole, as compared to tamoxifen (5.9% vs. 3.7%; $p < 0.0001$) (44). Furthermore, there are likely direct effects of chemotherapy upon bone, coupled with the induction of premature ovarian failure and menopause in premenopausal women leading to a state of rapid bone loss. In prostate cancer, patients receive agents that result in androgen deprivation including surgical orchiectomy or chemical orchiectomy by treatment with gonadotropin-releasing hormones (GnRH), which leads to a decline in bone density. Bisphosphonates have been the standard treatment for these indications and studies are underway to try and identify patients requiring therapy sooner to minimize the adverse effects of the treatment. While bisphosphonates are beneficial, there may be additional factors contributing to bone loss that require further investigation.

NOVEL MEDICAL THERAPIES

Bisphosphonates have been the cornerstone of therapy in treating metastatic cancer to bone for many years. Since their inception, the rate of skeletal-related events, including fractures related to bone involvement, have decreased by a factor of 50% (45,46). Further detailed information regarding the use of bisphosphonates in treating metastatic cancer to bone is covered in chapter 14. Despite their benefits, there have also been concerns over some of the serious adverse risks associated with the use of bisphosphonates, including the development of renal failure, nephrotic syndrome, or osteonecrosis of the jaw (47–50). Therefore, newer agents targeting bone destruction associated with tumor metastases are continually under investigation (Table 1).

Denosumab

Denosumab (Amgen) is a fully human monoclonal antibody raised against RANKL, which has been previously evaluated in women with postmenopausal osteoporosis as well as in patients with multiple myeloma or bone metastases from breast cancer. Initial studies demonstrated that a single dose of denosumab led to

Table 1 New Agents Under Development for Metastatic Bone Disease

RANK ligand monoclonal antibody
- Denosumab

PTHrP antibody
- CAL

Tyrosine kinase inhibition
- Tandutinib (MLN518)
- Imatinib mesylate (Gleevec®)
- Dasatinib (Sprycel®)
- AP23451
- AZD0530

Endothelin-1 inhibition
- Atrasentan (ABT-627)
- ZD4054

Cathepsin K inhibition
- MK 0822

TGF-β inhibition
- SD-208

Proteosome inhibition
- Bortezomib (Velcade®)

p38 MAP kinase inhibition

a dose-dependent, rapid, and sustained decline in markers of bone turnover [urinary N-telopeptide/creatinine (NTX), serum NTX, serum bone-specific alkaline phosphatase (BALP)] (51). Further studies identified an increase in bone mineral density, observed following a year of therapy, with results similar to those observed in studies using oral bisphosphonate therapy (52). A safety study conducted in patients with multiple myeloma or bone metastases from breast cancer comparing denosumab to pamidronate also demonstrated similar sustained suppression in markers of bone turnover (as in the initial postmenopausal studies) lasting up to 84 days (53). Currently, there is a multicenter, randomized, double-blind, placebo-controlled phase III trial comparing denosumab with Zometa® (Novartis) in patients with newly diagnosed breast cancer metastases to bone. Similar trials are also underway for prostate and lung cancer.

PTHrP Antibody

The role of PTHrP in promoting the "viscious cycle" of bone metastases, particularly in breast cancer, has been well established. Therefore, PTHrP represents an attractive target for therapeutic intervention. Chugai Pharmaceuticals, in conjunction with Roche, has developed a monoclonal antibody against PTHrP (CAL), which has completed a phase I trial in breast cancer metastatic to bone as compared to Zometa®. Phase II trials are currently underway for further development.

Tyrosine Kinase Inhibition

PDGF has been identified as having a potential role in osteoblast differentiation. Tandutinib (MLN518) is a quinazoline-based, fms-related tyrosine kinase 3 (FLT3) inhibitor that targets type III tyrosine kinase and the PDGF receptor (PDGF-R) (54). Tandutinib has demonstrated activity in hematological malignancies, including acute myelogenous leukemia and myelodysplastic syndrome (54). As PDGF is thought to be involved in the role of osteoblast differentiation, it is currently being studied in a phase II trial in patients with androgen-independent prostate cancer and progressive bone metastases.

Dasatinib (Sprycel®) is also a tyrosine kinase inhibitor that targets not only Bcr-Abl, PDGF-R, but also the Src family. Src has been shown to be important in osteoclast activity, as demonstrated in animal models where Src knock-outs developed osteopetrosis and inhibition of Src led to less bone destruction (55,56). Imantinib mesylate (Gleevec®) is the predecessor of dasatinib and is currently used in the treatment of chronic myeloid leukemia and gastrointestinal stromal tumors. It has been previously investigated as a potential modulator of osteoclast activity through modulation of PDGF-R (57). Dasatinib has also been approved by the FDA for treatment of chronic myeloid leukemia; however it is now under further investigation in the area of modulating tumor cell growth and bone metastases. The Southwest Oncology Group (SWOG) has a trial underway to investigate the activity of dasatinib in the second-line treatment of metastatic breast cancer to bone.

Additional Src tyrosine kinase inhibitors include AP23451, which also includes a bisphosphonate group, and AZD0530 (AstraZeneca), a Src kinase and Bcr-Abl small molecule inhibitor (58,59). Preclinical work involving AP23451 demonstrated a significant reduction in tumor volume within the marrow cavity of the treated animals, the prevention of osteolysis secondary to the metastases, and a decrease in osteolytic bone resorption and incidence of metastases (60,61). Thus, indicating that Src inhibition may be beneficial not only in inhibiting the associated bone resorption from cancer metastases to bone, but also in direct effects upon tumor cells. AZD0530 has demonstrated significant activity in phase I clinical trials involving healthy volunteers, in which there was a significant decrease in serum and urinary markers of bone turnover following treatment (59,62).

Endothelin-1 Inhibition

Endothelin-1 has been shown to stimulate metastases in both breast and prostate cancer. Following binding of endothelin-1 to its receptor endothelin-A (a G-protein-coupled receptor), a cascade of events follow, including vasoconstriction, bronchoconstriction, mitogenesis, antiapoptosis, neuropathic, and acute pain and an osteoblastic response (63). Atrasentan (ABT-627) is an endothelin-A receptor inhibitor. The area most widely studied for response to atrasentan is in prostate cancer.

Initial phase I studies demonstrated safety and tolerability of the agent. (64–66). An early glimpse into the activity of Atrasentan specifically for prostate cancer was also observed, resulting in further evaluation in larger phase II and III trials (64). Results of the larger studies have not been as robust, although an exploratory analysis in men with bone metastases at baseline demonstrated a significant delay in progression of their disease identifying a potential targeted area for further development (67,68). Also, a new endothelin receptor antagonist ZD4054 is also under development with both phase 1 and phase 2 studies currently underway (69).

Cathepsin K Inhibition

Cathepsin K is a cysteine protease enzyme important in collagen breakdown and is expressed almost entirely within osteoclasts (70). Through cathepsin K, osteoclasts are able to modulate bone resorption through the breakdown of type I collagen, which comprises the majority of the protein matrix in bone (70,71). Animal models with a complete lack of cathepsin K demonstrate an osteopetrotic phenotype, and inhibitors targeting cathepsin K have shown the ability to suppress bone resorption (72,73). A rare autosomal recessive human counterpart, pycnodysostosis, has been identified and characterized by increased bone mineral density associated with osteosclerosis and short statue, and arises form point mutations within the cathepsin K gene located on chromosome 1q21 (74). MK 0822 is a cathepsin K antagonist (Merck) that has been studied previously in the treatment of osteoporosis and is under phase III clinical trial development. There is a current phase II clinical trial that will evaluate the effects of treatment of MK 0822 on breast cancer metastatic to bone.

Tgf-β Inhibition

A small molecule inhibitor of TGF-β has been identified (SD-208) and acts by inhibiting downstream signals from the receptor. In an animal model of breast cancer, SD-208 decreased the development and progression of breast cancer bone metastases and also prolonged survival of the animals (75). A decline in the levels of osteoclytic factors PTHrP and IL-11 were also observed following treatment, as well as levels of TGF-β secreted from a common metastatic breast cancer cell line MD-MBA-231 (75). While still in preclinical development, targeting TGF-β may be beneficial in mitigating the effects of the "vicious cycle" that appears to be important in the propagation of bone metastases, particularly in breast cancer.

Proteosome Inhibition

Proteosome inhibitors, such as bortezomib, have been demonstrated to be regulators of osteoblast differentiation and bone formation through bone morphogenetic proteins (76). They also appear to have a role in the inhibition of osteoclast differentiation through inhibition of NF-κB (77). While preclinical data has been exciting for the possible role of protesome inhibition in modulating the effects of bone metastases, early clinical data has not been as convincing and further work is needed to fully define the role of proteosome inhibitors in metastatic bone disease (71,78).

p38 Mitogen-Activated Protein Kinase Inhibition

Activation of p38 mitogen-activated protein (MAP) kinase results in the upregulation of various growth factors and cytokines. Two particular cytokines include IL-1 and TNF, both of which are pro-inflammatory and contribute to osteoclast activation and, consequently, bone resorption (71). Inhibitors of p38 MAP kinase have demonstrated a reduction in osteoclast activity in animal models, and further development for clinical trials are underway (71,79).

ADDITIONAL TREATMENT OPTIONS

Bisphonsphonate therapy has been an important therapeutic intervention for patients with bone metastases. The additional agents outlined show promise in improving outcomes for those with metastatic disease of the bone. However, despite medical management, additional forms of therapy, including radiation and surgical management, are often required.

Radiation Therapy

Radiation therapy is effective in treating pathologic fractures and alleviating the pain of bone metastases. Some studies have cited effectiveness in nearly 80% of patients starting between 48 hours to four weeks following treatment, and lasting in 50% of patients for up to six months (80,81). Radiation therapy has also been shown to be beneficial following the surgical stabilization of pathologic fractures and for the prevention of spinal cord compression (80,81). It provides an important adjunct to both surgical and medical options for the management of bone metastases. Radiation is not without associated side effects including nausea/vomiting or diarrhea, alopecia, esophagitis, pneumonitis, and fatigue. However, the majority of side effects resolve shortly after completion of therapy (81).

External beam radiation therapy has been the standard of care for treatment of bone metastases; however, it is limited by its ability to target only one site at a time. In addition to external beam radiation, there are bone-seeking radiopharmaceuticals that deliver ionizing radiation to multiple areas of metastases simultaneously (82,83). They also have the advantage of less side effects, including nausea/vomiting/diarrhea and tissue damage, and can be administered intravenously (84). They are generally used for the palliation of pain, and not for spinal cord compression, peripheral nerve invasion by metastases, pathologic fractures, or pure osteolytic bone lesions. The most commonly used forms are the β-emitters including strontium chloride-89, sodium phosphate-32, and samarium-153 lexidronam. For example, strontium chorlide-89 has been demonstrated to improve symptoms of bone pain in nearly 80% of patients receiving therapy with a duration of response of approximately three to four months (85). The doses used generally result in pain relief, without significant compromise of the bone marrow; however, when used in treatment doses, more pronounced bone marrow effects can be observed (86). Radium-223 is an α-particle emitter currently under clinical trial development as an alternative radiopharmaceutical to the standard β-emitters and has shown promise in both the preclinical and clinical setting, including a more favorable side-effect profile with less myelosuppression observed (83).

Surgical Intervention

Common indications for surgical intervention of bone metastases include treatment or prevention of cord compression and pathologic fractures in the setting of metastatic cancer to bone (85). Other indications include surgical stabilization following pathologic fracture and for palliation of painful metastases. A general approach includes the utilization of an intramedullary rod, plate, or prosthetic device, resection of the affected area and reconstruction, and use of a prosthetic device or allograft (87). Retrospective studies looking at response rates following surgical intervention have demonstrated that 54% of patients required less analgesia, 65% requiring surgery to the lower extremities had full weight bearing, and 22% requiring surgery to the upper extremities regained use of their arms (88).

Less-invasive alternatives to standard surgical intervention include vertebroplasty or kyphoplasty. Their main indication is for treatment of pain that develops from compression fractures as a consequence of tumor involvement within the spine (89). In vertebroplasty, bone cement (polymethyl methacrylate) is injected by a radiologist percutaneously into the center of the collapsed vertebrae and allowed to harden, thus stabilizing the fractured area leading to improvement in pain that results from the compression (89). This treatment modality is often considered in patients who have failed conservative therapy and in whom radiation is not felt likely to provide significant benefit (89). Kyphoplasty is a variation of vetebroplasty, in which a balloon is inserted into the collapsed vertebral body and inflated to allow for expansion of the vertebrae and to create a cavity in which to instill bone cement (89–91). Retrospective evaluation has demonstrated improvement in pain in 84% of patients undergoing treatment with either vertebroplasty or kyphoplasty (89).

CONCLUSIONS

The effects of cancer upon bone are far-reaching and include not only treatment-related effect resulting in bone loss, but also the effects of metastatic cancer to bone. Bone metastases represent a significant source of morbidity and mortality for patients today with associated risks of pathologic fractures, bone pain, nerve impingement/compression, and side effects resulting from hypercalcemia. Bisphosphonates have been an important component of treatment for years; however, newer agents are being developed and explored as both adjuncts and alternatives for treatment. Understanding better the basic mechanisms of why cancer metastasizes to bone and the characteristics unique to the different type of metastases is important to better be able to treat this significant consequence of cancer.

REFERENCES

1. Coleman RE, Rubens RD. The clinical course of bone metastases from breast cancer. Br J Cancer 1987; 55(1):61–66.
2. Roodman GD. Mechanisms of bone metastasis. NEJM 2004; 350(16):1655–1664.
3. Coleman RE. Metastatic bone disease: clinical features, pathophysiology and treatment strategies. Cancer Treat Rev 2001; 27(3):165–176.
4. Ali SM, Harvey HA, Lipton A. Metastatic breast cancer: overview of treatment. Clin Orthop Relat Res 2003; (415 suppl):S132–S137.
5. Lipton A. Pathophysiology of bone metastases: how this knowledge may lead to therapeutic intervention. J Support Oncol 2004; 2(3):205–213; discussion 213–204, 216–207, 219–220.
6. Roodman GD. Cell biology of the osteoclast. Exp Hematol 1999; 27(8):1229–1241.
7. Kanis JA, McCloskey EV. Bone turnover and biochemical markers in malignancy. Cancer 1997; 80(8 suppl):1538–1545.
8. Riggs BL, Khosla S, Melton III, LJ. Sex steroids and the construction and conservation of the adult skeleton. Endocr Rev 2002; 23(3):279–302.
9. Vanderschueren D, Vandenput L, Boonen S, et al. Androgens and bone. Endocr Rev 2004; 25(3):389–425.
10. Hofbauer LC, Schoppet M. Clinical implications of the osteoprotegerin/RANKL/RANK system for bone and vascular diseases. JAMA 2004; 292(4):490–495.
11. Yasuda H, Shima N, Nakagawa N, et al. Osteoclast differentiation factor is a ligand for osteoprotegerin/osteoclastogenesis-inhibitory factor and is identical to TRANCE/RANKL. Proc Natl Acad Sci U S A 1998; 95(7):3597–3602.
12. Tsukii K, Shima N, Mochizuki S, et al. Osteoclast differentiation factor mediates an essential signal for bone resorption induced by 1 alpha,25-dihydroxyvitamin D3, prostaglandin E2, or parathyroid hormone in the microenvironment of bone. Biochem Biophys Res Commun 1998; 246(2):337–341.
13. Kodama H, Nose M, Niida S, et al. Essential role of macrophage colony-stimulating factor in the osteoclast differentiation supported by stromal cells. J Exp Med 1991; 173(5):1291–1294.
14. Dougall WC, Glaccum M, Charrier K, et al. RANK is essential for osteoclast and lymph node development. Genes Dev 1999; 13(18):2412–2424.
15. Lacey DL, Timms E, Tan HL, et al. Osteoprotegerin ligand is a cytokine that regulates osteoclast differentiation and activation. Cell 1998; 93(2):165–176.
16. Min H, Morony S, Sarosi I, et al. Osteoprotegerin reverses osteoporosis by inhibiting endosteal osteoclasts and prevents vascular calcification by blocking a process resembling osteoclastogenesis. J Exp Med 2000; 192(4):463–474.

17. Simonet WS, Lacey DL, Dunstan CR, et al. Osteoprotegerin: a novel secreted protein involved in the regulation of bone density. Cell 1997; 89(2):309–319.
18. Aubin JE. Bone stem cells. J Cell Biochem Suppl 1998; 30–31:73–82.
19. Yang X, Karsenty G. Transcription factors in bone: developmental and pathological aspects. Trends Mol Med 2002; 8(7):340–345.
20. Otto F, Thornell AP, Crompton T, et al. Cbfa1, a candidate gene for cleidocranial dysplasia syndrome, is essential for osteoblast differentiation and bone development. Cell 1997; 89(5):765–771.
21. Komori T, Yagi H, Nomura S, et al. Targeted disruption of Cbfa1 results in a complete lack of bone formation owing to maturational arrest of osteoblasts. Cell 1997; 89(5):755–764.
22. Mundy GR, Chen D, Zhao M, et al. Growth regulatory factors and bone. Rev Endocr Metab Disord 2001; 2(1):105–115.
23. Epstein RJ. The CXCL12-CXCR4 chemotactic pathway as a target of adjuvant breast cancer therapies. Nat Rev Cancer 2004; 4(11):901–909.
24. van der Pluijm G, Sijmons B, Vloedgraven H, et al. Monitoring metastatic behavior of human tumor cells in mice with species-specific polymerase chain reaction: elevated expression of angiogenesis and bone resorption stimulators by breast cancer in bone metastases. J Bone Miner Res 2001; 16(6):1077–1091.
25. Berruti A, Dogliotti L, Gorzegno G, et al. Differential patterns of bone turnover in relation to bone pain and disease extent in bone in cancer patients with skeletal metastases. Clin Chem 1999; 45(8 Pt 1):1240–1247.
26. Bendre MS, Gaddy-Kurten D, Mon-Foote T, et al. Expression of interleukin 8 and not parathyroid hormone-related protein by human breast cancer cells correlates with bone metastasis in vivo. Cancer Res 2002; 62(19):5571–5579.
27. Guise TA, Yin JJ, Taylor SD, et al. Evidence for a causal role of parathyroid hormone-related protein in the pathogenesis of human breast cancer-mediated osteolysis. J Clin Invest 1996; 98(7):1544–1549.
28. Pfeilschifter J, Mundy GR. Modulation of type beta transforming growth factor activity in bone cultures by osteotropic hormones. Proc Natl Acad Sci U S A 1987; 84(7):2024–2028.
29. Yin JJ, Selander K, Chirgwin JM, et al. TGF-beta signaling blockade inhibits PTHrP secretion by breast cancer cells and bone metastases development. J Clin Invest 1999; 103(2):197–206.
30. Buchs N, Manen D, Bonjour JP, et al. Calcium stimulates parathyroid hormone-related protein production in Leydig tumor cells through a putative cation-sensing mechanism. Eur J Endocrinol 2000; 142(5):500–505.
31. Coleman RE, Seaman JJ. The role of zoledronic acid in cancer: clinical studies in the treatment and prevention of bone metastases. Semin Oncol 2001; 28(2 suppl 6): 11–16.
32. Guise TA, Yin JJ, Mohammad KS. Role of endothelin-1 in osteoblastic bone metastases. Cancer 2003; 97(3 suppl):779–784.
33. Kasperk CH, Borcsok I, Schairer HU, et al. Endothelin-1 is a potent regulator of human bone cell metabolism in vitro. Calcif Tissue Int 1997; 60(4):368–374.
34. Nelson JB, Hedican SP, George DJ, et al. Identification of endothelin-1 in the pathophysiology of metastatic adenocarcinoma of the prostate. Nat Med 1995; 1(9): 944–949.

35. Yi B, Williams PJ, Niewolna M, et al. Tumor-derived platelet-derived growth factor-BB plays a critical role in osteosclerotic bone metastasis in an animal model of human breast cancer. Cancer Res 2002; 62(3):917–923.
36. Achbarou A, Kaiser S, Tremblay G, et al. Urokinase overproduction results in increased skeletal metastasis by prostate cancer cells in vivo. Cancer Res 1994; 54(9):2372–2377.
37. Rabbani SA, Desjardins J, Bell AW, et al. An amino-terminal fragment of urokinase isolated from a prostate cancer cell line (PC-3) is mitogenic for osteoblast-like cells. Biochem Biophys Res Commun 1990; 173(3):1058–1064.
38. Cramer SD, Chen Z, Peehl DM. Prostate specific antigen cleaves parathyroid hormone-related protein in the PTH-like domain: inactivation of PTHrP-stimulated cAMP accumulation in mouse osteoblasts. J Urol 1996; 156(2 Pt 1):526–531.
39. Maeda H, Koizumi M, Yoshimura K, et al. Correlation between bone metabolic markers and bone scan in prostatic cancer. J Urol 1997; 157(2):539–543.
40. Oades GM, Coxon J, Colston KW. The potential role of bisphosphonates in prostate cancer. Prostate Cancer Prostatic Dis 2002; 5(4):264–272.
41. Lee YP, Schwarz EM, Davies M, et al. Use of zoledronate to treat osteoblastic versus osteolytic lesions in a severe-combined-immunodeficient mouse model. Cancer Res 2002; 62(19):5564–5570.
42. Whang PG, Schwarz EM, Gamradt SC, et al. The effects of RANK blockade and osteoclast depletion in a model of pure osteoblastic prostate cancer metastasis in bone. J Orthop Res 2005; 23(6):1475–1483.
43. Geisler J, Haynes B, Anker G, et al. Influence of letrozole and anastrozole on total body aromatization and plasma estrogen levels in postmenopausal breast cancer patients evaluated in a randomized, cross-over study. J Clin Oncol 2002; 20(3): 751–757.
44. Baum M, Budzar AU, Cuzick J, et al. Anastrozole alone or in combination with tamoxifen versus tamoxifen alone for adjuvant treatment of postmenopausal women with early breast cancer: first results of the ATAC randomised trial. Lancet 2002; 359(9324):2131–2139.
45. Berenson JR, Lichtenstein A, Porter L, et al. Efficacy of pamidronate in reducing skeletal events in patients with advanced multiple myeloma. Myeloma Aredia Study Group. NEJM 1996; 334(8):488–493.
46. Petcu EB, Schug SA, Smith H. Clinical evaluation of onset of analgesia using intravenous pamidronate in metastatic bone pain. J Pain Symptom Manage 2002; 24(3):281–284.
47. Markowitz GS, Appel GB, Fine PL, et al. Collapsing focal segmental glomerulosclerosis following treatment with high-dose pamidronate. J Am Soc Nephrol 2001;12(6):1164–1172.
48. Desikan R, Veksler Y, Raza S, et al. Nephrotic proteinuria associated with high-dose pamidronate in multiple myeloma. Br J Haematol 2002; 119(2):496–499.
49. Ruggiero SL, Fantasia J, Carlson E. Bisphosphonate-related osteonecrosis of the jaw: background and guidelines for diagnosis, staging and management. Oral Surg Oral Med Oral Pathol Oral Radiol Endod 2006; 102(4):433–441.
50. Bamias A, Kastritis E, Bamia C, et al. Osteonecrosis of the jaw in cancer after treatment with bisphosphonates: incidence and risk factors. J Clin Oncol 2005; 23(34):8580–8587.

51. Bekker PJ, Holloway DL, Rasmussen AS, et al. A single-dose placebo-controlled study of AMG 162, a fully human monoclonal antibody to RANKL, in postmenopausal women. J Bone Miner Res 2004; 19(7):1059–1066.
52. McClung MR, Lewiecki EM, Bolognese MA, et al. AMG 162 increases bone mineral density (BMD) within 1 month in postmenopausal women with low BMD. J Bone Miner Res 2004; 19(Supp 1):S20; Abstract 1072.
53. Body JJ, Facon T, Coleman RE, et al. A study of the biological receptor activator of nuclear factor-kappaB ligand inhibitor, denosumab, in patients with multiple myeloma or bone metastases from breast cancer. Clin Cancer Res 2006; 12(4):1221–1228.
54. DeAngelo DJ, Stone RM, Heaney ML, et al. Phase 1 clinical results with tandutinib (MLN518), a novel FLT3 antagonist, in patients with acute myelogenous leukemia or high-risk myelodysplastic syndrome: safety, pharmacokinetics, and pharmacodynamics. Blood 2006; 108(12):3674–3681.
55. Missbach M, Jeschke M, Feyen J, et al. A novel inhibitor of the tyrosine kinase Src suppresses phosphorylation of its major cellular substrates and reduces bone resorption in vitro and in rodent models in vivo. Bone 1999; 24(5):437–449.
56. Sundaramoorthi R, Kawahata N, Yang MG, et al. Structure-based design of novel nonpeptide inhibitors of the Src SH2 domain: phosphotyrosine mimetics exploiting multifunctional group replacement chemistry. Biopolymers 2003; 71(6):717–729.
57. Dewar AL, Farrugia AN, Condina MR, et al. Imatinib as a potential antiresorptive therapy for bone disease. Blood 2006; 107(11):4334–4337.
58. Wang Y, Metcalf III, CA, Shakespeare WC, et al. Bone-targeted 2,6,9-trisubstituted purines: novel inhibitors of Src tyrosine kinase for the treatment of bone diseases. Bioorg Med Chem Lett 2003; 13(18):3067–3070.
59. Eastell R, Hannon RA, Gallagher N, et al. The effect of AZD0530, a highly selective, orally available Src/Abl kinase inhibitor, on biomarkers of bone resorption in healthy males. J Clin Oncol 2005; 3041.
60. Boyce BF, Xing L, Shakespeare W, et al. Regulation of bone remodeling and emerging breakthrough drugs for osteoporosis and osteolytic bone metastases. Kidney Int Suppl 2003; 85:S2–S5.
61. Rucci N, Recchia I, Angelucci A, et al. Inhibition of protein kinase c-Src reduces the incidence of breast cancer metastases and increases survival in mice: implications for therapy. J Pharmacol Exp Ther 2006; 318(1):161–172.
62. Hannon RA, Clack G, Gallagher N, et al. The effect of AZD0530, a highly selective Src inhibitor, on bone turnover in healthy males. Bone 2005; 36:S135.
63. Carducci MA, Jimeno A. Targeting bone metastasis in prostate cancer with endothelin receptor antagonists. Clin Cancer Res 2006; 12(20 Pt 2):6296s–6300s.
64. Carducci MA, Nelson JB, Bowling MK, et al. Atrasentan, an endothelin-receptor antagonist for refractory adenocarcinomas: safety and pharmacokinetics. J Clin Oncol 2002; 20(8):2171–2180.
65. Zonnenberg BA, Groenewegen G, Janus TJ, et al. Phase I dose-escalation study of the safety and pharmacokinetics of atrasentan: an endothelin receptor antagonist for refractory prostate cancer. Clin Cancer Res 2003; 9(8):2965–2972.
66. Ryan CW, Vogelzang NJ, Vokes EE, et al. Dose-ranging study of the safety and pharmacokinetics of atrasentan in patients with refractory malignancies. Clin Cancer Res 2004; 10(13):4406–4411.

67. Schulman C, Dearnaley D, Zonnenberg B, et al. Artrasentan delays disease progression in men presenting with metastatic hormone refractory prostate cancer. Presented at XIXth EAU Congress, Vienna; 2004:1057.
68. Carducci M, Nelson JB, Saad F, et al. Effects of atrasentan on disease progression and biological markers in men with metastatic hormone-refractory prostate cancer: Phase 3 study. Proceedings, 40th American Society of Clinical Oncology Annual Meeting, New Orleans; 2004: 4508.
69. Morris CD, Rose A, Curwen J, et al. Specific inhibition of the endothelin A receptor with ZD4054: clinical and pre-clinical evidence. Br J Cancer 2005; 92(12):2148–2152.
70. Gowen M, Lazner F, Dodds R, et al. Cathepsin K knockout mice develop osteopetrosis due to a deficit in matrix degradation but not demineralization. J Bone Miner Res 1999; 14(10):1654–1663.
71. Lipton A. Future treatment of bone metastases. Clin Cancer Res 2006; 12(20 Pt 2): 6305s–6308s.
72. Votta BJ, Levy MA, Badger A, et al. Peptide aldehyde inhibitors of cathepsin K inhibit bone resorption both in vitro and in vivo. J Bone Miner Res 1997; 12(9): 1396–1406.
73. Stroup GB, Lark MW, Veber DF, et al. Potent and selective inhibition of human cathepsin K leads to inhibition of bone resorption in vivo in a nonhuman primate. J Bone Miner Res 2001; 16(10):1739–1746.
74. Gelb BD, Shi GP, Chapman HA, et al. Pycnodysostosis, a lysosomal disease caused by cathepsin K deficiency. Science 1996; 273(5279):1236–1238.
75. Guise TA, Mohammad KS, Clines G, et al. Basic mechanisms responsible for osteolytic and osteoblastic bone metastases. Clin Cancer Res 2006; 12(20 Pt 2): 6213s–6216s.
76. Garrett IR, Chen D, Gutierrez G, et al. Selective inhibitors of the osteoblast proteasome stimulate bone formation in vivo and in vitro. J Clin Invest 2003; 111(11): 1771–1782.
77. Qin JZ, Ziffra J, Stennett L, et al. Proteasome inhibitors trigger NOXA-mediated apoptosis in melanoma and myeloma cells. Cancer Res 2005; 65(14):6282–6293.
78. Peles S, Fisher NM, Gao F, et al. A prospective study of the effects of once weekly bortezomib on markers of bone metabolism in patients with multiple myeloma. J Clin Oncol 2006; 24(18 suppl): 7548.
79. Badger AM, Bradbeer JN, Votta B, et al. Pharmacological profile of SB 203580, a selective inhibitor of cytokine suppressive binding protein/p38 kinase, in animal models of arthritis, bone resorption, endotoxin shock and immune function. J Pharmacol Exp Ther 1996; 279(3):1453–1461.
80. Falkmer U, Jarhult J, Wersall P, et al. A systematic overview of radiation therapy effects in skeletal metastases. Acta Oncol 2003; 42(5–6):620–633.
81. Frassica DA. General principles of external beam radiation therapy for skeletal metastases. Clin Orthop Relat Res 2003; 415 (suppl):S158–S164.
82. Silberstein EB. Systemic radiopharmaceutical therapy of painful osteoblastic metastases. Semin Radiat Oncol 2000; 10(3):240–249.
83. Bruland OS, Nilsson S, Fisher DR, et al. High-linear energy transfer irradiation targeted to skeletal metastases by the alpha-emitter 223Ra: adjuvant or alternative to conventional modalities? Clin Cancer Res 2006; 12(20 Pt 2): 6250s–6257s.

84. Smith H, Navani A, Fishman SM. Radiopharmaceuticals for palliation of painful osseous metastases. Am J Hosp Palliat Care 2004; 21(4):303–313.
85. Lipton A. Bisphosphonate therapy in the oncology setting. Expert Opin Emerg Drugs 2003; 8(2):469–488.
86. Atkins HL. Overview of nuclides for bone pain palliation. Appl Radiat Isot 1998; 49(4): 277–283.
87. Weber KL, Lewis VO, Randall RL, et al. An approach to the management of the patient with metastatic bone disease. Instr Course Lect 2004; 53:663–676.
88. Katzer A, Meenen NM, Grabbe F, et al. Surgery of skeletal metastases. Arch Orthop Trauma Surg 2002; 122(5):251–258.
89. Fourney DR, Schomer DF, Nader R, et al. Percutaneous vertebroplasty and kyphoplasty for painful vertebral body fractures in cancer patients. J Neurosurg 2003, 98(1 suppl), 21–30.
90. Dudeney S, Lieberman IH, Reinhardt MK, et al. Kyphoplasty in the treatment of osteolytic vertebral compression fractures as a result of multiple myeloma. J Clin Oncol 2002; 20(9):2382–2387.
91. Lane JM, Hong R, Koob J, et al. Kyphoplasty enhances function and structural alignment in multiple myeloma. Clin Orthop Relat Res 2004; (426):49–53.

14

The Role of Bisphosphonates to Preserve Bone Health in Patients with Breast Cancer

Allan Lipton
*Penn State Cancer Center,
Milton S. Hershey Medical Center,
Hershey, Pennsylvania, U.S.A.*

INTRODUCTION

The incidence of cancer-related deaths (including those related to breast cancer) in the United States is projected to decrease in 2006 for the first time in history (1). This milestone suggests that oncologists now have tools to prevent, diagnose, and treat cancer more effectively than ever before. However, the increase in survival for patients comes with an increased risk of long-term complications from cancer and cancer treatments. An area in which improved patient management can make an important difference is bone health. An estimated 65% to 75% of patients with advanced breast cancer develop bone metastases (2), which can have devastating consequences for their quality of life (QOL) and functional independence (3). Metastatic bone disease from breast cancer typically involves the ribs, spine, pelvis, skull, and proximal limbs (4,5), and can result in skeletal complications, termed skeletal-related events (SREs), including pathologic fracture, the need for palliative radiotherapy to bone, spinal cord compression, the need for surgery to bone to stabilize an impending fracture, and hypercalcemia of malignancy (HCM) (6).

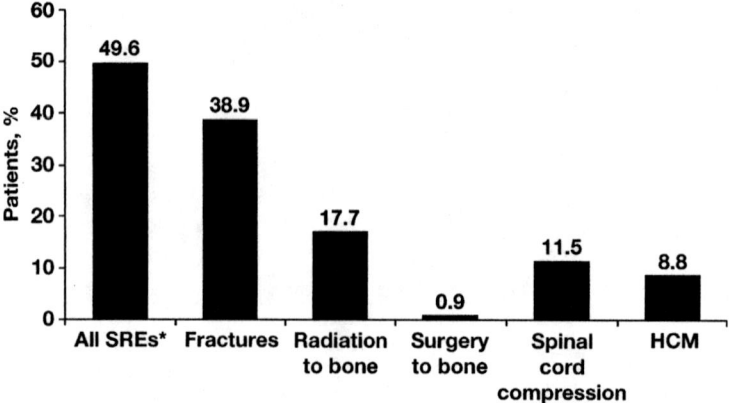

Figure 1 Skeletal-related events (SREs) in patients with advanced breast cancer who did not receive bisphosphonate therapy in a one-year trial. *Source*: Adapted with permission from Ref. 7. *Excluding hypercalcemia of malignancy (HCM).

In a one-year trial in patients with bone metastases from breast cancer, approximately half of the patients who received standard anticancer therapy but no bisphosphonate treatment developed at least one SRE, and each type of SRE occurred (Fig. 1) (7). Moreover, median survival for this population is approximately two years (2,8,9). Therefore, patients typically survive long enough to experience multiple SREs from their bone lesions (2).

Although the natural history of skeletal morbidity is highly variable, patients who experience SREs typically suffer multiple SREs over the course of their disease. In a two-year clinical trial in patients with osteolytic bone lesions from breast cancer, the annual incidence of SREs was four events/year among patients who did not receive bone-specific therapies (9). As metastatic disease progresses, the risk of skeletal complications increases, and patients often experience clusters of events that can have a devastating effect on their QOL (10). Moreover, patients who have had one event are at higher risk of developing subsequent events (11,12). In a recent retrospective analysis, pathologic fracture was reported to be associated with significantly reduced survival in patients with bone metastases from advanced breast cancer (13). These data suggest that SREs from bone metastases may add to the erosion in QOL that patients with breast cancer experience during the course of their disease (2,14,15). The introduction and international regulatory approval of the intravenous (IV) bisphosphonates pamidronate (Aredia®; Novartis Pharma AG, Basel, Switzerland; Novartis Pharmaceuticals Corporation, East Hanover, NJ, USA) and zoledronic acid (ZOMETA®; Novartis Pharma AG, Basel, Switzerland; Novartis Pharmaceuticals Corporation, East Hanover, NJ, USA) has provided oncologists with a powerful tool to help protect patients from skeletal morbidity. Monitoring and enacting therapies to maintain skeletal health may help to preserve QOL for patients with advanced breast cancer (16,17). Research in this area is ongoing.

METASTASIS TO BONE

Metastasis to bone is a complex and multistep process that occurs in the majority of patients with advanced breast cancer (Fig. 2) (2,6). Intervention at each step in the metastatic process is currently being investigated in preclinical model systems using currently available therapeutic agents, including the bisphosphonates and novel targeted therapies. However, we have made significant progress in interfering with the interactions between the bone microenvironment and metastatic tumor cells. Our increased understanding of the interactions between tumor and bone has allowed for the development of treatments to reduce skeletal morbidity associated with malignant bone lesions, and future research may allow us to prevent metastasis to bone in patients with breast cancer.

The interactions between breast cancer cells and the bone microenvironment were first postulated in 1889 by Sir Stephen Paget, who compared breast cancer cells to seeds and bone to a fertile soil in which these seeds could flourish (18). The skeleton is the site of ongoing remodeling activity that includes the balanced and locally coupled processes of removal of old or damaged bone (osteolysis) by osteoclasts and new bone formation by osteoblasts (19). Osteoclast-mediated osteolysis releases minerals and growth factors from the bone matrix (20), and these factors can foster the growth of metastatic tumor cells that arrest in the bone microenvironment. Furthermore, breast cancer cells have a predilection for interactions with bone-remodeling cells (6,19,21). As the tumor cells proliferate in the bone, they release factors such as parathyroid hormone-related protein (PTHrP) and interleukin-6 (IL-6), which stimulate osteoclast differentiation, recruitment to the bone surface, and osteolysis (22–24). Increases in osteoclast-mediated osteolysis result in further

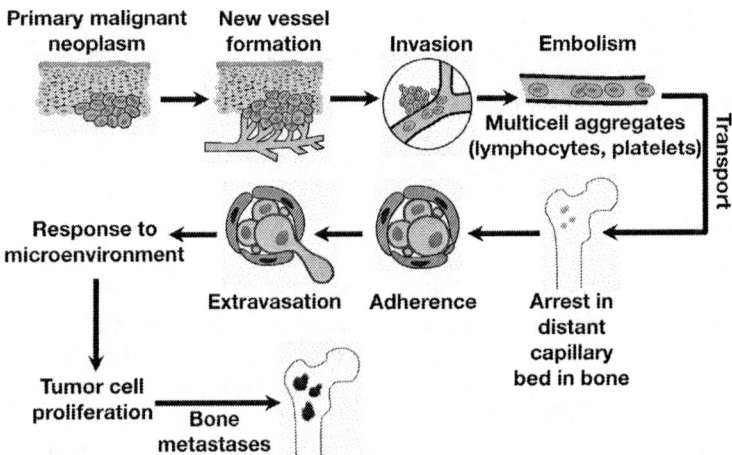

Figure 2 Multiple steps involved in breast cancer metastasis to the skeleton. *Source*: Reprinted with permission from Ref. 6.

release of growth factors from the bone matrix, which can further stimulate the metastatic tumor cells. The result is a vicious cycle of tumor growth and bone destruction (2). Other factors released from breast cancer cells can lead to the stimulation of osteoblasts, which results in increased bone matrix production (25,26). The resulting bone lesions are described as osteoblastic. Although new bone is formed in association with these lesions, the increased osteoblastic activity stimulates adjacent osteoclasts and releases paracrine signaling molecules that increase osteoclast activity, resulting in localized and generalized increase in osteolysis (described in the following section) (26). Therefore, osteoblastic lesions also increase the release of growth factors from bone and stimulate further tumor cell growth.

Osteolytic and Osteoblastic Bone Lesions

The osteolytic or osteoblastic nature of metastatic bone lesions is dictated by factors secreted by the tumor cells. Osteoclast-mediated osteolysis is directly stimulated by factors, such as PTHrP and IL-6, whereas transforming growth factor-beta (TGF-β) and endothelin-1 (ET-1) promote bone formation by osteoblasts (6). Although bone lesions are typically described based on their radiographic appearance as either osteolytic or osteoblastic, they often exhibit characteristics of both. Purely osteolytic bone lesions appear as areas of radiolucency and are characterized by an abnormally high rate of bone resorption without concomitant formation of new bone (27). In contrast, osteoblastic lesions appear as areas of increased bone density or abnormal new bone growth and are characterized by increased bone formation around tumor cell deposits. However, osteoblastic lesions are also associated with markedly increased osteolysis and bone turnover.

Pathophysiology of Bone Metastases from Breast Cancer

Most bone lesions from breast cancer are primarily osteolytic. However, many breast cancer cells have the propensity to induce osteoblastic lesions. Therefore, bone metastases secondary to breast cancer often have a mixed radiologic appearance (Fig. 3A and B) (28,29). Although osteoblastic regions exhibit radiographic evidence of increased bone formation, they are also associated with significant increases in biochemical markers of bone resorption (29–32). A study examining biochemical markers of bone resorption [urinary excretion of *N*-telopeptide (NTX) of type-I collagen, a breakdown product of the bone matrix that is produced during osteolysis] and bone formation [bone-specific alkaline phosphatase (BALP), an enzyme expressed by osteoblasts] in patients with various types of bone lesions showed that both of these markers of bone metabolism were highest in patients with osteoblastic lesions (Fig. 3C and D) (28,29). Indeed, a body of histomorphometric and biochemical evidence suggests that osteoblastic lesions are associated with markedly increased osteolysis in addition to their characteristic increases in bone formation (30,31,33–36). However, these two processes are uncoupled; bone resorption and formation occur at different sites. Therefore, the aberrant bone formation does not contribute to bone strength, and patients often suffer from generalized bone loss (27,30,37). In summary, regardless of their radiographic appearance, malignant bone lesions compromise the integrity of bone and place patients at risk of skeletal complications.

THE ROLE OF BISPHOSPHONATES FOR THE TREATMENT OF BONE METASTASES SECONDARY TO BREAST CANCER

Bisphosphonates are synthetic analogs of naturally occurring pyrophosphate that have become an integral component in the treatment of patients with advanced breast cancer. Benefits in this setting include the treatment of HCM, prevention of skeletal complications, and palliation of bone pain, all of which are based on the same underlying mechanism of action (7,9,16,38–43). Bisphosphonates bind avidly to the bone at sites of active bone remodeling and potently inhibit osteoclast-mediated osteolysis, thereby breaking the vicious cycle of bone destruction associated with bone metastases (44).

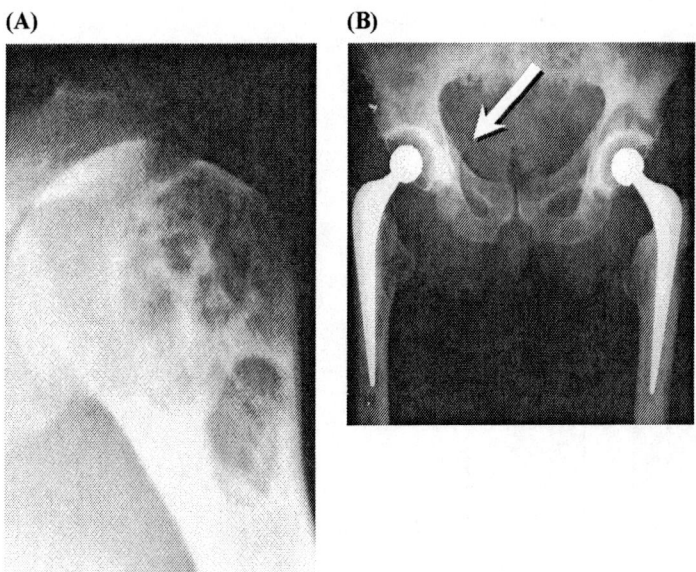

Figure 3 Plain radiograph showing a lytic (panel A) and blastic (panel B) bone lesion. Levels of bone markers in 77 patients with bone metastases grouped according to the radiologic appearance of the bone lesions. Panel C (see page 246): serum bone-specific alkaline phosphatase. Panel D: urinary N-telopeptide/creatinine ratio expressed as bone collagen equivalents (BCE) per mole creatinine (Cr). *Source*: Reprinted with permission from Ref. 29.

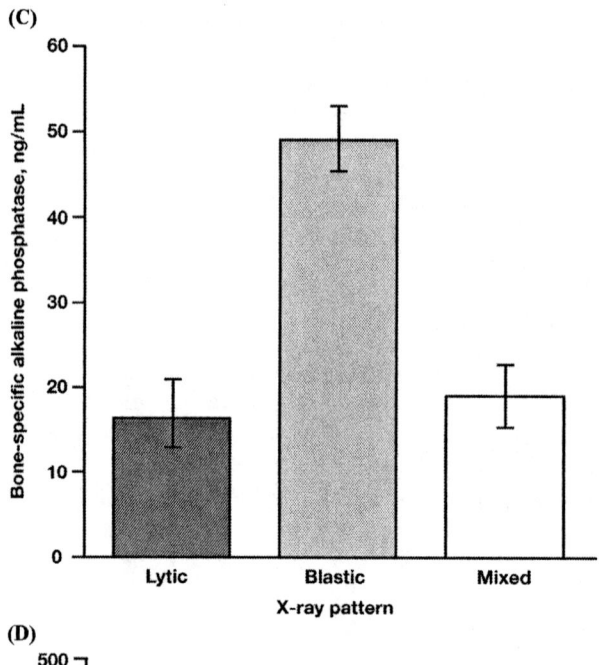
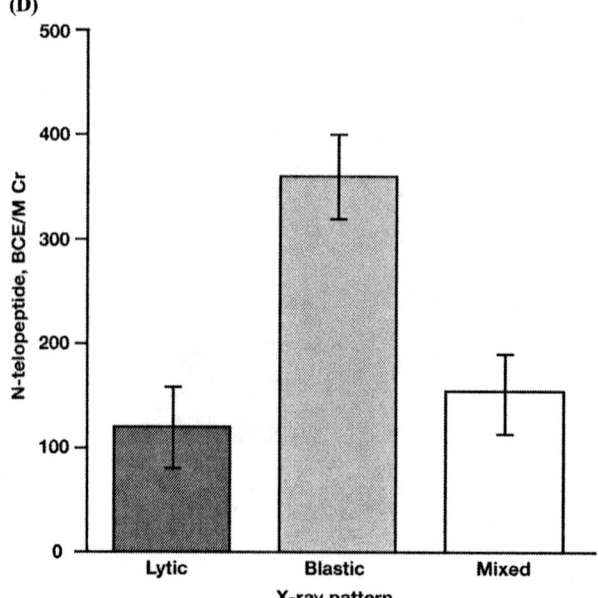

Figure 3 (Continued)

During the past 30 years, several successive generations of bisphosphonates have been developed, and each generation has demonstrated improved clinical activity (45). The majority of bisphosphonates in clinical use today have nitrogen-containing side chains. These agents are ingested by osteoclasts during osteolysis and disrupt protein prenylation via the mevalonate pathway (44,46,47), which effectively blocks the G-protein–mediated signal transduction that stimulates osteolysis (48,49). Bisphosphonates can also induce apoptosis of osteoclasts (48,50), and some agents have also been shown to have antitumor effects both in vitro and in animal model systems (51). In these systems, zoledronic acid has demonstrated the most potent antitumor effects. All of these activities may contribute to the clinical activity of bisphosphonates in patients with bone metastases from breast cancer.

Bisphosphonates Significantly Reduce Skeletal Morbidity from Malignant Bone Lesions

Clinical trials of bisphosphonates have utilized a composite endpoint, the SRE, to capture multiple clinical events that result from the same underlying pathophysiologic processes. The SRE is defined as pathologic fracture, HCM, the requirement for palliative radiotherapy, spinal cord compression, and the need for surgery of bone to treat or prevent a pathologic fracture (10,52). Both IV and oral bisphosphonates have been shown to produce significant reductions in the rate or risk of SREs in patients with bone metastases secondary to breast cancer in randomized placebo-controlled trials (Table 1) (7,9,42,53–55). In addition to their beneficial effects on objective endpoints such as risk of an SRE, bisphosphonates have also been reported to reduce bone pain and preserve QOL in patients with advanced breast cancer (16,17). Among the bisphosphonates tested in this setting, IV nitrogen-containing bisphosphonates have demonstrated the most consistent efficacy and patient compliance with therapy as compared to oral agents, and only pamidronate and zoledronic acid have been approved for the treatment of patients with bone lesions from breast cancer. Therefore, the American Society of Clinical Oncology (ASCO) consensus treatment guidelines specifically recommend that treatment with 90 mg pamidronate or 4 mg zoledronic acid be used for breast cancer patients with radiologic evidence of bone destruction (56,57). Few clinical trials have directly compared the relative efficacy of the different bisphosphonates. However, the current data suggest that zoledronic acid may provide additional benefits as compared to other agents.

Comparative Trial of Intravenous Bisphosphonates

Pamidronate was the first bisphosphonate approved for the prevention of skeletal morbidity in patients with osteolytic lesions from breast cancer and established bisphosphonates as a standard of care in this setting. Zoledronic acid is the only

Table 1 Clinical Endpoints of Bisphosphonates in Placebo-Controlled Trials for the Treatment of Bone Metastases and Breast Cancer

Agent	N	Dose (mg)	Study (Ref. no.)	Patients with ≥1 SRE (%)	Time to first SRE	SMR	SMPR	Multiple event analysis
Oral clodronate	185	1600	(53,42)	–	0.022	<0.001[a]	–	NS
Oral ibandronate	564	50	(54)	0.122	0.089	–	0.004	<0.0001[b]
IV pamidronate	367	90	(9)	<0.001	<0.001	<0.001	–	–
IV zoledronic acid	228	4	(7)	0.003	0.007	0.027	–	0.009[c]
IV ibandronate	466	6	(55)	0.052	0.018	–	0.004	–

Abbreviations: SRE, skeletal-related event; SMR, skeletal morbidity rate; SMPR, skeletal morbidity period rate; NS, not significant; IV, intravenous.
[a]Expressed as total events per 100 patient-years.
[b]By Poisson's regression analysis.
[c]By Andersen-Gill multiple event analysis.

bisphosphonate to be directly compared with pamidronate for efficacy and safety in patients with advanced breast cancer in a large-scale randomized, phase III, international, noninferiority trial (58,59). In this study, patients with either osteolytic lesions from multiple myeloma or bone metastases (osteolytic, mixed, or osteoblastic) from breast cancer were treated with 4 mg zoledronic acid or 90 mg pamidronate every three to four weeks for up to 24 months (58,59). Overall, 4 mg zoledronic acid was at least as effective as 90 mg pamidronate in the overall trial population and was significantly more effective than pamidronate in reducing the overall risk of developing an SRE over the two year study period based on multiple event analysis (59). Both agents had similar overall and renal safety profiles. In the subset of 766 breast cancer patients treated with either 4 mg zoledronic acid or 90 mg pamidronate, the benefits of zoledronic acid over pamidronate were even more apparent. Although the study was not statistically powered to detect differences between the proportion of patients who experienced at least 1 SRE in the 4 mg zoledronic acid and 90 mg pamidronate treatment groups, zoledronic acid consistently reduced the percentage of patients with each type of SRE as compared to pamidronate (60). Notably, significantly fewer patients treated with zoledronic acid required radiation therapy to bone (19% for zoledronic acid vs. 27% for pamidronate; $p = 0.011$) (60), suggesting that zoledronic acid may delay the onset of intractable bone pain. Zoledronic acid (4 mg) also produced a 42% reduction in the mean annual incidence of SREs beyond that produced by pamidronate, which represents a trend toward reduced skeletal morbidity (0.91 SRE/year for 4 mg zoledronic acid vs. 1.57 SREs/year for 90 mg pamidronate; $p = 0.102$) (59). Moreover, zoledronic acid significantly reduced the risk of developing an SRE (including HCM) by an additional 20% over the benefit provided by pamidronate in patients with breast cancer (hazard ratio $= 0.799$; $p = 0.025$) (60).

This trial enrolled patients with osteolytic and osteoblastic bone lesions, whereas earlier trials of pamidronate had enrolled only patients with osteolytic lesions (38–40). In a post hoc analysis of this trial that assessed skeletal morbidity patterns in patients with at least 1 primarily osteolytic bone lesion ($n = 528$), zoledronic acid produced a reduction in the proportion of patients who experienced an SRE that approached statistical significance as compared to pamidronate (48% for 4 mg zoledronic acid vs. 58% for 90 mg pamidronate; $p = 0.058$) (43). Moreover, zoledronic acid significantly prolonged the time to first SRE beyond that produced by pamidronate (median, 310 days for 4 mg zoledronic acid vs. 174 days for 90 mg pamidronate; $p = 0.013$) and produced an additional 30% reduction in the ongoing risk of SREs as compared to pamidronate ($p = 0.010$). Therefore, zoledronic acid has demonstrated superior efficacy compared with pamidronate in patients with osteolytic lesions from breast cancer. Zoledronic acid has also demonstrated broad clinical utility in patients with both osteolytic and osteoblastic metastases and has received widespread regulatory approval for use in patients with multiple myeloma and a broad range of solid tumors. Moreover, in a patient preference study, almost all of the participants (92%) preferred the 15 minute infusion of zoledronic acid over the two hour infusion of pamidronate (61).

Meta-Analyses of Bisphosphonate Efficacy

Although the trial comparing zoledronic acid with pamidronate is the only randomized double-blind trial comparing the two bisphosphonates, a recent meta-analysis of placebo-controlled trials of bisphosphonates in the Cochrane system database provides some insight into the relative efficacy of the different agents (Fig. 4) (42). This analysis of 21 randomized controlled studies in patients with bone metastases from breast cancer concluded that, overall, bisphosphonates reduced the risk of developing an SRE by 17% ($p < 0.00001$) and the median rate of SREs by 29%. Overall, oral and IV bisphosphonates had similar efficacy in the clinical trial setting, but the results for oral bisphosphonates were more variable. Of the assessed bisphosphonates, 4 mg IV zoledronic acid reduced the risk of SREs by 41%, as compared with 23% for 90 mg IV pamidronate, 18% for 6 mg IV ibandronate, 14% for 50 mg oral ibandronate, and 16% for 1600 mg oral clodronate (42). Each of these agents has also demonstrated significant pain reduction compared with placebo in patients with painful osseous lesions. The results from this analysis confirm the utility of bisphosphonates overall in this setting and suggest that zoledronic acid may have

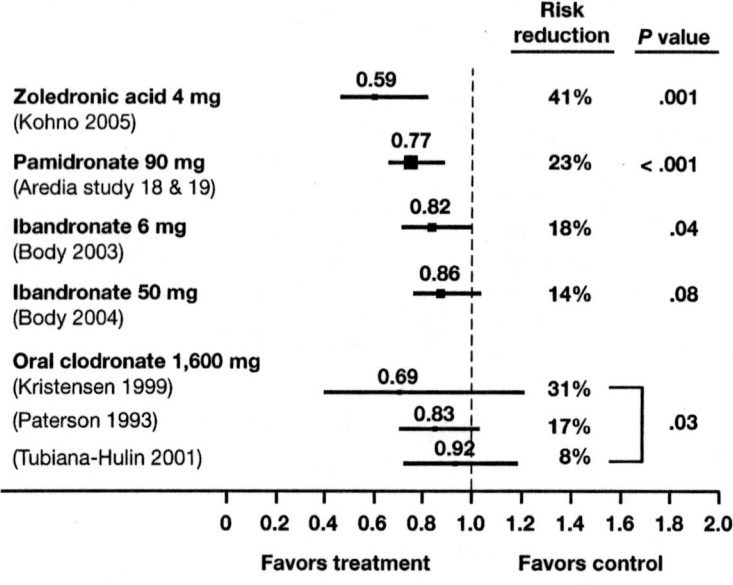

Figure 4 Cochrane Database analysis of the SRE risk reduction for bisphosphonates in patients with bone metastases from breast cancer. *Source*: Adapted with permission from Ref. 42.

an efficacy benefit when compared with other agents. Furthermore, a recent analysis comparing the associated healthcare costs per quality-adjusted life-year during IV or oral bisphosphonate therapy concluded that across multiple analyses zoledronic acid was consistently the most cost-effective therapy, and that zoledronic acid treatment of patients with bone metastases from breast cancer would actually result in cost savings to the healthcare system (14).

INVESTIGATIONAL INDICATIONS AND THERAPIES

Our current understanding of the pathophysiology of bone metastases provides us with the tools to investigate new applications for available agents and to develop new therapeutic modalities. Bisphosphonates are currently investigational for the prevention of metastasis to bone, and investigational therapies are targeting signaling factors in the bone. Therefore, in the future, combination therapies may further extend treatment benefits.

Bisphosphonates are currently investigational for the treatment of bone loss during hormonal therapy and for the prevention of bone metastases in patients with high-risk solid tumors. Previous trials with oral clodronate suggested that adjuvant therapy with bisphosphonates may delay the time to onset of skeletal metastases; however, results with this first-generation, relatively weak bisphosphonate have been inconsistent (62–65). Therefore, more active new agents may provide additional benefits. For example, in a pilot study in patients with a variety of high-risk solid tumors, zoledronic acid treatment significantly delayed metastasis to bone (66). An ongoing trial, titled the Adjuvant Zoledronic Acid to Reduce Recurrence in Patients With High-Risk Localized Breast Cancer (AZURE), is currently investigating whether administering zoledronic acid to patients with high-risk stage II/III breast cancer can delay the onset of bone metastases. This trial has currently finished accrual ($N = 3360$), and an interim analysis is planned after 470 events have occurred, which is projected to happen in late 2007. Molecular markers of bone resorption, such as NTX, are currently being investigated as prognostic indicators of patients who are at high risk of SRE. Persistently elevated NTX levels have been found to correlate with an increased risk of SRE and death. Recent analyses indicate that zoledronic acid-mediated normalization of NTX levels within three months significantly reduces the risk of death as compared to patients with refractory NTX elevations (67). Targeting high-risk patients with early intervention will likely improve their overall clinical outcome.

Signal transduction intermediates within the bone metabolism signaling pathways have recently been targeted by investigational therapies in an attempt to more effectively block the vicious cycle of bone destruction and tumor growth. One of these molecular targets is receptor activator of nuclear factor kappa B (RANKL), which plays a pivotal role in the differentiation and activation of osteoclasts (68). Denosumab (AMG162) is a fully humanized monoclonal antibody directed against RANKL (68,69). This agent has recently shown significant benefits for the treatment of postmenopausal osteoporosis, although there was a slight increase in infections and cancer rates for the patients treated with denosumab compared with placebo (69). Preliminary results from trials in malignant bone disease presented at the 2006 ASCO meeting suggest that this agent has utility for the prevention of SREs (70). Further investigations are necessary to determine the role of this agent alone or in combination with bisphosphonates for the treatment of bone metastases in patients with breast cancer.

CONCLUSIONS

Patients with bone metastases from breast cancer are at risk for SREs that can undermine their QOL and functional independence. However, the introduction of bone-specific therapies has provided an important tool for the maintenance of skeletal health in this setting. Currently, only two bisphosphonates have been approved in the United States for the treatment of bone metastases: pamidronate and zoledronic acid. Of these agents, zoledronic acid has the shortest infusion time and broadest clinical utility. Recent analyses suggest that zoledronic acid may be the most efficacious bisphosphonate in this setting. The addition of other bone-specific therapies into the therapeutic repertoire may allow for greater control over the interactions between tumor and bone by use of combination therapy approaches. This is currently an area of active research, and additional benefits including possible reductions in the rate of metastasis to bone are possible.

REFERENCES

1. Jemal A, Siegel R, Ward E, et al. Cancer statistics, 2006. CA Cancer J Clin 2006, 56(2), 106–130.
2. Coleman RE. Metastatic bone disease: clinical features, pathophysiology and treatment strategies. Cancer Treat Rev 2001; 27(3):165–176.
3. Cheville AL. Cancer rehabilitation. Semin Oncol 2005; 32(2):219–224.
4. Coleman RE. Skeletal complications of malignancy. Cancer 1997; 80(8 suppl): 1588–1594.
5. Coleman RE. Efficacy of zoledronic acid and pamidronate in breast cancer patients: a comparative analysis of randomized phase III trials. Am J Clin Oncol 2002; 25 (6 suppl 1):S25–S31.
6. Guise TA, Mundy GR. Cancer and bone. Endocr Rev 1998, 19(1), 18–54.
7. Kohno N, Aogi K, Minami H, et al. Zoledronic acid significantly reduces skeletal complications compared with placebo in Japanese women with bone metastases from breast cancer: a randomized, placebo-controlled trial. J Clin Oncol 2005; 23(15): 3314–3321.
8. Domchek SM, Younger J, Finkelstein DM, et al. Predictors of skeletal complications in patients with metastatic breast carcinoma. Cancer 2000; 89(2):363–368.
9. Lipton A, Theriault RL, Hortobagyi GN, et al. Pamidronate prevents skeletal complications and is effective palliative treatment in women with breast carcinoma and osteolytic bone metastases: long term follow-up of two randomized, placebo-controlled trials. Cancer 2000; 88(5):1082–1090.

10. Major PP, Cook R. Efficacy of bisphosphonates in the management of skeletal complications of bone metastases and selection of clinical endpoints. Am J Clin Oncol 2002; 25(6 suppl 1):S10–S18.
11. Zheng M, Rosen L, Gordon D, et al. Continuing benefit of zoledronic acid for the prevention of skeletal complications in breast cancer patients with bone metastases. Poster presented at Primary Therapy of Early Breast Cancer 9th International Conference, St. Gallen, Switzerland, 26–29 January 2005.
12. Conte P, Rosen LS, Gordon D, et al. Zoledronic acid is superior to pamidronate in patients with breast cancer and multiple myeloma: analysis of patients at high risk for skeletal complications. Poster presented at 29th European Society for Medical Oncology Congress, Vienna, Austria, 29 October–2 November 2004. Abstract 463PD.
13. Hei Y-J, Saad F, Coleman R, et al. Fractures negatively affect survival in patients with bone metastases from breast cancer. Poster presented at the 28th Annual San Antonio Breast Cancer Symposium (SABCS), San Antonio, Texas, Dec 8–11, 2005. Abstract 6036.
14. Botteman M, Barghout V, Stephens J, et al. Cost effectiveness of bisphosphonates in the management of breast cancer patients with bone metastases. Ann Oncol 2006; 17(7):1072–1082.
15. Wedin R, Bauer HC, Rutqvist LE. Surgical treatment for skeletal breast cancer metastases: a population-based study of 641 patients. Cancer 2001; 92(2):257–262.
16. Wardley A, Davidson N, Barrett-Lee P, et al. Zoledronic acid significantly improves pain scores and quality of life in breast cancer patients with bone metastases: a randomised, crossover study of community vs hospital bisphosphonate administration. Br J Cancer 2005; 92(10):1869–1876.
17. Weinfurt KP, Castel LD, Li Y, et al. Health-related quality of life among patients with breast cancer receiving zoledronic acid or pamidronate disodium for metastatic bone lesions. Med Care 2004; 42(2):164–175.
18. Paget S. The distribution of secondary growths in cancer of the breast. Lancet 1889; 1:571–572.
19. Mundy GR. Metastasis to bone: causes, consequences and therapeutic opportunities. Nat Rev Cancer 2002; 2(8):584–593.
20. Saad F. Zoledronic acid: past, present and future roles in cancer treatment. Future Oncol 2005; 1(2):149–159.
21. Barnes GL, Javed A, Waller SM, et al. Osteoblast-related transcription factors Runx2 (Cbfa1/AML3) and MSX2 mediate the expression of bone sialoprotein in human metastatic breast cancer cells. Cancer Res 2003; 63(10):2631–2637.
22. Hunt NC, Fujikawa Y, Sabokbar A, et al. Cellular mechanisms of bone resorption in breast carcinoma. Br J Cancer 2001; 85(1):78–84.
23. Roodman GD. Biology of osteoclast activation in cancer. J Clin Oncol 2001, 19(15), 3562–3571.
24. Thomas RJ, Guise TA, Yin JJ, et al. Breast cancer cells interact with osteoblasts to support osteoclast formation. Endocrinology 1999; 140(10):4451–4458.
25. Lipton A, Small E, Saad F, et al. The new bisphosphonate, Zometa (zoledronic acid), decreases skeletal complications in both osteolytic and osteoblastic lesions: a comparison to pamidronate. Cancer Invest 2002; 20(suppl 2):45–54.
26. Guise TA, Kozlow WM, Heras-Herzig A, et al. Molecular mechanisms of breast cancer metastases to bone. Clin Breast Cancer 2005; 5(2 suppl):S46–S53.

27. Vinholes J, Coleman R, Eastell R. Effects of bone metastases on bone metabolism: implications for diagnosis, imaging and assessment of response to cancer treatment. Cancer Treat Rev 1996; 22(4):289–331.
28. Lipton A. Bisphosphonate therapy for patients with osteolytic and osteoblastic bone metastases from breast or prostate cancer. In: Yao AP, ed. Trends in Breast Cancer Research. New York: Nova Science Publishers Inc.2005:157–180.
29. Demers LM, Costa L, Lipton A. Biochemical markers and skeletal metastases. Cancer 2000; 88(12 suppl):2919–2926.
30. Berruti A, Dogliotti L, Tucci M, et al. Metabolic bone disease induced by prostate cancer: rationale for the use of bisphosphonates. J Urol 2001; 166(6):2023–2031.
31. Garnero P, Buchs N, Zekri J, et al. Markers of bone turnover for the management of patients with bone metastases from prostate cancer. Br J Cancer 2000; 82(4):858–864.
32. Mundy GR. Mechanisms of bone metastasis. Cancer 1997; 80(8 suppl):1546–1556.
33. Clarke NW, McClure J, George NJ. Morphometric evidence for bone resorption and replacement in prostate cancer. Br J Urol 1991; 68(1):74–80.
34. Clarke NW, McClure J, George NJ. Disodium pamidronate identifies differential osteoclastic bone resorption in metastatic prostate cancer. Br J Urol 1992; 69(1):64–70.
35. Percival RC. Skeletal effects of carcinoma of the breast and prostate. Ann R Coll Surg Engl 1986; 68(5):267–270.
36. Taube T, Kylmala T, Lamberg-Allardt C, et al. The effect of clodronate on bone in metastatic prostate cancer. Histomorphometric report of a double-blind randomised placebo-controlled study. Eur J Cancer 1994; 30A(6):751–758.
37. Kanis JA, McCloskey EV, Taube T, et al. Rationale for the use of bisphosphonates in bone metastases. Bone 1991; 12(suppl 1):S13–S18.
38. Hortobagyi GN, Theriault RL, Lipton A, et al. Long-term prevention of skeletal complications of metastatic breast cancer with pamidronate. Protocol 19 Aredia Breast Cancer Study Group. J Clin Oncol 1998; 16(6):2038–2044.
39. Hortobagyi GN, Theriault RL, Porter L, et al. Efficacy of pamidronate in reducing skeletal complications in patients with breast cancer and lytic bone metastases. Protocol 19 Aredia Breast Cancer Study Group. NEJM 1996; 335(24):1785–1791.
40. Theriault RL, Lipton A, Hortobagyi GN, et al. Pamidronate reduces skeletal morbidity in women with advanced breast cancer and lytic bone lesions: a randomized, placebo-controlled trial. Protocol 18 Aredia Breast Cancer Study Group. J Clin Oncol 1999; 17(3):846–854.
41. Major PP, Lipton A, Berenson J, et al. Oral bisphosphonates: A review of clinical use in patients with bone metastases. Cancer 2000; 88(1):6–14.
42. Pavlakis N, Schmidt RL, Stockler M. Bisphosphonates for breast cancer (review). Cochrane Database Syst Rev 2005; 3:CD003474.
43. Rosen LS, Gordon DH, Dugan Jr., W, et al. Zoledronic acid is superior to pamidronate for the treatment of bone metastases in breast carcinoma patients with at least one osteolytic lesion. Cancer 2004; 100(1):36–43.
44. Russell RG, Rogers MJ. Bisphosphonates: from the laboratory to the clinic and back again. Bone 1999; 25(1):97–106.
45. Fleisch H. Development of bisphosphonates. Breast Cancer Res 2002; 4(1):30–34.
46. Luckman SP, Hughes DE, Coxon FP, et al. Nitrogen-containing bisphosphonates inhibit the mevalonate pathway and prevent post-translational prenylation of GTP-binding proteins, including Ras. J Bone Miner Res 1998; 13(4):581–589.

47. Rogers MJ, Frith JC, Luckman SP, et al. Molecular mechanisms of action of bisphosphonates. Bone 1999; 24(5 suppl):73S–79S.
48. Coxon FP, Helfrich MH, Van't Hof R, et al. Protein geranylgeranylation is required for osteoclast formation, function, and survival: inhibition by bisphosphonates and GGTI-298. J Bone Miner Res 2000; 15(8):1467–1476.
49. Alakangas A, Selander K, Mulari M, et al. Alendronate disturbs vesicular trafficking in osteoclasts. Calcif Tissue Int 2002; 70(1):40–47.
50. Benford HL, McGowan NW, Helfrich MH, et al. Visualization of bisphosphonate-induced caspase-3 activity in apoptotic osteoclasts in vitro. Bone 2001; 28(5):465–473.
51. Clezardin P. The antitumor potential of bisphosphonates. Semin Oncol 2002; 29(6 suppl 21):33–42.
52. Johnson JR, Williams G, Pazdur R. End points and United States Food and Drug Administration approval of oncology drugs. J Clin Oncol 2003; 21(7):1404–1411.
53. Paterson AH, Powles TJ, Kanis JA, et al. Double-blind controlled trial of oral clodronate in patients with bone metastases from breast cancer. J Clin Oncol 1993; 11(1):59–65.
54. Body JJ, Diel IJ, Lichinitzer M, et al. Oral ibandronate reduces the risk of skeletal complications in breast cancer patients with metastatic bone disease: results from two randomised, placebo-controlled phase III studies. Br J Cancer 2004; 90(6): 1133–1137.
55. Body JJ, Diel IJ, Lichinitser MR, et al. Intravenous ibandronate reduces the incidence of skeletal complications in patients with breast cancer and bone metastases. Ann Oncol 2003; 14(9):1399–1405.
56. Hillner BE, Ingle JN, Berenson JR, et al. American Society of Clinical Oncology guideline on the role of bisphosphonates in breast cancer. J Clin Oncol 2000; 18(6): 1378–1391.
57. Hillner BE, Ingle JN, Chlebowski RT, et al. American Society of Clinical Oncology 2003 update on the role of bisphosphonates and bone health issues in women with breast cancer. J Clin Oncol 2003; 21(21):4042–4057.
58. Rosen LS, Gordon D, Kaminski M, et al. Zoledronic acid versus pamidronate in the treatment of skeletal metastases in patients with breast cancer or osteolytic lesions of multiple myeloma: a phase III, double-blind, comparative trial. Cancer J 2001; 7(5): 377–387.
59. Rosen LS, Gordon D, Kaminski M, et al. Long-term efficacy and safety of zoledronic acid compared with pamidronate disodium in the treatment of skeletal complications in patients with advanced multiple myeloma or breast carcinoma: a randomized, double-blind, multicenter, comparative trial. Cancer 2003; 98(8):1735–1744.
60. Coleman RE, Rosen LS, Gordon D, et al. Zoledronic acid significantly reduces the risk of developing a skeletal-related event compared with pamidronate in breast cancer patients with bone metastases. Poster presented at 25th Annual San Antonio Breast Cancer Symposium, San Antonio, Tex, December 11–14, 2002. Poster 355.
61. Chern B, Joseph D, Joshua D, et al. Bisphosphonate infusions: patient preference, safety and clinic use. Support Care Cancer 2004; 12(6):463–466.
62. Diel IJ, Solomayer EF, Costa SD, et al. Reduction in new metastases in breast cancer with adjuvant clodronate treatment. NEJM 1998; 339(6):357–363.
63. Jaschke A, Bastert G, Solomayer E, et al. Adjuvant clodronate treatment improves the overall survival of primary breast cancer patients with micrometastases to bone marrow: a longtime follow-up. J Clin Oncol 2004; 23(14S suppl):9. Abstract 529.

64. Powles T, Paterson S, Kanis JA, et al. Randomized, placebo-controlled trial of clodronate in patients with primary operable breast cancer. J Clin Oncol 2002; 20(15):3219–3224.
65. Saarto T, Blomqvist C, Virkkunen P, et al. Adjuvant clodronate treatment does not reduce the frequency of skeletal metastases in node-positive breast cancer patients: 5-year results of a randomized controlled trial. J Clin Oncol 2001; 19(1):10–17.
66. Mystakidou K, Katsouda E, Parpa E, et al. Randomized, open label, prospective study on the effect of zoledronic acid on the prevention of bone metastases in patients with recurrent solid tumors that did not present with bone metastases at baseline. Med Oncol 2005; 22(2):195–201.
67. Lipton A, Cook RJ, Coleman RE, et al. Prognostic significance of persistently elevated N-telopeptide levels in patients with bone metastases from solid tumors. Poster presented at 31st European Society for Medical Oncology (ESMO) Congress, Istanbul, Turkey, 29 September–3 October 2006. Abstract 870P.
68. Whyte MP. The long and the short of bone therapy. NEJM 2006; 354(8):860–863.
69. McClung MR, Lewiecki EM, Cohen SB, et al. Denosumab in postmenopausal women with low bone mineral density. NEJM 2006; 354(8):821–831.
70. Lipton A, Alvarado C, De Boer R, et al. Randomized, active-controlled study of denosumab (AMG 162) in breast cancer patients with bone metastases not previously treated with intravenous (IV) bisphosphonates (BP). J Clin Oncol 2006; 24(18S suppl):6S. Abstract 512.

15

Supportive Care for Older Cancer Patients

Michelle Shayne
James P. Wilmot Cancer Center, University of Rochester, Rochester, New York, U.S.A.

Lodovico Balducci
H. Lee Moffitt Cancer Center, University of South Florida, Tampa, Florida, U.S.A.

INTRODUCTION

Supportive care refers to the management of symptoms or side effects for patients who carry a diagnosis of cancer. The term encompasses a broad range of meaning as in "best supportive care," which generally implies an alternative to disease management employing chemotherapy, hormonal therapy, or targeted therapies. Supportive care instead focuses on management of symptoms that develop as a result of disease progression. Such usage of the term is synonymous with palliative care. In addition, supportive care suggests aggressive management of disease-related symptoms as well as side effects from treatment employed to reduce the risk of disease recurrence. In the case of incurable malignancies, supportive care measures enhance quality of life and minimize symptoms of chemotherapy used to control disease progression. Supportive care can vary in approach and the level of complexity. Older cancer patients have unique needs that can impact the approach to maintaining optimal supportive care. Malignancy-related symptoms can negatively impact quality of life, and in some cases can also serve as critical determinants in assessing prognosis (1). The decline in organ function, along with multiple comorbidities, can make the treatment of cancer as well as the administration of palliative care a significant challenge for the healthcare team. Furthermore, communication may be compromised by auditory, visual, or cognitive deficits. Nevertheless, the goals of supportive care in older cancer patients are not unlike those of their younger counterparts, specifically, to prolong the duration of life, while optimizing quality of life.

This chapter will address the variety of strategies available not only to manage the side effects of cancer treatment in patients 65 years of age and older, but also to control the problems that arise from malignancy itself in this unique population of patients. The principles presented here are applicable to older patients who develop symptoms in the setting of cancer treatment administered with intent to cure, as well as to those for whom chemotherapy and other medical therapies are no longer an option.

Symptom Assessment and Clinical Decision Making

The initial series of clinical decisions made to determine the optimal approach to an individual older cancer patient's care should always employ a comprehensive geriatric assessment (CGA) to estimate life expectancy and potential tolerance to treatment (2,3). The primary domains in the CGA include functional status, gait, fall risk, cognition, affective status, nutritional status, pain, and social interaction (4). One strategy to allow for a more patient-tailored approach to treatment employs a CGA that includes the activities of daily living (ADL) as well as the instrumental activity of daily living (IADL) scales (5). A determination of benefit to risk for any potential treatment should include the identification of conditions that could increase the risk of treatment-related complications. Certain conditions may be reversible before treatment initiation. Other conditions can be anticipated and mitigated with prophylactic measures so as to minimize overall toxicity.

A symptom assessment tool, such as the validated Edmonton Symptom Assessment Score (6,7), can be employed to readily ascertain both the major problems and the relative severity of each issue as determined by the patient on a 10-point scale.

Clinicians who routinely employ these assessment tools can better identify specific issues affecting their older cancer patients. Problems can then be stratified with respect to level of severity and a targeted approach to management promptly initiated. Significant overlap between major issues such as fatigue, depression, and pain in many cancer patients may be further complicated in older patients in whom multiple comorbidities, polypharmacy, and unique psychosocial stressors coexist. Therefore, this systematic approach to palliative care is well suited to older cancer patients.

MANAGEMENT OF CANCER-RELATED SYMPTOMS

Pain

Cancer-related pain is experienced by over 70% of patients during the course of their illness (8), and over 40% of older cancer patients have reported poorly controlled pain (9). The prevalence of pain appears to vary with respect to situational context and is age-associated. For individuals who live independently, pain is more commonly observed over the age of 60 (10). Prevalence rates of pain as high as 80% have been reported for those living in alternative care settings (11). Yet, older individuals are less likely to receive appropriate pain management as compared to their younger counterparts (9,12). The reasons for this may stem from some patients' inability to effectively communicate their symptoms. Furthermore, there may be age-related variability in pain perception. An increase in pain threshold and decline in pain tolerance have been observed in older patients (13,14). Under-reporting of pain by older patients may be related to a number of factors including concerns regarding addiction, misconception that pain is a common consequence of aging, and also atypical manifestations of pain, such as delirium. Thus, differences in perception and reporting can potentially lead to under-diagnosis of pain or misinterpretation of pain severity by treating clinicians (15). Furthermore, clinicians may undertreat pain due to concerns regarding side-effect profiles of specific analgesics or drug interactions (16). In addition to patient- and clinician-generated barriers to effective pain control, economic barriers should be considered. The cost of drugs and insurance coverage limitations are critical variables for older patients on limited or fixed incomes.

The major barrier to effective pain management is suboptimal pain assessment (17). To appropriately assess and treat pain in the older cancer patient, the intensity, quality, and distribution of the pain are essential characteristics to define. One common means of assessing pain severity is the visual analog scale (VAS), a 10-point scale in which the extremes are defined as "no pain" corresponding to a level of 0/10 and "the worst possible pain" corresponding to a level of 10/10 (18). While unidimensional scales such as this one only measure pain intensity, multidimensional scales such as the McGill Pain Questionnaire (MPQ) offer a more comprehensive assessment (19). Reliability and suitability of these scales in older patients have been questioned (20). A higher rate of incorrect responses on the VAS has been associated with increasing age (21). It is, therefore, best to couple the use of such pain assessment scales with questions directed at ascertaining the specific impact of the patient's pain on day-to-day functioning.

The clinician must also consider general age-associated physiologic alterations in pharmacokinetics as well as comorbid illnesses and current medications of the individual patient. While a parsimonious approach to prescribing is favored, the clinician should always bear in mind the possibility that various types of pain may coexist, necessitating different analgesic agents for effective control (22).

Nonpharmacologic approaches to pain control include physical and cognitive methods. Physical methods, such as physical therapy, massage, acupressure, acupuncture, transcutaneous electrical nerve stimulation (TENS), and exercise, are some of the options available to patients. Cognitive methods include the use of imagery, music therapy, and behavioral therapies such as relaxation techniques (23). In the outpatient setting, pain education intervention has been shown to provide valuable support for the older cancer patient and family members (24).

The three types of analgesic drugs employed for the management of cancer pain include the non-opioid, opioid, and adjuvant agents. The World Health Organization "analgesic ladder" approach is advised for appropriate drug selection (25).

Opioids

Opioids are considered the mainstay of cancer pain management. A combination of opioid and non-opioid should be used to control mild to moderate cancer pain (25). Stronger opioids, such as morphine or oxycodone, should be used to manage more severe cancer pain. Low-dose, short-acting, or immediate-release forms of these drugs should be used initially over 24 to 48 hours. For opioid-naïve patients, the suggested initial dose for morphine is 5 to 10 mg every 4 hours. The total 24-hour dose should then be calculated and converted to a long-acting sustained release form to maintain more uniform levels. Ongoing titration is often required to maintain optimal pain control. Older patients are not necessarily more susceptible to opioid effects during opioid titration as compared to younger patients. As such, individual response should guide titration efforts regardless of age (26). In situations where pain is inadequately controlled and accompanied by unacceptable toxicity, substitution with another opioid should be attempted (27). The optimal dose is that which confers adequate pain relief without unmanageable side effects. Once a long-acting optimal pain regimen has been determined, most patients will also require fast-acting pain control for the intermittent acute pain exacerbation known as "breakthrough" pain. The fast-acting narcotic dose should be between 10% and 20% of the long-acting, 24-hour narcotic dose.

Side effects of opioids most often include constipation, sedation, and nausea. Older patients treated with opioids can also develop confusion, hallucinations, seizures, and respiratory depression. The symptom of constipation should be anticipated and managed prophylactically with increased dietary fiber and fluid intake (28,29). Medications, such as senna, docusate, and bisacoldyl, can be incorporated into the prophylactic bowel regimen (see below). Nausea can be exacerbated by constipation. A promotility agent such as metoclopramide can sometimes be used to manage both nausea and constipation, particularly in older patients with impaired gastrointestinal motility related to long-standing diabetes.

Opioid-induced delirium in older patients can be effectively managed with low-dose haloperidol; however, other causes of delirium should always be ruled out first.

A number of routes of administration exist for opioid delivery. Oral tablets are convenient and the least costly; however, an alternative oral form is the transmucosal approach. Fentanyl is available as a lollipop for breakthrough pain control. Transdermal Fentanyl is a long-acting drug available for patients who have difficulty in swallowing. Time to peak delivery of this drug is 12 hours with a steady state achieved in 48 to 72 hours (30). As such, a short-acting opioid is needed in conjunction for pain management when initiating this drug.

Opioids that are not recommended for older patients include meperidine and propoxyphene because of potential accumulation of toxic metabolites that can cause central nervous system toxicity.

Non-Opioid Analgesics

The non-opioid analgesics, such as nonsteroidal anti-inflammatory agents (NSAIDs), acetaminophen, and aspirin, can be used in conjunction with opioids to manage moderate-level cancer pain. As the mechanism of action of these drugs is independent of opioid receptor activation, these agents can confer synergy and allow, in some cases, for lower doses of opioids while still conferring adequate pain control. Caution should be exercised when using NSAIDs in older patients due to multiple potential adverse side effects, such as gastritis or renal insufficiency (31).

Analgesic Adjuvants

Analgesic adjuvants include tricyclic antidepressants, anticonvulsants, and steroids. These drugs can be used to target specific types of pain, such as neuropathic pain or pain that is exacerbated by inflammation. Occasionally, an opioid-sparing advantage can be had by using these alagesics. While tricyclic antidepressants, such as amitriptyline, nortriptyline, and desipramine, are effective for some patients in conferring relief of neuropathic pain, these drugs should be used with caution in older patients, given the primarily anticholinergic side-effect profile that includes sedation, orthostatic hypotension, constipation, urinary retention, and agitation. Tricyclic antidepressants should be avoided in older patients with cardiac conduction abnormalities, such as bundle branch block and bifascicular block (32).

The anticonvulsant drug gabapentin has been shown to be effective for the management of neuropathic cancer pain in conjunction with opioids (33). The drug is generally well tolerated, but side effects may include sedation, dizziness, and ataxia.

Corticosteroids are effective at controlling pain in the setting of advanced malignancy, particularly when pain is associated with nerve compression, increased intracranial pressure, or bone metastases (34). In addition to providing pain relief, corticosteroids can enhance mood and appetite. Adverse side effects include water retention, impaired glucose tolerance, and, with prolonged use, myopathy and avascular bone necrosis.

Fatigue and Weakness

Fatigue is one of the most common symptoms experienced by cancer patients and has been reported in more than 78% of these individuals, particularly those undergoing active treatment (35,36). Individual perception of fatigue is highly variable. As such, defining, characterizing, and quantifying fatigue can be challenging. This, in turn, can make the determination of the specific etiology of fatigue, as well as the approach to treatment, equally daunting. Cancer-associated fatigue differs qualitatively from tiredness that results from stress or exercise. Fatigue, by definition, is not responsive to sleep or rest. Yet, even when controlling for hemoglobin level, fatigue in cancer patients is significantly more severe than fatigue experienced in the general, healthy population (37). In the setting of malignancy, fatigue can be progressive over time and may produce physical, cognitive, psychological, and emotional sequelae including diminished energy and activity, compromised mental concentration, and decreased motivation (38). Several validated instruments are available to assist the clinician in characterizing fatigue and ascertaining its impact on the quality of life (39–44). While these instruments have not been validated in a population strictly comprised of older patients, another assessment tool has, the Fatigue Symptom Inventory (FSI) (45,46).

Management of fatigue should initially involve ascertaining the specific cause and correcting this whenever possible. In addition, both pharmacologic and nonpharmacologic approaches exist to further optimize intervention. Nonpharmacologic approaches include patient education; (47) addressing the issues pertaining to sleep hygiene (48), instituting exercise, and rehabilitation; (49) and encouraging proper nutrition (50).

Pharmacologic management of fatigue includes the use of drugs to address the possible contributing variables such as narcotics and anti-inflammatory agents to palliate pain, exogenous erythropoietin and or blood transfusions to address anemia, and antidepressants to control depression. Medications should be reviewed routinely to eliminate drug duplications, or nonessential medications should be discontinued as they may exert a sedating effect. If these approaches are ineffective in managing fatigue, psychostimulants such as methylphenidate and dextroamphetamine can be employed. While patient-controlled methylphenidate has been studied for management of cancer-related fatigue, the study population was not relegated specifically to older patients (51). We recommend using these agents only after an exhaustive effort has been attempted to control fatigue through other means as psychostimulants can be associated with anorexia, delirium, anxiety, and tachycardia.

Depression

Depression in patients with malignancy is a common problem having prevalence rates between 17% and 33% (52,53). The prevalence of depression in cancer patients also varies with respect to cancer type (pancreas 50%, breast 10–26%, and colon 13–32%) and may be affected by the specific antineoplastic agents used in disease management (54). Depression in older cancer patients may be further complicated by diverse psychosocial issues, such as the deaths of spouse and/or siblings and close friends, retirement, gradual loss of independence, and the impact of comorbid diseases. Identifying depression in older cancer patients can be challenging as numerous signs and symptoms—such as decreased appetite, weight loss, difficulty in sleeping, fatigue, and decreased social interaction—used to make the diagnosis may also result from the malignancy itself, related symptoms, or medications.

The assessment of depression may be facilitated by the use of several screening instruments, such as the Geriatric Depression Scale (GDS) (55) and the Center for Epidemiologic Studies-Depression Scale (CES-D) (56). While reasonably sensitive and specific for identifying depression in older patients, these instruments have yet to be validated in a population of older cancer patients.

The management of depression in older patients with cancer includes both pharmacologic and psychotherapeutic interventions. Education has been shown to be an effective means of reducing depressive symptoms in the general population of cancer patients (57); however, studies on psychoeducational interventions in older cancer patients are lacking.

The class of drugs known as selective serotonin reuptake inhibitors (SSRIs) includes fluoxetine, paroxetine, and sertraline. These drugs are safe to use for older cancer patients as they are nonsedating and have few anticholignergic side effects (58). These drugs are also an appropriate first choice for management of depression in older patients who have cardiac conduction defects, prostatic hypertrophy, or poorly controlled glaucoma (59,60). The disadvantages of these drugs are possible side effects of anorexia, nausea, diarrhea, and anxiety. The onset of action is at least two weeks and the half-life may be prolonged in older patients.

Numerous antidepressants, such as tricyclic antidepressants including amitriptyline, amoxapine, clomipramine, desipramine, doxepin, imipramine, and nortiptyline, should generally be avoided in older persons as these drugs may cause severe cardiovascular or central nervous system events (58,61).

Anorexia and Cachexia

Anorexia is characterized by loss of appetite or interest in eating. Over time, this can result in significant weight loss and contribute to generalized weakness. The cause of anorexia in older cancer patients is often multifactorial and related to nausea, vomiting, mucositis, depression, pain, dysphagia, odynophagia, and dysguesia.

Difficulty swallowing may be a direct side effect of chemotherapy or a secondary symptom of infection such as by *Candida albicans*. Such yeast infections may arise in the setting of steroid use and/or poor oral hygiene. The rate of depressive symptomatology was inversely correlated with nutritional status in a study of older men with prostate cancer (62).

The best approach to managing anorexia is to identify the specific etiology responsible for this problem and address it as soon as possible. The mininutritional assessment (MNA) is a commonly used screening tool. Good oral hygiene is an important first step in improving nutritional status, but this may be hampered by painful oral lesions secondary to chemotherapy (approach to management of oral mucositis below). In the setting of oral mucositis, patients should be encouraged to try softer foods. Moist and bland foods are likewise appropriate in this setting. Nutritional assessment with a dietician is often beneficial. Diet plans and food choice can be addressed in detail during these consultations, and a multitargeted strategy geared towards optimizing nutritional status can be initiated. The added complexities of comorbidities, such as diabetes or renal failure, which are more common in older patients, and may impact dietary choices, can likewise be addressed.

Appetite stimulation is an additional therapeutic approach for management of anorexia in the older cancer patient that is not without its own unique set of challenges. Early identification of poor nutrition and implementation of corrective measures is important as recovery of lean body mass may be a slower process in these patients (63).

Numerous studies have demonstrated the benefits of megestrol acetate in the setting of cancer-related anorexia and cachexia (64–66). Benefits of this drug include improved appetite, increased caloric intake, and weight gain. There may also be antiemetic benefits associated with megestrol acetate use (64). Older, less active patients, however, may be particularly vulnerable to potential thromboembolic complications associated with the use of this agent. In addition, adrenal insufficiency as a result of adrenal-axis suppression may further complicate this approach to anorexia.

Corticosteroids such as prednisone and dexamethasone may be used to ameliorate anorexia. The benefit of these drugs may include optimizing caloric intake or overall nutritional status (67). The use of these drugs may also be associated with potential inhibition of the hypothalamic-pituitary-adrenal axis as well as increased risk for the development of gastrointestinal irritation with exacerbation of reflux symptoms. To avoid complications, steroids should be administered in the morning with food. A concomitant proton pump inhibitor or H2 blocker should be taken. Added benefits of corticosteroid use include the control of symptoms related to inflammation such as bronchospasm and bone pain. Mood elevation occurs in some patients. This may result in activation that can compromise sleep.

Cancer cachexia is characterized by decreased nutrient consumption and disproportionate loss of lean body mass along with increased resting energy expenditure. This state is the result of inflammatory cytokine abnormalities and resultant metabolic alterations (68). Tumor necrosis factor, interleukin-1 and -6, and interferon-alpha (69,70) are some of the inflammatory cytokines thought to play a role.

Nutritional supplementation with parenteral feeding is a controversial issue. Metabolic cachexia cannot be reversed by nutritional supplementation alone (71). Parantaral nutrition seldom influences the course of the disease. Furthermore, elderly patients may be at increased risk for some of the complications of parantaral feeding such as catheter-related infections (72). Other complications of artificial nutrition include catheter-related thrombosis, metabolic imbalances, and hepatic dysfunction. At present, the American Society for Parenteral and Enteral Nutrition does not support the routine implementation of parenteral nutrition for individuals with advanced malignancy. Nevertheless, the European Organization for Research and Treatment of Cancer has demonstrated survival and quality of life advantages for the use of parenteral nutrition (73). These findings await validation as well as confirmation in older cancer patients.

Constipation

A decrease in the number of bowel movements, along with a harder stool consistency, characterizes constipation. Older cancer patients may be at an increased risk of developing this problem on the basis of physiologic loss of colonic cells and decreased gastrointestinal mucosal growth with age, comorbidities (such as diabetes that may contribute to delayed gastrointestinal motility), dietary changes (such as decreased fiber intake), and medications (such as narcotics for pain control that may compromise gastrointestinal motility). Furthermore, older patients, in general, may have difficulty in physically accessing the toilet or may require assistance with toileting, which may result in avoidance or decreased frequency of bowel movements. Cancer-associated causes of constipation, such as hypercalcemia, spinal cord compression, or obstructive colorectal tumors, can further exacerbate these existing issues.

An assessment of bowel function should be included in each routine physical and history for the older cancer patient. When constipation is identified as a problem, this should be further characterized by the number of bowel movements per day, frequency, and stool consistency. The approach to management includes nonpharmacologic and pharmacologic interventions. The nonpharmacologic means of optimizing bowel function includes recommendations for increased physical activity where possible, increasing dietary fiber content, and encouraging ingestion of fluids. Physical activity promotes gastrointestinal motility; dietary fiber increases stool bulk and volume to facilitate evacuation.

Stool softeners such as docusate sodium are anionic surfactants that facilitate water uptake of stool by reducing stool surface tension. Safe and gentle-acting, these agents are often used in combination with stimulant laxatives to maximize the effect.

Simulant laxatives have a wide range of action. Mild-acting agents as represented by senna, cascara, and aloe are best to try in the initial management of constipation for older persons. Moderate-acting drugs such as bisacodyl can be used if the desired effect is not achieved with the frontline drugs. The mechanism of action involves the initiation of peristalsis directly through myenteric plexus stimulation as well as promotion of water and electrolyte secretion. Stronger-acting stimulant laxatives such as castor oil are not recommended for older persons as these drugs can cause marked electrolyte and fluid imbalances and exert direct toxic effects on the intestinal epithelium.

Osmotic laxatives also work by stimulating peristalsis through water retention. This class of drugs includes lactulose, glycerin, and polyethylene glycol. These drugs can be effective for problematic constipation not responsive to stool softeners and mild-acting stimulant laxatives.

Bulk-forming agents, such as psyllium mucilloid, methylcellulose, and carboxymethylcellulose, are crude fiber products that absorb water and produce intestinal bulk (74). Fluid intake is essential to avoid intestinal obstruction. The effects of these agents may be delayed in older patients.

The use of enemas should be reserved for specific indications such as fecal impaction. Milk and molasses enemas and soap suds enemas should not be used for older patients as these can cause severe irritation and occasionally colitis.

Diarrhea

Diarrhea is characterized by frequent and numerous stools of liquid consistency. If severe, there may be incontinence of stool. Diarrhea may have numerous causes, such as drugs including laxatives, antibiotics, and antineoplastic agents. Infectious etiologies, such as *Clostridium difficile, Escherichia coli,* or viral pathogens, can cause severe diarrhea. Changes in diet may significantly affect bowel patterns as well.

It is important to grade the severity of chemotherapy-related diarrhea in order to select an optimal management strategy as well as understand when chemotherapy dose reductions are needed. Opioid-related drugs, such as loperamide and diphenoxylate, are effective first-line agents for the management of grade 2 or higher diarrhea. Opium tincture, while often useful, should be used with great caution in older patients as this population may be more sensitive to its effects. For persistent or grade 3 or 4 diarrhea, subcutaneous octreotide can be employed. Often IV hydration is necessary as well for optimal management.

Dyspnea

Dyspnea in older cancer patients is a factor that may affect long-term survival (75,76). There are numerous potential etiologies to account for dyspnea in cancer patients. These causes may be associated with concurrent illnesses, such as chronic obstructive pulmonary disease and congestive heart failure. Pleural or pericardial effusion, superior vena cava obstruction, ascites, progressive anemia, or pneumothorax as a complication of the underlying malignancy can also cause dyspnea. Treatment, such as chemotherapy- or radiation-induced pneumonitis or fibrosis can cause dyspnea. Further complicating matters of diagnosis in older patients is the potential for unusual presentations of cancer-related complications such as pulmonary embolus (77). Elucidating the etiology of dyspnea in any patient is necessary since this will affect the approach to its management. Interventions such as thoracentesis or paracentesis may be indicated. Medical management of nontreatable dyspnea can be quite effective and can have a significant benefit in terms of optimizing the quality of life. Morphine may function to relieve dyspnea by reducing excessive respiratory drive due to a direct effect on the brainstem respiratory center (78). There may also be mechanistic contributions from anxiolytic and antitussive effects as well as pain relief.

MANAGEMENT OF CANCER TREATMENT-RELATED COMPLICATIONS

Mucositis

Musositis, an inflammation of the tissue lining the mouth and gastrointestinal tract, is associated with use of specific cytotoxic chemotherapeutic agents, such as flurouricil, methotrexate, and doxorubicin. Mucositis can also occur in the setting of radiation therapy. This symptom can contribute to decreased oral intake with resultant weight loss and fatigue. When severe, this side effect can result in chemotherapy dose reduction and delay, which, in turn, can compromise the effectiveness of treatment. Mucositis can also lead to infectious complications as well as significantly influence analgesic and parenteral nutrition use. Clinical studies have demonstrated that mucositis in older cancer patients may be particularly severe (79), possibly as a result of compromised repair of mucosal damage that occurs with aging (80).

A variety of prophylactic and treatment approaches exist to address mucositis. One method to decrease the risk of mucositis involves the replacement of intravenous fluorinated pyrimidine with oral capecitabine. Since capecitabine is the prodrug of 5-fluorouracil with activation in the liver and neoplastic cells, the use of this drug effectively minimizes exposure of normal cells to the active metabolite (81). When this approach is not possible and bolus infusional fluorinated pyrimidines must be employed, oral cryotherapy, having patients hold ice chips in their mouths during chemotherapy infusion, has been shown to reduce oral mucositis by about 50%. The ice produces local vasoconstriction that limits the exposure of the oral mucosa to the circulating cytotoxic drug (82,83). This approach is not an option for patients receiving concomitant oxaliplatin, given the propensity for cold-induced neuropathy associated with this drug.

Keratinocyte growth factors such as palifermin have been shown to reduce mucositis severity and duration following stem cell transplantation for hematologic malignancies. Yet, the double-blind study that demonstrated these findings did not include patients of 70 years of age and older (84). Further research is ongoing in the role of this agent in patients with solid tumors and radiation-induced mucositis (85).

AES-14, which concentrates L-glutamine in the oral mucosa, has been found to reduce the risk of mucositis in a phase III trial. AES-14 reduced the first cycle incidence of grade 2 to 4 oral mucositis by 22%. Of 326 chemotherapy patients randomized in the study, the mean age was 51 years (86).

The management of existing mucositis should include good oral hygiene. Rinsing with salt water or a solution of salt water with baking soda can be soothing. To control pain associated with severe cases, the use of viscous lidocaine alone or in combination with diphenhydramine and Maalox, is effective for some patients. Dentures may cause further irritation particularly if ill-fitting, and removal of these may temporarily ease oral discomfort. Avoidance of acidic and spicy foods should also be encouraged.

Nausea and Vomiting

Age is a determinant in developing chemotherapy-induced nausea and vomiting (87), with older patients generally experiencing less severe immediate and anticipatory nausea and vomiting with respect to the administration of treatment as compared to younger patients.

Delayed nausea and vomiting following chemotherapy may be more common and severe in older cancer patients (88). Delayed emesis is well controlled with corticosteroids and 5-HT3-receptor antagonists. However, comorbidity and polypharmacy in the elderly may contribute to underutilization of steroids for management of nausea and vomiting in this population of patients (89). While 5-HT3-receptor antagonists may cause dehydration and impaired cognition in older patients, palonosetron, a second generation 5-HT-3 antagonist, has been studied in elderly patients. This drug was shown to provide effective antiemetic control as well as demonstrate a favorable safety profile (90).

Myelosuppression

Multiple risk models for neutropenic complication in cancer patients undergoing systemic chemotherapy have identified increasing age as a significant independent predictor of such risk (91). The neutropenic infection incidence in a study of 500 unselected large-cell lymphoma patients in the community treated with cyclophosphamide, adriamycin/mitoxantrone, vincristine, prednisone (CHOP/CNOP) was 38% for patients 65 years of age and older as compared to 18% for younger patients. The duration of hospitalization for neutropenic complications was 25% (4 days) longer for the older patients (92). Furthermore, more neutropenia-related deaths occur in older patients (93,94). Yet, the resultant compensatory reductions in chemotherapy relative dose intensity in older cancer patients may compromise the outcome in these patients (95).

The use of prophylactically administered myeloid growth factor represents an alternative approach to chemotherapy dose reduction in supportive management of neutropenic complications in cancer treatment. A reduction in risk of febrile neutropenia among older patients has been demonstrated in several randomized clinical trials employing the prophylactic myeloid growth factor strategy (96–98). Nevertheless, prophylactic myeloid growth factor support is offered to only a minority of older cancer patients initiating systemic chemotherapy. The more common approach to reducing risk of neutropenia in older cancer patients has been the reduction in relative dose intensity of chemotherapy (99,100).

Variables associated with increased risk of neutropenic complications of chemotherapy in older cancer patients include cancer type, planned relative dose intensity of chemotherapy $\geq 85\%$, body surface area ≤ 2 m^2, previous chemotherapy, anthracycline- or platinum-based chemotherapy, elevated baseline alkaline phosphatase, and blood urea nitrogen (101). A validated risk model for predicting early chemotherapy-related neutropenic events in cancer patients 65 years of age and older has demonstrated good discrimination between those patients at decreased risk for neutropenic complications and those at increased risk, who may derive significant benefit from prophylactic myeloid growth factor use (102). These findings await prospective confirmation in a cohort of older cancer patients.

Cost Effectiveness of Myeloid Growth Factors

Half of cancer healthcare expenditures are for patients 65 years of age and older (103). As such, the cost of preventive strategies such as the use of prophylactic myeloid growth factors to limit potentially costly hospitalizations for neutropenic complications have been analyzed (104–106). Clinical decision models have repeatedly demonstrated economic as well as clinical benefits to be had by patients receiving myeloid growth factors. Benefits of cancer treatment are also assessed in terms of disease-free and overall survival. Limited life expectancy and less treatment-responsive malignancy are factors that contribute to less cost-effective management in older as compared to younger cancer patients (107). To offset these limitations in treatment benefits, significant gains must be observed in reduction of treatment-related toxicity. Significant benefits in cost effectiveness of targeted granulocyte colony–stimulating factor use have been observed in a study of early-stage breast cancer patients receiving adjuvant chemotherapy.

A group of women at highest risk for neutropenic complications, in whom growth factors were employed to sustain chemotherapy dose intensity, were compared with women who received a standard chemotherapy dose reduction (108). The use of prophylactic growth factors thus proved effective not only in terms of cost effectiveness but also in terms of maintaining chemotherapy standard dose intensity, which has been shown to improve disease-free and overall survival (109).

Presently the American Society of Clinical Oncology (ASCO), European Organisation for Research and Treatment of Cancer (EORTC), and National

Comprehensive Cancer Network (NCCN) guidelines are consistent in the recommendation for the use of prophylactic growth factors when the risk of developing chemotherapy-related neutropenia is greater than 20%. The use of growth factors is also recommended for secondary prophylaxis in response to chemotherapy reaction, to sustain chemotherapy dose intensity, and in the management of patients 65 years of age and older (110–112).

Cardiomyopathy

Anthracyclines and the monoclonal antibody traztuzumab are associated with rates of cardiotoxicity as high as 1% and 4%, respectively (113,114). Older age is a significant independent risk factor for development of anthracycline-induced subclinical cardiomyopathy even at moderate doses (115). Approaches to mitigating risk of anthracycline-induced cardiomyopathy include the substitution of epirubicin for doxorubicin in the adjuvant setting. In the metastatic setting, the liposomal form of doxorubicin can be used as an alternative to standard doxorubicin. The antidote desrazoxane has been used to reduce the cardiotoxicity of anthracyclines. The use of sequential traztuzumab following chemotherapy, as opposed to concomitant use, has been shown to decrease potential cardiotoxicity, though possibly at the price of diminished efficacy (116). For older patients with existing cardiac compromise, avoidance of anthracyclines may be necessary. No specific precautions against chemotherapy-related cardiotoxicity are recommended for older cancer patients at this time. A tailored approach is suggested in incorporating each unique patient's cardiac history, cancer type, and stage in decision making with respect to the use of potentially cardiotoxic agents. Ongoing monitoring of cardiac function with echocardiogram or radionuclide scan is appropriate.

Neuropathy

Peripheral Neuropathy

Numerous antineoplastic agents are associated with peripheral neuropathy including taxanes (paclitaxel, docetaxel, and abraxane), vinca alkaloids (vincristine and vinblastine), synthetic alkaloids (vindesine and vinorelbine), epipodophyllotoxins (etoposide and teniposide), and platinum-containing drugs cisplatin, carboplatin, and oxaliplatin. In addition, thalidomide and borteomib, both used to treat myeloma, are associated with neuropathy. As a result of exposure to these drugs, patients may develop dysesthesias including numbness and tingling, weakness, compromise in fine motor skills, dysphagia, odynophagia, high-frequency hearing loss, and decrease in deep tendon reflexes. In addition, autonomic neuropathy characterized by postural hypotension, bradycardia, bladder atony, and obstipation may develop.

Advanced age alone may not be associated with increased incidence or severity of peripheral neuropathy (117,118). Nevertheless, with incidence rates between 16% (117) and 50% (118), depending upon the chemotherapy regimen used, the effects can be devastating in this population of patients. Chemotherapy-induced peripheral neuropathy may exacerbate pre-existing diabetic neuropathy and negatively impact mobility or diminish fine motor skills so as to negatively impact ADL.

Approaches to minimizing chemotherapy-related neuropathy include modifying the dosing schedule of drugs wherever possible, such as substituting weekly taxanes for every three-weekly taxanes (119).

Central Neurotoxicity

Older patients may be at increased risk for development of chemotherapy-induced CNS toxicity as a result of age-related decline in neurons (120). In addition, age-related effects on the blood–brain barrier may enhance susceptibility to drugs in older patients (121). A number of antineoplastic agents, such as fludarabine and fluorouracil, may cause neurotoxicity, particularly in elderly cancer patients. Older cancer patients are more likely to sustain cerebellar toxicity from high-dose cytarabine (3 g/m^2) (122). Yet, one study demonstrated no association between neurotoxicity and age following the adjustment for renal insufficiency (123). The neurotoxic effects of cytarabine may thus be exacerbated when excretion of its toxic metabolite uracil arabinoside is impaired in the setting of a reduced glomerular filtration rate. Neurologic evaluations should be performed at scheduled intervals throughout the course of high-dose cytarabine administration, and the drug discontinued at the first sign of CNS toxicity. While cerebellar toxicity secondary to fluorouracil is uncommon, the effects can be devastating. The necessity to discontinue fluorouracil following such toxicities poses a significant clinical dilemma for management of gastrointestinal malignancies where fluorouracil constitutes the "backbone" of multiagent therapy.

SUMMARY

Aggressive symptom control for cancer patients, whether on active treatment or facing the end of life, can have a substantial effect on improving quality of life. Supportive care of older patients with cancer may be particularly challenging due to the complex interplay between comorbidities, polypharmacy, and psychosocial issues. While validated instruments for assessing and characterizing complex symptoms do exist, many have not been specifically validated in older persons. Research in supportive measures, specifically tailored to the needs of older cancer patients, is ongoing and should eventually contribute to enhanced quality of life.

REFERENCES

1. Laussaniere J, Vinant P. Prognostic factors, survival, and advanced cancer. J Palliat Care 1992; 8(4):52–54.
2. Extermann M, Hurria A. Comprehensive geriatric assessment for older patients with cancer. JCO 2007; 25(14):1824–1829.
3. Repetto L, Balducci L. A case for geriatric oncology. Lancet Oncol 2002; 3(5):289–297.
4. Monfardini S, Balducci L. A comprehensive geriatric assessment (CGA) is necessary for the study and the management of cancer in the elderly. Eur J Cancer 1999; 35:1771–1772.
5. Bernardi D, Milan I, Balzarotti M, et al. Comprehensive geriatric evaluation in elderly patients with lymphoma: feasibility of a patient-tailored treatment plan. J Clin Oncol 2003; 21:754.
6. Bruera E, Kuehn N, Miller MJ, et al. The Edmonton Symptom Assessment System (ESAS): a simple method for the assessment of palliative care patients. J Palliat Care 1991; (Summer, 7):6–9.
7. Chang VT, Hwang SS, Feuerman M. Validation of the edmonton symptom assessment Scale. Cancer 2000; 88:2164–2171.
8. Cleeland C, Gonin R, Hatfield AK, et al. Pain and its treatment in outpatients with metastatic cancer. NEJM 1994; 330:592–596.
9. Cleeland CS. Undertreatment of cancer pain in elderly patients. JAMA 1998; 279:1914–1915.
10. Crook J, Rideout E, Browne G. The prevalence of pain complaints among a general population. Pain 1984; 18:299–302.
11. Ferrell BA, Ferrell BR, Osterweil D. Pain in the nursing home. J Am Griatr Soc 1990; 38:409–414.
12. Bernabei R, Gambassi G, Lapane K, et al. Management of pain in elderly patients wit cancer. SAGE Study Group. Systematic Assessment of Geriatric Drug Use via Epidemiology. JAMA 1998; 279:1877–1882.
13. Gagliese L, Melzack R. Chronic pain in elderly people. Pain 1997; 70:3–14.
14. Gibson SJ, Helme RD. Age-related differences in pain perception and report. Clin Geriatr Med 2001; 17:433–456.
15. Cohen-Mansfield J, Marx MS. Pain and depression in the nursing home. Corroborating results. J Gerentol 1993; 48:906–907.
16. Gloth FM. Geriatric pain. Factors that limit pain relief and increased complication. Geriatrics 2000; 55:46–54.
17. von Roenn J, Cleeland C, Gonin R, et al. Physician attitudes and practice in cancer pain management: a survey from the Eastern Cooperative Oncology Group. Ann Intern Med 1993; 119:121–126.
18. Huskisson EC. Measurement of pain. Lancet 1974; 2:1127–1131.
19. Melzack, R. The McGill Pain Questionnaire: major properties and scoring methods. Pain 1975; 1:277–299.
20. Herr KA, Mobily PR. Comparison of selected pain assessment tolls for use with the elderly. Appl nurs Res 1993; 6:39–46.
21. Jensen, MP, Karoly P, Braver S. The measurement of clinical pain intensity: a comparison of six methods. Pain 1986; 27:117–126.
22. Jensen, MP, Karoly P, Braver S. The measurement of clinical pain intensity: a comparison of six methods. Pain 1986; 27:117–126.

23. Urba SG. Nonpharmacologic pain management in terminal care. Glin Geriatr Med 1996; 12:301–311.
24. Ferrell BR, Ferrell BA, Ahn C, Tran K. Pain management for elderly patients with cancer at home. Cancer 1994; 74:2139–2146.
25. World Health Organization. Cancer Pain Relief and Palliative Care: a Report of a WHO Expert Committee. Geneva: World Health Organization, 1990.
26. Mercadante S, Ferrera P, Villari P, et al. Opioid Escalation in patients with cancer patients: The effect of age. J Pain Symptom Manage 2006; 32:413–419.
27. Mercadante S. Opioid rotation for cancer pain. Cancer 1999; 86:1856–1866.
28. Portenoy R, Miransky J, Thaler K, et al. Pain in ambulatory patients with lung or colon cancer: prevalence, characteristics, and effect. Cancer 1992; 70:1616–1624.
29. Grossman S, Benedetti C, Payne R, et al. NCCN practice guidelines for cancer pain. Oncology 1999; 13:33–44.
30. Payne R, Mathias S, Pasta D. Quality of life and cancer pain; satisfaction and side effects with transdermal fentanyl versus oral morphine. J Clin Oncol 1998; 16:1588–1593.
31. AGS Panel on Chronic Pain in Older Persons. The management of chronic pain in older persons. J Am Geriatr Soc 1998; 46:653–651.
32. Dietch JT, Fine M. The effect of nortriptylline in elderly patients with cardiac conduction disease. J Clin Psychiatry 1990; 51:65–67.
33. Caraceni A, Zecca E, Bonezzi C, et al. Gabapentin for neuropathic cancer pain: a randomized controlled trial from the Gabpentin Cancer Pain Study Group. J Clin Oncol 2004; 22:2909–2917.
34. Twycross R. The risks and benefits of corticosteroids in advanced cancer. Drug Saf 1994; 11:163–178.
35. Curt GA. The impact of Fatigue on patients with cancer: overview of FATIGUE 1 and 2. The Oncologist 2000; 5:9–12.
36. Vogelzang NJ, Breitbart W, Cella D, et al. Patient, caregiver and oncologist perceptions of cancer-elated fatigue: results of a tripart assessment survey. Semin Hematol 1997; 34:4–12.
37. Cella D, Lai JS, Chang CH, et al. Fatigue in cancer patients compared with fatigue in the general United States population. Cancer 2002; 94:528–538.
38. Cella D, Lai JS, Chang CH, et al. Fatigue in cancer patients compared with fatigue in the general United States population. Cancer 2002; 94:528–538.
39. Yellen SB, Cella DR, Webster K, et al. Measuring fatigue and other anemia-related symptoms with the Functional Assessment of Cancer Therapy (FACT) measurement system. J Pain Symptom Manage 1997; 13:63–74.
40. Piper BF, Dibble SL, Dodd MJ, et al. The revised Piper Fatigue Scale: psychometric evaluation in women with breast cancer. Oncol Nurs Forum 1998; 25:677–684.
41. Schwartz AL. The Schwartz Cancer Fatigue Scale: testing reliability and validity. Oncol Nurs Forum 1998; 25:711–717.
42. Hann DM, Jacobsen PB, Azzarello LM, et al. Measurement of fatigue in cancer patients: development and validation of the Fatigue Symptom Inventory. Qual Life Res 1998; 7:301–310.
43. Mendoza TR, Wang XS, Cleeland CS, et al. The rapid assessment of fatigue severity in cancer patients: use of the Brief Fatigue Inventory. Cancer 1999; 85:1186–1196.

44. Okuyama T, Akechi T, Kugaya A, et al. Development and validation of the cancer fatigue scale: a brief, three-dimensional, self-rating scale for assessment of fatigue in cancer patients. J Pain Symptom Manage 2000; 19:5–14.
45. Hann DM, Jacobsen PB, Azzarello LM, et al. Measurement of fatue in cancer patients: development and validation of the fatigue symptom inventory. Qual Life Res 1998; 7:301–310.
46. Respini D, Jacobsen PB, Thors C, et al. The prevalence and correlates of fatigue in older cancer patients. Crit Rev in Oncol Hematol 2003; 47:273–279.
47. Stacey D. Coping with fatigue: an education session for cancer patients. Can Oncol Nurs J 1998; 8:S15.
48. Berger AM, VonEssen S, Khun BR, et al. Feasibility of a sleep intervention during adjuvant breast cancer chemotherapy. Oncol Nurs Forum 2002; 29:1431–1441.
49. Dimeo F, Stieglitz RD, Novelli-Fischer U, et al. Effects of physical activity on the fatigue in cancer patients. Cancer 2001; 92:1694–1698.
50. Kalman D, Villani LJ. Nutritional aspects of cancer-related fatigue. J Am Diet Assoc 1997; 97:650–654.
51. Bruera E, Driver L, Barnes EA, et al. Patient-controlled methylphenidate for the management of fatigue in patients with advanced cancer: a preliminary report. J Clin Oncl 2003; 21:4439–4443.
52. Bukberg J, Penman D, Holland JC. Depression in hospitalized cancer patients. Psychomsom Med 1984; 46:199–212.
53. Hopweel P, Stephens RJ. Depression in patients with lung cancer: prevalence and risk factors derived from quality-of-life data. J Clin Oncol 2000; 18(4):893–903.
54. Newport DJ, Nemeroff CB. Assessment and treatment of depression in the cancer patient. J Psychosom Res 1998; 45:215–237.
55. Montorio I, Izal M. The Geriatric Depression Scale: a review of its development and utility. Int Psychogeriatr 1996; 8:103–112.
56. Roberts RE, Vernon SW. The Center for Epidemiologic Studies Depression Scale: its use in a community sample. Am J Psychiatr 1983; 140:41–46.
57. Barsevick AM, Sweeney C, Haney E, et al. A systematic qualitative analysis of psychoeducational interventions for depression in patients with cancer. Oncol Nurs Forum 2002; 29:73–84.
58. Berney A, Stiefel F, Mazzacato C, et al. Psychopharmacology in supportive care of cancer: a review for the clinician. III Antidepressants. Support Care Cancer 2000; 8:278–286.
59. Reynolds III, CF., depression: making the diagnosis and using SSRIs in the older patient. Geriatrics 1996; 51:28–34.
60. Flint AJ. Choosing appropriate antidepressant therapy in the elderly. A risk-benefit assessment of available agent. Drugs Aging 1998; 13:269–280.
61. Beers MH, Explicit criteria for determining potentially inappropriate medication use by the elderly. An update. Arch Intern Med 1997; 157:1531–1536.
62. Toliusiene J, Lesauskaite V. The nutritional status of older men with advanced prostate cancer and factors affecting it. Support Care Cancer 2004; 12:716–719.
63. Hardy C, Wallace C, Khansur T, et al. Nutrition, cancer, and aging: an annotated review. II. Cancer cachexia and aging. J Am Geriatr Soc 1986; 34:219–228.
64. Loprinzi CL, Ellison NM, Schaid DJ, et al. A controlled trial of megestrol acetate in patients with cancer anorexia and/or cachexia. J Natl Cancer Inst 1990; 82: 1127–1132.

65. Rowland Jr., KM, Loprinzi CL, Shaw EF, et al. Randomized double blind placebo controlled trial of cisplatin and etoposide plus megestrol acetate. Placebo in extensive stage small cell lung cancer. J Clin Oncol 1996; 14:135–141.
66. Loprinzi CL, Kugler JW, Sloan JA, et al. Randomized comparison of megestrol acetate verses dexamethasone versus fluoxymesterone for the treatment of cancer anorexia/cachexia. J Clin Oncol 1999; 17:3299–3306.
67. Puccio M, Nathanson L. The cancer cachexia syndrome. Semin Oncol 1997; 24:277–287.
68. Falconer JS, Fearon KC, Plester CE, et al. Cytokines, the acute-phase response, and resting energy expenditure in cachectic patients with pancreatic cancer. Ann Surg 1994; 219:325–331.
69. Mantovani G, Maccio A, Mura L, et al. Serum levels of leptin and proinflammatory cytokines in patients with advanced: stage cancer at different sites. J Mol Med 2000; 78:554–561.
70. Staal-van den Brekel AJ, Dentener MA, Schols AM, et al. Increased resting energy expenditure and weight loss are related to a systemic inflammatory response in lung cancer patients. J Clin Oncol 1995; 13:2600–2605.
71. Tisdale MJ. Cancer cachexia. Nutrition 1997; 13:1–7.
72. Andris DA, Krzywda EA. Central venous access: clinical practice issues. Nurs Clin North Am 1997; 32:719–740.
73. Shang E, Weiss C, Post S, et al. The influence of early supplementation of parenteral nutrition on quality of life and body composition in patients with advanced cancer. J Parenter Enteral Nutr 2006; 30:222–230.
74. Cheskin Lj, Kamal N, Crowell MD, et al. Mechanisms of constipation in older persons and effects of fiver compared to placebo. J Am Geriatr Soc 1995; 43: 666–669.
75. Dominguez-Ventura A, Cassivi SD, Allen MS, et al. Lung cancer in octogenarians: factors affecting long-term survival following resection Eur J Cardiothorac Surg 2007 Jun 5(E-ub ahead of print).
76. Volpino P, Cangemi R, Fiori E, et al. Risk of mortality from cardiovascular and respiratory causes in patients with chronic obstructive pulmonary disease submitted to follow-up after lung resection for non-small cell lung cancer. J Cardiovasc Surg 2007; 48:375–383.
77. Rogers RL. Venous thromboembolic disease in the elderly patient: atypical, subtle, and enigmatic. Clin Geriatr Med 2007; 23:413–423.
78. Goodman and Gilman. The Pharmacological Basis of Therapeutics, 10th ed. New York: McGraw Hill, 2001.
79. Petrelli N, Douglass HO, Herrera L, et al. The modulation of fluorouracil with leucovorin in metastatic colorectal carcinoma: a prospective randomized phase III trila. J Clin Oncol 1989; 7:1419–1496.
80. Gelman RS, Raylor SG. Cyclophosphamide, methotrexate and 5-fluorouracil chemotherapy in women more than 65 years old with advanced breast cancer. The elimination of age trends in toxicity by using doses based on creatinine clearance. J Clin Oncol 1984; 2:1406–1414.
81. Carreca I, Balducci L. Oral chemotherapy for the older cancer patient. Am J Cancer 2002; 1:101–108.
82. Mahood DA, Dose AM, Loprinzi CL, et al. Inhibition of fluroruracil-induced stomatitis by oral cryotherapy. J Clin Oncol 1991; 9:449–452.

83. Cascinu S, Fedeli A, Fedeli SL, et al. Oral cooling (cryotherapy), an effective treatment for the prevention of 5-fluorouracil-induced stomatitis. Eur J Cancer B Oral Oncol 1994; 30B:234–236.
84. Spielberger R, Stiff P, Bensinger W, et al. Palifermin for oral mucositis after intensive therapy for hemtologic cancers. NEJM 2004; 351:2590–2598.
85. Beaven AW, Shea TC. Palifermin: a keratinocyte growth factor that reduces oral mucositis after stem cell transplant for haematological malignancies. Exper Opin Pharmacother 2006; 7:2287–2299.
86. Peterson DE, Petit RG. Phase III study: AES-14 in patients at risk for mucositis secondary to anthracycline-based chemotherapy. J Clin Oncol 2004; 22(14s):8008.
87. Pollera CF, Giannarelli D. Prognostic factors influendcing cisplatin-induced emesis. Definition and validation of a predictive logistic model. Cancer 1989; 64: 1117–1122.
88. Kris MG, Gralla RJ, Tyson LB, et al. Controlling delayed vomiting: double-blind, randomized trial comparing placebo, dexamethasone alone, and metoclproamide plus dexamethasone in patients receiving cisplatin. J Clin Oncol 1989; 7:108–114.
89. Gridelli C, Maione P, Rossi A. Corticosteroids underemployment in delayed chemotherapy-induced nausea and emesis with poor adherence to American Society of Clinical Oncology guidelines: is this a reasonable clinical choice for the elderly? J Clin Oncol 2003; 21:4066–4067.
90. Aapro MS, Macciocchi A, Gridelli C. Palonosetron improves prevention of chemotherapy-induced nausea and vomiting in elderly patients. J Support Oncol 2005; 3:369–374.
91. Lyman GH, Lyman C, Ogboola Y. Risk models for the prediction of chemotherapy induced neutropenia. Neutropneia Oncol 2001; 1:2–7.
92. Chrischilles E, Delgado DI, Stolshek BS, et al: Impact of age and colony stimulating factor use in hospital length of stay for febrile neutropenia in CHOP treated non-Hodgkin's lymphoma patients. Cancer Control 2002; 9:203–221.
93. Kuderer NM, Dale D, Crawford J, et al. The morbidity, mortality and cost of febrile neutopenia in cancer patients. Cancer 2006; 106:2258–2266.
94. Kuderer NM, Dale DC, Crawford J, Lyman GH. Impact of primary prophylaxis with granulocyte colony-stimulating factor on febrile neutropenia and mortality in adult cancer patients receiving chemotherapy: a systematic review. J Clin Oncol 2007; 25:3158–3167.
95. Lyman GH, Dale D, Crawford J. Incidence, practice patterns, and predictors of low dose intensity in adjuvant breast cancer chemotherapy: results of a nationwide study of community practices. J Clin Oncol 2003; 21:4524–4531.
96. Zinzani PG, Storti S, Zaccaria A, et al. Elderly aggressive histology non-Hodgkin's lymphoma. Firtst line VNCOP-B regimen: experience in 350 patients. Blood 1999; 94:33–38.
97. Osby E, Hagberg, Kvaloy S, et al. CHOP is superior to CNOP in elderly patients with aggressive lymphoma while outcome is unaffected by filgrastim treatment: results of a Nordic Lymphoma Group randomized trial. Blood 2003; 101:3840–3848.
98. Doorduijn JK, van der Holt B, can Imhoff GW, et al. CHOP compared with CHOP plus granulocyte colony-stimulating factor in elderly patients with aggressive on-Hodgkin's lymphoma. J Clin Oncol 2003; 21:3041–3050.

99. Lyman GH, Dale D, Friedberg J, et al. Incidence and predictors of low chemotherapy dose intentsity in aggressive non-Hodgkin's lymphoma: a nationwide study. J Clin Oncol 2004; 22:4302–4311.
100. Shayne M, Crawford J, Dale DC, et al. Predictors of reduced dose intensity in patients with early-stage breast cancer receiving adjuvant chemotherapy. Breast Cancer Res Treat 2006; 100:255–262.
101. Shayne M, Culakova E, Poniewierski M, et al. Dose intensity and hematologic toxicity in older cancer patients receiving systemic chemotherapy. Cancer 2007; 1; 110(7):1611–1620.
102. Shayne M, Culakova E, Dale D, et al. A validated risk model for early neutropenic events in older cancer patients receiving systemic chemotherapy. J Clin Oncol 2007; 25(18S):9036.
103. Brown ML, Fintor L. The economic burden of cancer. Cancer Prevention and Control. New York: Marcel Dekker, 1995.
104. Lyman GH, Lyman CG, Sanders RA, et al. Decision analysis of hematopoietic growth factor use in patients receiving cancer chemotherapy. J Natl Cancer Inst 1993; 85:488–493.
105. Lyman GH, Balducci L. A cost analysis of hematopoietic colony-stimulating factors. Oncology 1995; 9:85–91.
106. Galspy JA, Bleecker G, Crawford J, et al. The impact of therapy with filgrastim (recombinant granulocyte colony-stimulating factor) on the health care costs associated with cancer chemotherapy. Eur J Cancer 1993; 29A: S23–S30.
107. Lyman GH, Kuderer N, Balducci L. Cancer care in the elderly: cost and quality of life considerations. Cancer Control 1998; 5:347–354.
108. Silber JH, Friedman M, DiPaula RS, et al. Modeling the cost-effectiveness of granulocyte-stimulating factor use in early-stage breast cancer. J Clin Oncol 1998; 16:2435–2444.
109. Bonnadonna G, Valagussa P, Moliterni A, et al. Adjuvant cyclophosphamide, methotrexate, and fluorouracil in node-positive breast cancer: the results of 20 years of follow-up. NEJM 1995; 332:901–906.
110. Smith TJ, Khatcheressian J, Lyman GH, et al. Update of recommendations for the use of white blood cell growth factors: an evidence-based clinical practice guideline. J Clin Oncol 2006; 24:3187–3205.
111. Repetto L, Bigansoli L, Koehne CH, et al. EORTC Cancer in the Elderly Task Force Guidelines for the use of the colony-stimulating factors in elderly patients with cancer. Eur J Cancer 2003; 39:2264–2272.
112. Lyman GH. Guidelines of the National Comprehensive Cancer Network on the use of myeloid growth factors with cancer chemotherapy: a review of the evidence. J NCCN 2005; 3:557–571.
113. Hortobagyi GN, Buzdar AU, Marcus CE, et al. Immediate and long-term toxicity of adjuvant chemotherapy regimens containing doxorubicin in trials at M.D. Anderson Hospital and Tumor Institute. NCI Monogr 1986; 1:105–109.
114. Romond EH, Perez EA, Bryant J, et al. Traztuzumab plus adjuvant chemotherapy for operable HER2-positive breast cancer. NEJM 2005; 252:1673–1683.
115. Hequet O, Le QH, Moullet I, et al. Subclinical late cardiomyopathy after doxorubicin therapy for lymphoma in adults. J Clin Oncol 2004; 22:1864–1871.
116. Hortobagyi GN. Trastuzumab in the treatment of breast cancer. NEJM 2005; 353:1734–1736.

117. Hensing TA, Peterman AH, Schell MJ, et al. The impact of age on toxicity, response rate, quality of life and survival in patients with advanced, stage IIIB or IV nonsmall cell lung carcinoma treated with carboplatin and paclitaxel. Cancer 2003; 98: 779–788.
118. Argyrio AA, Polychronopoulos P, Koutras A, et al. Is advanced age associated with increased incidence and severity of chemotherapy-induced peripheral neuropathy? Support Care Cancer 2006; 14:223–229.
119. Wildiers H, Paridaens R. Taxanes in elderly breast cancer patients. Cancer Treat Rev 2004; 30:333–342.
120. Katzman R. Human nervous system. In: Masoro EJ, ed. Handbook of Physiology. Section 11: Aging. Oxford: Oxford University Press, 1995:325–344.
121. Shah GN, Mooradian AD. Age-related changes in the blood-brain barrier. Exp Gerontol 1997; 32:501–519.
122. Rubin EH, Andersen JW, Berg DR, et al. Risk factors for high-dose cytarabine neurotoxictiy: an analysis of a Cancer and Leukemia Group B trial in patients with acute myeloid leukemia. J Clin Oncol 1992; 10:948–953.
123. Damon LE, Mass R, Linker CA, The association between high-dose cytarabine neurotoxicity and renal insufficiency. J Clin Oncol 1989; 7:1563–1568.

16

Care of the Cancer Survivor

Craig C. Earle and Ann H. Partridge
Dana Farber Cancer Institute, Center for Outcomes/Policy Research, Harvard Medical School, Boston, Massachusetts, U.S.A.

INTRODUCTION

Improvements in screening, detection, and treatment of various malignancies, as well as the aging of the American population, has lead to a burgeoning number of cancer survivors over the last three decades. It has been estimated that there are now over 10 million people with a personal history of cancer in the United States alone. While there are thousands of children and young adult survivors, over 60% of the cancer survivors in the United States are 65 years or older, the majority of whom have a history of the common solid tumor malignancies, such as breast and prostate cancer.

Cancer and cancer treatment have profound implications for individuals and society, including physical, psychological, social, vocational, spiritual, and economic effects. In a landmark treatise highlighting the issues of cancer survivorship, Fitzhugh Mullan declared, "The challenge in overcoming cancer is not only to find therapies that will prevent or arrest the disease quickly, but also to map the middle ground of survivorship and minimize medical and social hazards." (1). Cancer survivors are a very large, heterogeneous group of individuals. Their needs and concerns vary by personal attributes and experiences, disease and treatment, and time since treatment. Nevertheless, some general recommendations for their management can be made. The essential components of survivorship care include (1) surveillance for local and distant recurrence of cancer, (2) management of medical and psychosocial long-term and late effects, and (3) coordination of care between providers to ensure that cancer as well as non-cancer-related health needs are met. In this chapter, we will give an overview of each of these areas.

SURVIVORSHIP CARE PLANNING

When patients are undergoing primary cancer treatment, they have the comfort and reassurance of seeing their providers regularly. Many find that their anxiety levels increase, however, as they approach the completion of therapy. "Survivorship care plans" as envisioned by the Institute of Medicine (IOM) in its recent report *From cancer patient to cancer survivor: Lost in transition* (2), are designed to address this by explicitly laying out a plan for surveillance and other care going forward for patients and all involved providers. Ideally, patients would undergo a visit dedicated specifically to reviewing a summary of their diagnosis and the treatment they received, recommendations for surveillance of cancer recurrence, recommendations for routine health maintenance unrelated to their cancer, and education about psychosocial support and other resources available for cancer survivors. A document would be prepared for the patient as well as for their providers for future reference (Table 1). The purpose of the survivorship care plan is to make sure that everyone knows what has been done, what should be done going forward, and who should do what.

Treatment Summary

The IOM report made the recommendation that after completion of primary treatment for cancer, patients should receive a *treatment summary*. The treatment summary would indicate the cancer diagnosis, histology, and stage, and list the different primary treatments given. It should also identify and provide contact information for those who provided care. Patients often receive care from a number of providers during the course of cancer treatment. A primary care physician (PCP) may refer a patient with hematochezia to a gastroenterologist, who diagnoses a rectal cancer and refers the patient to medical and radiation oncologists for neoadjuvant chemoradiotherapy, then resection by a surgeon, and finishing up with the medical oncologist for more chemotherapy. There may also have been involvement by a psychosocial provider and nutritionist. Not uncommonly, these different aspects of care take place in different locations with different forms of medical record keeping. At the end of treatment, a summary of the care given is not consistently created by anyone, and some providers may have been left off from the cc list at some point. This is a problem because the knowledge of the preceding diagnosis and treatment can be crucial to the patient's subsequent medical care.

Table 1 The Institute of Medicine Survivorship Care Plan

Upon discharge from cancer treatment, including treatment of recurrences, every patient should be given a record of all care received and important disease characteristics. This should include, at a minimum:

1. Diagnostic tests performed and results
2. Tumor characteristics (e.g., site(s), stage and grade, hormone receptor status, marker information)
3. Dates of treatment initiation and completion
4. Surgery, chemotherapy, radiotherapy, transplant, hormonal therapy, or gene or other therapies provided, including agents used, treatment regimen, total dosage, identifying number and title of clinical trials (if any), indicators of treatment response, and toxicities experienced during treatment
5. Psychosocial, nutritional, and other supportive services provided
6. Full contact information on treating institutions and key individual providers
7. Identification of a key point of contact and coordinator of continuing care

Upon discharge from cancer treatment, every patient and his/her primary healthcare provider should receive a written follow-up care plan incorporating available evidence-based standards of care. This should include, at a minimum:

1. The likely course of recovery from acute treatment toxicities as well as the need for ongoing health maintenance or adjuvant therapy
2. A description of recommended cancer screening and other periodic testing and examinations, and the schedule on which they should be performed (and who should provide them)
3. Information on possible late and long-term effects of treatment and symptoms of such effects
4. Information on possible signs of recurrence and second tumors.
5. Information on the possible effects of cancer on marital/partner relationship, sexual functioning, work, and parenting, and the potential future need for psychosocial support
6. Information on the potential insurance, employment, and financial consequences of cancer and, as necessary, referral to counseling, legal aid, and financial assistance
7. Specific recommendations for healthy behaviors (e.g., diet, exercise, healthy weight, sunscreen use, immunizations, smoking cessation, and osteoporosis prevention); when appropriate, recommendations that first-degree relatives be informed about their increased risk and the need for cancer screening (e.g., breast cancer, colorectal cancer, prostate cancer)
8. As appropriate, information on genetic counseling and testing to identify high-risk individuals who could benefit from more comprehensive cancer surveillance, chemoprevention, or risk-reducing surgery
9. As appropriate, information on known effective chemoprevention and behavioral strategies for secondary prevention (e.g., tamoxifen in women at high risk for breast cancer; smoking cessation after lung cancer) and monitoring of adherence to these recommendations
10. Referrals to specific follow-up care providers (e.g., rehabilitation, fertility, psychology), support groups, and/or the patient's primary care provider
11. A listing of cancer-related resources and information (e.g., Internet-based sources and telephone listings for major cancer support organizations).

Source: Adapted from Ref. 2 (Box 3–16, pp. 152–153).

SURVEILLANCE FOR LOCAL RECURRENCE OF CANCER

Local recurrence of cancer either means that the primary therapy failed to eradicate it, or that because of a predisposition, whether genetic or due to environmental exposures, an entirely new occurrence of cancer has developed in the residual organ. Local surveillance usually addresses both mechanisms.

Surveillance for local recurrence only makes sense in those cases where salvage treatment can still affect a cure, or have a substantial impact of future symptoms or quality of life. Examples include examination and mammograms of a breast after breast conserving surgery, anoscopy after primary chemoradiotherapy for anal cancer, and clinical evaluation of a prior site of head and neck cancer. In these cases, patients treated with surgery can often be salvaged by either another surgical procedure or radiation, while those treated initially with primary radiotherapy may have surgical salvage options. Unfortunately, this is not the case for all cancers. Local recurrence of pancreatic cancer after surgery, for example, cannot be cured.

Surveillance for New Primary Cancers

Surveillance practices focused on finding new primaries in an organ with a predisposition to forming cancer include mammography of the uninvolved breast after breast cancer, surveillance colonoscopy after colorectal cancer, skin exam after melanoma, cystoscopy after bladder cancer, or ultrasound following resection of a hepatoma. In such cases, the predisposition can come from genetic factors, such as the Hereditary Non-Polyposis Colorectal Cancer (HNPCC) syndrome, "field cancerization" caused by environmental exposures like the effect of smoking on the lungs, head, neck, or bladder, or cirrhosis from any cause in the liver. For example, patients cured of head and neck cancer remain at a 3% to 6% risk per year of developing lung cancer (3–6).

SURVEILLANCE FOR DISTANT RELAPSE

"Relapse" is really a misnomer because in reality, it means that the cancer had already spread by hematogenous, lymphatic, or serosal routes beyond the primary organ prior to primary therapy for solid tumors and/or was resistant to systemic therapy for both solid and hematologic malignancies. The term relapse just means that the disease is again detectable. It is surveillance for distant relapse in solid tumors that engenders the most angst and controversy. Patients understandably extrapolate the idea that early detection of cancer is important to infer that detecting metastatic disease early is useful. In order for such surveillance to be of benefit, though, the following criteria must be met:

1. It must detect recurrences earlier than it would otherwise become apparent from symptoms.
2. Treatment of asymptomatic disease must improve patient outcomes.
3. Whatever benefit is realized should be obtained within accepted bounds of cost-effectiveness.

Most surveillance strategies can probably find distant recurrence earlier than they would become clinically apparent from signs and symptoms. Consequently, there is little disagreement that periodic clinical evaluation with history and physical examination is reasonable as recurrences detected in this way are either symptomatic, or will likely soon become symptomatic and are consequently important to recognize. Periodic scheduled visits are justified because studies have shown that patients do not always initiate contact with their physicians when symptoms that could portend recurrence arise (7). The question then becomes, how intensively to pursue additional testing to screen for asymptomatic recurrences. Tumor markers are available for many cancers (breast, colorectal, pancreatic, liver, ovarian, prostate, and testicular (8)) and can detect asymptomatic diseases. Imaging studies can increase this sensitivity. However, the marginal benefit may be small. For example, by the time recurrent lymphoma is detectable by imaging studies, a combination of symptoms, signs, and lactate dehydrogenase (LDH) would also have picked up almost all lymphoma relapses (9). Thus, addition of more expensive surveillance modalities often come with diminishing returns.

In most cases, especially in solid tumor oncology, the early treatment of distant recurrence does not improve patient outcome. Most distant diseases cannot be cured, and early treatment of asymptomatic incurable diseases do not provide benefit (10). For example, it has been shown in two large randomized trials of breast cancer surveillance that intensive monitoring for distant relapse does not improve survival or quality of life (11–13). Similarly, second-look surgeries for ovarian and pancreatic cancers have not been associated with improved outcomes (14). Such procedures simply alert patients (and providers) a little earlier that they have terminal cancer (lead-time bias). Perhaps, this allows them to start planning for and accepting their situation, but such a benefit has not been detectable on measures of health-related quality of life. Any diagnostic test or procedure also carries with it the possibility of false positive results, with ensuing anxiety, expense, and risk of complications from subsequent investigation.

However, there are some exceptions to this rather nihilistic view of surveillance for recurrent disease. For example, surgical resection of colorectal or renal cell oligometastases can be curative, as can chemotherapy or salvage bone marrow transplantation for low-volume metastases from testicular cancer or some lymphomas and leukemias (15). In these cases, intensive surveillance at least has a rationale. The challenge is to identify those situations for which routine screening for recurrent disease is both cost-effective and improves patient outcomes. For example, looking at the role of imaging following primary treatment of stage II and III colon cancer, if we assume that 50% of the patients will relapse and that perhaps 10% of those (or 5% of all patients) will recur in such a way that potentially curative surgery could be undertaken, we know that up to 40% of these (2% of all patients) may be cured. The Carcino-Embryonic Antigen (CEA) will rise with recurrence approximately 70% of the time, so it becomes clear that imaging could only possibly affect the outcome of less than

1% of patients. Debates about imaging recommendations need to recognize the escalating incremental cost for very marginal possible benefit with more frequent routine scans. In fact, it may very well be that those recurrences requiring more frequent scanning to pick up at a potentially curable stage may be too aggressive to actually be cured (length-time bias). Consequently, trials to detect these small differences must be very large (16), and it has required meta-analysis of several trials to suggest any benefit from imaging (17,18).

Ideally, the content of a survivorship care plan should be based on evidence from high-quality studies that show that different forms of cancer surveillance and survivorship care have a real impact on hard endpoints. Unfortunately, at present, such evidence exists only in relatively few settings. Thus, survivorship care is often based on clinical judgment and expert consensus. As a result, there is wide variation in surveillance recommendations, even among experts (19), and the American Society of Clinical Oncology (ASCO) only has surveillance guidelines for two cancer sites: breast (8,20) and colorectal cancers (8,21).

SURVEILLANCE FOR LONG-TERM AND LATE EFFECTS OF CANCER TREATMENT

Another rationale for follow up after cancer is to detect long-term or late effects of treatment. Table 2 lists common late effects following exposures to surgery, radiation, and chemotherapy during cancer treatment. For example, hypothyroidism and dental issues are common after neck irradiation. Lymphedema can be a sequela of local surgical management or radiation. Accelerated cardiovascular disease can accompany chest irradiation or certain drugs. Bone marrow transplant patients are at risk for cataracts and effects of Graft Versus Host Disease (GVHD). They also may have lost a significant amount of their immunity and require re-administration of their routine vaccinations. Patients who have had either surgical or functional splenectomy require immunization against encapsulated organisms. Hormonal treatments for cancer, including steroids, can result in impaired bone health, sexual dysfunction, and menopausal symptoms. Iatrogenic cancers include a new cancer developing in a radiation field, such as lung, breast, or upper gastrointestinal cancers after mantle radiation for Hodgkin's Disease, myelodysplasia, or acute leukemia following adjuvant chemotherapy for breast cancer, or endometrial cancer from tamoxifen. Radiation-induced tumors typically occur at the edge of a radiation field where normal tissue is damaged but not killed by radiation, and usually present 8 to 20 years after radiation.

The survivorship care plan should describe the common late effects of a patient's treatment. Long-term effects are those that first occur during cancer treatment and persist after completion of primary therapy, like the functional consequences of a limb amputation. Late effects are those that were not apparent during primary treatment, but become apparent at some later time, such as

Table 2 Common Long-Term and Late Effects of Cancer Treatment

Surgery
- Cosmetic effects
- Functional disability from removal of a limb or organ
- Damage to an organ (bowel, bladder, sexual organs)
- Pain
- Scarring/adhesions
- Incisional hernia
- Lymphedema
- Systemic effects (removal of endocrine organs, infection risk postsplenectomy)

Radiation
- Second malignancies
- Neurocognitive deficits
- Xerophalmia, cataracts
- Xerostomia, dental caries
- Hypothyroidism
- Pneumonitis, pulmonary fibrosis
- Coronary artery, valvular, conduction, cardiomyopathic, and pericardial disease
- Bowel stricture
- Radiation proctitis
- Bladder scarring
- Infertility, impotence, premature menopause
- Lymphedema
- Bone fractures

Systemic therapy
- Second malignancies (myelodysplasia and leukemia)
- Chronic graft-versus-host disease
- Ototoxicity (e.g., cisplatin)
- Cardiomyopathy (e.g., anthracyclines)
- Pulmonary fibrosis (e.g., bleomycin)
- Renal toxicity (e.g., cisplatin)
- Premature menopause and infertility (e.g., alkylating agents)
- Menopausal symptoms and sexual dysfunction (e.g., hormonal therapy)
- Osteoporosis (e.g., hormonal therapy, chemotherapy via premature menopause)
- Neuropathy (e.g., taxanes, platinums)
- Cognitive dysfunction (Chemobrain)
- Weight gain
- Fatigue

coronary artery disease after mantle radiation. Unfortunately, there is little evidence on which to base surveillance strategies for most of these, and consensus guidelines are lacking for adult patients. The Children's Oncology Group (www.survivorshipguidelines.org) has developed consensus recommendations for late-effect screening based on the exposures received by a patient, many of which can be extrapolated to the adult population. While being aware of the risk of a potential late effect is helpful, it is also important to be judicious and not over-investigate in the absence of symptoms. It is also prudent not to overly distress patients about things they cannot prevent, such as the small risk of leukemia that may follow the treatment with certain chemotherapy drugs.

MANAGEMENT OF SPECIFIC LONG-TERM AND LATE EFFECTS

Many of the repercussions of cancer and cancer treatment in survivors are treated in the same way that they would be treated in a patient without cancer. For example, a patient with hypothyroidism after local irradiation for lymphoma or head and neck cancer should receive appropriate replacement thyroid hormone and monitoring. A patient with congestive heart failure following anthracycline-based chemotherapy or trastuzumab therapy is generally treated according to the standard practice for patients with cardiac dysfunction. Physical disability and disfiguration is also a common problem for cancer survivors for which there are available management options. Physical therapy can substantially improve strength and use of a limb after it has been damaged secondary to cancer or cancer treatment. Prostheses and reconstructive surgery are also important components of the management of various malignancies including, for example, after mastectomy for breast cancer or amputation for sarcoma. Still, there are a number of complications of cancer and cancer treatment that have been studied primarily in survivor populations because they are particularly common or relatively unique to cancer survivors or present unique challenges in survivor populations.

Lymphedema

Much of the research on treatment of lymphedema has been conducted among breast cancer survivors who develop or are at risk for lymphedema following axillary surgery or radiation, although lymphedema can occur in the setting of any cancer or treatment that interferes with normal lymph flow. Management of lymphedema may include elevation of an affected body part, compression garments, pneumatic compression pumps, massage and physical therapies, and more rarely surgery and diuretics (22). Prior to beginning any treatment for lymphedema, it is important to consider and evaluate for the possibility of tumor recurrence, infection, or venous thrombosis in the area when lymph nodes have been removed or irradiated (e.g., the axilla) causing the swelling. To minimize the chances of lymphedema, protection of the affected limb from infection, compression, venipuncture, exposure to intense heat, and abrasion may be prudent, although the utility of such measures has not been formally evaluated (23). Further, because obesity is a risk factor for lymphedema, maintenance of a healthy weight and weight loss as needed may prevent or treat lymphedema. Ongoing studies are evaluating the role of local compression (i.e., compression sleeves) and exercise for lymphedema prevention.

Osteoporosis

Men and women receiving endocrine therapy or women who develop chemotherapy-induced ovarian failure are at risk for osteopenia, and subsequently osteoporosis, and should consider having their bone density monitored. Bone loss may be offset to some degree in postmenopausal women with breast cancer by the use of tamoxifen through its proestrogenic effects. In premenopausal women, however, tamoxifen use has been associated with a *decrease* in bone mineral density (24). Lifestyle modifications including weight-bearing exercise, smoking cessation, and avoidance of excess alcohol intake, and supplementation of dietary calcium and vitamin D as needed should be considered. In addition, there are several available non-hormonal interventions to attenuate bone loss in both men and women, including bisphosphonates (25).

Fertility and Children after Cancer

Infertility is a dreaded consequence of cancer and cancer treatment for many young patients facing a cancer diagnosis and treatment decisions. In 2006, guidelines published by the ASCO recommended that oncologists address the possibility of infertility with all patients treated for cancer during their reproductive years, and be prepared to discuss possible fertility preservation options or refer interested patients to reproductive specialists as early as possible (26). Ideally, strategies should be considered for all young patients interested in future fertility to prevent or avoid infertility. However, there are several limitations to the available options for both men and women when considering fertility preservation. Thus, many patients will face the problem of infertility in survivorship. The treatment of infertility in female cancer survivors is not well-studied. Ovarian stimulation medications (e.g., clomid), in vitro fertilization (IVF), or egg donation and surrogate carriers can be considered. However, the use of techniques such as IVF with the resulting high hormonal levels in women with a history of a hormone-sensitive cancer is of unclear safety (e.g., in estrogen receptor-positive breast cancer). Research to evaluate alternative methods of ovarian stimulation in this setting using tamoxifen or aromatase inhibition is promising (27). Actual fertility outcomes after adult cancer treatment are not well documented. Previous studies among select populations have suggested that between 5% and 15% of young women with breast cancer will have a subsequent pregnancy (28,29).

In women with history of a hormone-sensitive tumor (e.g., breast cancer), there have been concerns that pregnancy will increase the risk of cancer recurrence because of the high hormonal levels surrounding a pregnancy. To date, however, there is no clear evidence for a negative effect of subsequent pregnancy on the prognosis of young women with breast cancer (29). Nonetheless, available studies are all limited by significant biases, and so concerns remain (30). A common recommendation is that that women wait at least two years after treatment is completed before attempting conception, primarily because this is the time of highest rate of aggressive recurrence, and treatment for recurrent breast cancer may be quite complicated during a pregnancy. However, it is unclear whether a shorter wait has any effect on prognosis in a patient who does not plan to take hormonal breast cancer treatment during that time (e.g., tamoxifen). It is also important to recognize that rates of recurrence in women with breast cancer are significant long beyond the two-year point and that fertility will decline with aging during that time. Another issue facing young female cancer survivors may be difficulty in carrying a pregnancy, particularly if a woman has a history of gynecologic surgery or radiation (e.g., uterus-sparing surgery for early cervical cancer). In light of these and other concerns that might arise among pregnant women with a history of cancer, such patients should consider high-risk obstetrical management.

Men facing infertility should also seek consultation with fertility specialists. Patients with impotence and ejaculation problems (e.g., retrograde ejaculation) can undergo alternative methods of sperm extraction including testicular aspiration or extraction and electroejaculation (26). For patients with oligospermia, intracytoplasmic sperm injection (ICSI) may be used to improve the likelihood of fertilization of an oocyte.

Although an increased rate of birth defects might be expected in offspring conceived from the eggs or sperm of patients exposed to potentially mutagenic drugs, none has been found. In three large studies including nearly 4000 offspring of both male and female survivors of childhood cancer, when clearly hereditary cancers like retinoblastoma were excluded, no statistically significant increase in cancers or malformations was detected in the offspring (31). However, it is generally recommended that survivors wait at least several months at a minimum to try to have a biologic child after systemic therapy or radiation therapy that may have short-term effects on developing oocytes or spermatozoa.

Hormonal Symptoms and Sexual Dysfunction

Many patients with cancer experience symptoms of hormonal manipulation, such as hot flashes, genitourinary problems, and sexual difficulties (32–34). For women who undergo premature menopause, hormone replacement therapy (HRT) is a reasonable option. HRT has traditionally been discouraged, however, among women with a history of hormone-sensitive tumors (e.g., breast cancer and endometrial cancer) because of theoretical risks of hormonal stimulation of cancer cells, epidemiologic evidence that HRT increases the risk of developing these cancers, and the evidence of benefits of antiestrogen therapies for these diseases. The Women's Health Initiative, a prospective randomized study of HRT compared with placebo in healthy women, recently revealed that at five years follow-up the overall health risks exceeded benefits from use of combined estrogen plus progestin for healthy women (35). In this study, there was no evidence that HRT prevents cardiac disease, and further evidence that HRT increases the risk of breast cancer. Furthermore, there are now other treatments available that have been shown to prevent and treat cardiovascular disease as well as osteoporosis. At present, the consideration of HRT seems most reasonable in the small subgroup of survivors with a favorable breast cancer prognosis who have severe symptoms of estrogen deficiency, not amenable to other available treatments. In Europe, HRT has been used to treat menopausal symptoms in women taking tamoxifen, and has provided some relief (36); however, the effects of this combination on breast cancer prognosis is not known and so it is not routinely recommended in the United States.

A variety of non-estrogenic options are available, which may attenuate hot flashes and night sweats (37). Alternative therapies like vitamin E have been shown to have modest effectiveness in women with breast cancer. Antidepressants such as venlafaxine significantly reduce hot flash frequency and intensity in women with breast cancer as compared to a placebo (38). Gabapentin, an anti-seizure medication, has also been shown to reduce hot flashes substantially (39). Hot flashes are also common in men receiving androgen deprivation therapy (ADT) for prostate cancer. Pilot studies have revealed some effect of selective serotonin reuptake inhibitors (SSRIs) in this setting as well.

For vaginal dryness caused by treatment-induced menopause or aromatase inhibitor therapy in women with a history of a hormone-sensitive cancer, non-hormonal treatments include over-the-counter water-based lubricants. Intravaginal estrogen therapy with estrogen creams or estrogen-impregnated rings may relieve genitourinary symptoms and may be associated with minimal systemic absorption of estrogen. Women with vaginal atrophy or stenosis may benefit from vaginal dilatation as well as lubricants. For men with erectile dysfunction, prosthetic devices and prescription medications, including sildenafil citrate, are available. Both male and female cancer survivors may have difficulty with libido secondary to the psychosocial effects of the diagnosis as well as disease and treatment effects. Attention to ruling out and treating medical causes like hormonal deficiencies as well as couples therapy and psychotherapy may be of benefit for some patients. However, the use of testosterone did not appear to improve libido in one randomized trial of postmenopausal female cancer survivors (40).

Fatigue

Cancer-related fatigue (CRF) is a very common phenomenon among survivors, which may have a significant impact on an individual's quality of life. The National Comprehensive Cancer Network (NCCN, www.nccn.org) has recently made recommendations for the assessment and management of CRF. It is prudent to rule out other causes of fatigue including pain, malnutrition, hypothyroidism, anemia, insomnia, and depression, and treat these maladies accordingly when discovered. However, for many survivors there is no other clear etiology for their fatigue. Research has revealed that non-pharmacologic interventions, such as exercise and psychotherapy, are effective in relieving CRF. Most other treatments for fatigue remain experimental, including psychostimulants such as modafinil, buspirone as well as complementary therapies, such as ginseng, coenzyme Q10, yoga, and mindfulness meditation (41,42). Recent preliminary data suggest that the psychostimulant modafinil may also improve symptoms of "Chemobrain," such as memory problems and difficulties in concentrating, although further research is warranted (43).

PSYCHOSOCIAL CONCERNS

Although most cancer patients cope well with their illness and treatment, there is a subset with emotional and social distress that can actually become more severe as the frequency of contact with their oncology providers decreases. Whether surveillance visits themselves provide psychological benefit is debatable (44,45) and probably patient-specific. The fear of recurrence is a dominant psychological sequela of cancer (46). As a result, reassurance that there is no sign of the cancer at follow-up can understandably ameliorate anxiety (47). However, the inconvenience and often discomfort of surveillance testing, and the stress of waiting for test results and visits with clinicians can themselves generate anxiety (48). Moreover, if all of the tests are not completely normal, the patient will not be reassured (49). Although patients report in surveys that they prefer routine follow-up and derive reassurance from clinic visits (11), Muss et al. found that this is often because they incorrectly assume that early detection of recurrence will improve their chance of cure, or at least prolong survival (50). Randomized trials of surveillance after breast cancer have not found any overall positive psychological effects with more intensive surveillance strategies.(11,45)

Because of the high prevalence of anxiety and depression in cancer survivors, appropriate psychosocial support including referral to a mental health professional may be necessary upon detection of symptoms of distress during follow-up. There have been numerous psychosocial interventions that have been studied among cancer survivors, particularly in women with a history of breast cancer. Studies have revealed that individual and group therapy, relaxation, and meditation therapy, and drug interventions with antidepressants and antianxiety medications can improve psychosocial distress (51). Management of patients with clinical psychiatric diagnoses like anxiety, depression, or posttraumatic stress disorder is similar to that in patients without a history of cancer. An important part of survivorship care planning is to be sensitive to and recognize such distress, and to make available to patients services like counseling, support groups, stress management, or referrals to mental health providers when appropriate.

NON-CANCER-RELATED CARE

Given that 70% of cancer patients now survive their disease, it is important that general medical care should not be ignored. There is evidence that cancer survivors may be less likely to receive recommended care for chronic conditions across a wide range of diseases (52). For example, five-year colorectal cancer survivors with angina, congestive heart failure, and chronic lung disease have been observed to be less likely than matched controls to have recommended follow-up care. Diabetic survivors are less likely to have preventive eye examination, and there has been a trend toward less intensive monitoring of the HbA1c (52). It is important that cancer patients maintain a relationship with a PCP, as this has been a strong predictor of receiving high-quality general medical care (52,53). While some oncologists are willing and able to act as a PCP, surveys have shown that most are not (54).

PREVENTION

Surviving cancer provides several opportunities to actually improve health. Cancer survivors usually have more medical contacts than people without a history of cancer, and consequently, have more opportunity to receive recommended health maintenance interventions like screenings (cholesterol, bone density, other cancers) and immunizations (53). In addition, patients faced with a life-threatening illness may be more receptive to messages about improving health behaviors, making the development of cancer a potential "teachable moment" (55). For example, physicians can counsel patients at surveillance visits on lifestyle modifications, such as smoking and alcohol cessation and decreasing sun exposure. Recently, chemoprevention has become available in some circumstances, such as tamoxifen for breast cancer (56) and aspirin for colorectal cancer (57). There is also emerging evidence that lifestyle factors, like diet and exercise, may play a role in preventing recurrence (58), though randomized confirmation is needed. The transition off of primary cancer treatment is also another chance to consider whether genetic assessment might be necessary. If a hereditary predisposition to cancer is suspected, genetic counseling and testing may lead to interventions that could prevent future cancers in the cancer survivor and the survivor's relatives. The survivorship care plan should include recommendations on these issues.

EMPLOYMENT, INSURANCE, AND ECONOMIC ISSUES

The IOM report also recommends that the survivorship care plan direct patients to sources of information on how to deal with the potential insurance, employment, and financial consequences of cancer, and refer as necessary to providers of legal aid and financial assistance. This can largely be achieved by giving them a directory of online or telephone resources made available by several advocacy organizations.

DELIVERY OF SURVIVORSHIP CARE

There is no single best way that survivorship care must be provided. Whether follow-up is carried out by specialists, generalists, a combination of the two in a "shared care" model, or in a specialized survivorship clinic, is likely unimportant as long as there is clarity about what should be done for individual patients and which provider has responsibility for each aspect of care. Randomized trials have shown that PCPs that have been given what amounts to a brief survivorship care plan with explicit directions achieve the same outcomes as specialists (59–63). Moreover, PCPs are generally willing to take on this role (64) and patients may prefer it (45). As the general population ages over the next few decades, the number of cancer patients is projected to grow rapidly. Coupled with advances, which mean that there is increasingly more that can be done for many patients with cancer, the United States appears to be headed for a manpower shortage within oncology (65). While there is also a need for more physicians in primary care, it is likely that shared care models will be most feasible for managing these patients.

CONCLUSIONS AND FUTURE DIRECTIONS

The number of cancer survivors is growing exponentially. Survivorship is just now being recognized as an important and unique part of the cancer care continuum. Optimal care of cancer survivors will require *routine* attention to their issues and coordination of care among multiple providers. There is a huge need for research in survivorship that ranges from basic science and clinical interventions to prevent and treat long-term and late effects of treatment, through evaluating strategies for cancer surveillance and screening for late effects, to health services research questions about the optimal format, content, and resultant effects of formal survivorship care plans and different models of care. Research to evaluate both the utility and cost-effectiveness of various strategies of surveillance, intervention, and overall delivery of survivorship care is necessary from both individual and societal perspectives. In the meantime, practitioners are faced with this ever-growing population. Attention to survivorship care planning is necessary to optimize communication with patients and with other providers in order to provide the highest quality of care to cancer survivors.

REFERENCES

1. Mullan F. Seasons of survival: reflections of a physician with cancer. NEJM 1985; 313:270–273.
2. Institute of Medicine. From Cancer Patient to Cancer Survivor: Lost in Transition. Washington: National Academies Press, 2005.
3. Wynder EL, Mushinski MH, Spivak JC. Tobacco and alcohol consumption in relation to the development of multiple primary cancers. Cancer 1977; 40:1872–1878.

4. Vikram B. Changing patterns of failure in advanced head and neck cancer. Arch Otolaryngol 1984; 110:564–565.
5. Vikram B, Strong EW, Shah JP, et al. Second malignant neoplasms in patients successfully treated with multimodality treatment for advanced head and neck cancer. Head Neck Surg 1984.6:734–737.
6. Vikram B, Strong EW, Shah JP, et al. Failure at distant sites following multimodality treatment for advanced head and neck cancer. Head Neck Surg 1984; 6:730–733.
7. Walsh GL, O'Connor M, Willis KM, et al. Is follow-up of lung cancer patients after resection medically indicated and cost-effective? Ann Thorac Surg 1995; 60: 1563–1570.
8. Bast RCJ, Ravdin P, Hayes DF, et al. 2000 update of recommendations for the use of tumor markers in breast and colorectal cancer: clinical practice guidelines of the American Society of Clinical Oncology. J Clin Oncol 2001; 19:1865–1878.
9. Weeks JC, Yeap BY, Canellos GP, et al. Value of follow-up procedures in patients with large-cell lymphoma who achieve a complete remission. J Clin Oncol 1991; 9:1196–1203.
10. Nordic Gastrointestinal Tumor Adjuvant Therapy Group. Expectancy or primary chemotherapy in patients with advanced asymptomatic colorectal cancer: a randomized trial. J Clin Oncol 1992; 10:904–911.
11. The GIVIO Investigators. Impact of follow-up testing on survival and health-related quality of life in breast cancer patients. A multicenter randomized controlled trial. JAMA 1994; 271:1587–1592.
12. Rosselli DT, Palli D, Cariddi A, et al. Intensive diagnostic follow-up after treatment of primary breast cancer: a randomized trial. National Research Council Project on Breast Cancer follow-up. JAMA 1994; 271:1593–1597.
13. Rojas MP, Telaro E, Russo A, et al. Follow-up strategies for women treated for early breast cancer. Cochrane Database Syst Rev 1905; CD001768.
14. NIH Consensus Development Panel on Ovarian Cancer. NIH consensus conference. Ovarian cancer. Screening, treatment, and follow-up. JAMA 1995; 273: 491–497.
15. Anderson JE, Litzow MR, Appelbaum FR, et al. Allogeneic, syngeneic, and autologous marrow transplantation for Hodgkin's disease: the 21-year Seattle experience. J Clin Oncol 1993; 11:2342–2350.
16. Northover JM, Houghton J, Lennon T. CEA to detect recurrences of colon cancer (letter). JAMA 1994; 272:31.
17. Rosen M, Chan L, Beart RWJ, et al. Follow-up of colorectal cancer: a meta-analysis. Dis Colon Rectum 1998; 41:1116–1126.
18. Renehan AG, Egger M, Saunders MP, et al. Impact on survival of intensive follow up after curative resection for colorectal cancer: systematic review and meta-analysis of randomised trials. BMJ 2002; 324:813–816.
19. Johnson FE. Overview. In: Johnson FE, Virgo KS, eds. Cancer Patient Follow-Up. St. Louis: Mosby, 1997:4.
20. Smith TJ, Davidson NE, Schapira DV, et al. American Society of Clinical Oncology 1998 update of recommended breast cancer surveillance guidelines. J Clin Oncol 1999; 17:1080–1082.
21. Desch CE, Benson AB, Somerfield MR, et al. Colorectal cancer surveillance: 2005 update of an American Society of Clinical Oncology practice guideline. J Clin Oncol 2005; 23:8512–8519.

22. Harris SR, Hugi MR, Olivotto IA, et al. Clinical practice guidelines for the care and treatment of breast cancer: 11. Lymphedema. CMAJ 2001; 164:191–199.
23. Burstein HJ, Winer EP. Primary care for survivors of breast cancer. N Eng J Med 2000; 343:1086–1094.
24. Osborne CK. Tamoxifen in the treatment of breast cancer. NEJM 1998; 339:1609–1618.
25. Hillner BE, Ingle JN, Chlebowski RT, et al. American Society of Clinical Oncology 2003 update on the role of bisphosphonates and bone health issues in women with breast cancer. J Clin Oncol 2003; 21:4042–4057.
26. Lee SJ, Schover LR, Partridge AH, et al. American Society of Clinical Oncology recommendations on fertility preservation in cancer patients. J Clin Oncol 2006; 24:2917–2931.
27. Oktay K. Further evidence on the safety and success of ovarian stimulation with letrozole and tamoxifen in breast cancer patients undergoing in vitro fertilization to cryopreserve their embryos for fertility preservation. J Clin Oncol 2005; 23:3858–3859.
28. Partridge AH, Gelber S, Peppercorn J, et al. Web-based survey of fertility issues in young women with breast cancer. J Clin Oncol 2004; 22:4174–4183.
29. Ives A, Saunders C, Bulsara M, et al. Pregnancy after breast cancer: population based study. BMJ 2007; 334:194.
30. Petrek JA. Pregnancy safety after breast cancer. Cancer 1994; 74:528–531.
31. Hawkins MM. Pregnancy outcome and offspring after childhood cancer. BMJ 1994; 309:1034.
32. Krychman ML, Pereira L, Carter J, et al. Sexual oncology: sexual health issues in women with cancer. Oncology 2006; 71:18–25.
33. Stead ML, Fallowfield L, Selby P, et al. Psychosexual function and impact of gynaecological cancer. Best Pract Res Clin Obstet Gynaecol 2007; 21:309–320.
34. Donatucci CF, Greenfield JM. Recovery of sexual function after prostate cancer treatment. Curr Opin Urol 2006; 16:444–448.
35. Rossouw JE, Anderson GL, Prentice RL, et al. Risks and benefits of estrogen plus progestin in healthy postmenopausal women: principal results from the Women's Health Initiative randomized controlled trial. JAMA 2002; 288:321–333.
36. Powles TJ, Hickish T, Casey S, et al. Hormone replacement after breast cancer. Lancet 1993; 342:60–61.
37. Bordeleau L, Pritchard K, Goodwin P, et al. Therapeutic options for the management of hot flashes in breast cancer survivors: An evidence-based review. Clin Ther 2007; 29:230–241.
38. Loprinzi CL, Kugler JW, Sloan JA, et al. Venlafaxine in management of hot flashes in survivors of breast cancer: a randomised controlled trial. Lancet 2000;356:2059–2063.
39. Loprinzi CL, Kugler JW, Barton DL, et al. Phase III trial of gabapentin alone or in conjunction with an antidepressant in the management of hot flashes in women who have inadequate control with an antidepressant alone: NCCTG N03C5. J Clin Oncol 2007; 25:308–312.
40. Barton DL, Wender DB, Sloan JA, et al. Randomized controlled trial to evaluate transdermal testosterone in female cancer survivors with decreased libido; North Central Cancer Treatment Group protocol N02C3. J Natl Cancer Inst 2007; 99:672–679.
41. Mustian K, Morrow G, Carroll J, et al. Integrative nonpharmacologic behavioral interventions for the management of cancer-related fatigue. Oncologist 2007; 12(suppl1):52–67.

42. Carroll J, Kohli S, Mustian K, et al. Pharmacologic treatment of cancer-related fatigue. Oncologist 2007; 12(suppl.1):43–51.
43. Kohli S, Fisher SG, Tra Y, et al. The cognitive effects of modafinil in breast cancer survivors: A randomized clinical trial. Proc Am Soc Clin Oncol 2007; 25:abstr 9004.
44. Stiggelbout AM, de Haes JC, Vree R, et al. Follow-up of colorectal cancer patients: quality of life and attitudes towards follow-up. British Journal of Cancer 1997; 75:914–920.
45. Grunfeld E, Mant D, Yudkin P, et al. Routine follow-up of breast cancer in primary care: randomised trial. BMJ 1996; 313:665–669.
46. Wolfe SN, Nichols C, Ulman D, et al. Survivorship: An unmet need of the patient with cancer: implications of a survey of the Lance Armstrong Foundation (LAF). Proc Am Soc Clin Oncol 2005; 23:abstr 6032.
47. Kjeldsen BJ, Thorsen H, Whalley D, et al. Influence of follow-up on health-related quality of life after radical surgery for colorectal cancer. Scand J Gastroenterol 1999; 34:509–515.
48. Lampic C, Wennberg A, Schill JE, et al. Anxiety and cancer-related worry of cancer patients at routine follow-up visits. Acta Oncol 1994; 33:119–125.
49. Loprinzi CL, Hayes D, Smith T: Doc, shouldn't we be getting some tests? J Clin Oncol 2000; 18:2345–2348.
50. Muss HB, Tell GS, Case LD, et al. Perceptions of follow-up care in women with breast cancer. Am J Clin Oncol 1991; 14:55–59.
51. Stanton AL: Psychosocial concerns and interventions for cancer survivors. J Clin Oncol 2006; 24:5132–5137.
52. Earle CC, Neville BA: Underuse of necessary care among elderly colorectal cancer survivors. Cancer 2004; 101:1712–1719.
53. Earle CC, Burstein HJ, Winer EP, et al. Quality of non-breast cancer health maintenance among elderly breast cancer survivors. J Clin Oncol 2003; 21:1447–1451.
54. American Society of Clinical Oncology. Status of the medical oncology workforce. J Clin Oncol 1996; 14:2612–2621.
55. Ganz PA. A teachable moment for oncologists: cancer survivors, 10 million strong and growing! J Clin Oncol 2005; 23:5458–5460.
56. Chlebowski RT, Collyar DE, Somerfield MR, et al. American Society of Clinical Oncology technology assessment on breast cancer risk reduction strategies: tamoxifen and raloxifene. J Clin Oncol 1999; 17:1939–1955.
57. Fuchs C, Meyerhardt JA, Heseltine DL, et al. Influence of regular aspirin use on survival for patients with stage II colon cancer: Findings from Intergroup trial CALGB 89803. Proc Am Soc Clin Oncol 2005; 23:abstr 3530.
58. Meyerhardt JA, Heseltine DL, Niedzwiecki D, et al. The impact of physical activity on patients with stage III colon cancer: findings from intergroup trial CALGB 89803. Proc Am Soc Clin Oncol 2005; 23.
59. Grunfeld E, Levine MN, Julian JA, et al. Randomized trial of long-term follow-up for early-stage breast cancer: a comparison of family physician versus specialist care. J Clin Oncol 2006; 24:848–855.
60. Grunfeld E, Mant D, Yudkin P, et al. Routine follow up of breast cancer in primary care: randomised trial. BMJ 1996; 313:665–669.
61. Grunfeld E, Yudkin P, Adewuyl-Dalton R, et al. Follow up in breast cancer. Quality of life unaffected by general practice follow up. BMJ 1995; 311:54.

62. Grunfeld E, Mant D, Vessey MP, et al. Evaluating primary care follow-up of breast cancer: methods and preliminary results of three studies. Ann Oncol 1995; 6(suppl 2): 47–52.
63. Grunfeld E, Fitzpatrick R, Mant D, et al. Comparison of breast cancer patient satisfaction with follow-up in primary care versus specialist care: results from a randomized controlled trial. Br J Gen Pract 1999; 49:705–710.
64. Grunfeld E, Mant D, Vessey MP, et al. Specialist and general practice views on routine follow-up of breast cancer patients in general practice. Fam Pract 1995; 12:60–65.
65. Erikson C, Salsberg E, Forte G, et al. Future supply and demand for oncologists: Challenges to assuring access to oncology services. J Oncol Practice 2007; 3:79–86.

17

Pain and Palliation

Jeanne-Marie Maher
Home Health and Hospice Care, Nashua, New Hampshire, U.S.A.

Ann Berger
Bethesda, Maryland, U.S.A.

PAIN AND PALLIATION

Pain is an integral part of human experience. It is the single most frequent reason for physician consultation in the United States (1). Many cancer patients do not present with pain, but ultimately experience it as a result of progressive disease, diagnostic or therapeutic treatments, palliative interventions (surgery, radiation, chemotherapy) (2), complications of the same, and from other comorbid disease states.

EPIDEMIOLOGY

In 2000, there were 10.9 million new (incident) cases of cancer, 6.7 million deaths, and 24.6 million people living with cancer (prevalence) (3). Pain is the most feared symptom (4,5) with an impact estimate of 30% to 50% (6) of patients in active therapy suffering from pain, increasing to 70% to 90% with advanced progressive disease (7,8).

DEFINING PALLIATION AND PAIN

Palliation is defined by Webster as "reducing the violence of a disease, to abate" from the Latin word *palliare,* meaning to cloak or shield (from pain and suffering).

Pain is "an unpleasant sensory and emotional experience associated with actual or potential tissue damage, or described in terms of such damage" (9). Furthermore, "it is always subjective. Each individual learns the application of the word through experiences related to injury early in life" (10). "The inability to communicate verbally does not negate the possibility that an individual is experiencing pain and is in need of appropriate pain-relieving treatment" (11). Function and quality of life (QOL) are significantly impacted by the persistence of pain. This, in turn, increases the risk of anxiety and depression, and may increase the risk of suicidal ideation. To provide relief, one must first recognize the individual's experiences. It is critical to successful therapeutic management.

"Only when the sense of the pain of others begins does man begin." Yevgeny Yevtushenko

Contrary to the often-held clinical opinion, there may not be changes in vital signs, which were previously believed to be markers of pain (12). In addition to acknowledging an individual's pain, the astute clinician is familiar with the various types of pain as well as the appropriate interventions.

ACCURATELY ASSESSING THE ETIOLOGIES OF DIFFERENT PAIN PATTERNS

Acute vs. Chronic Cancer Pain

Acute cancer pain is caused by noxious or tissue-damaging stimulation resulting from bodily insult or disease. Anxiety may play a prominent role. Cancer patients may react with anxiety to acute painful therapeutic interventions (bone marrow, spinal taps, etc.) and have an amplified perception of the pain induced by actual insult. In general, because acute pain is said to be a direct discrete time-limited response to nociceptive stimuli, the task of assessment is more straightforward than that of chronic pain (13).

When pain persists beyond the point when healing would have expected to occur (usually 3–6 months) it is considered chronic, and it may occur in the absence of tissue damage (14).

Chronic cancer pain is longer standing, may be intractable, and caused by progressive disease. If therapeutic interventions for cancer symptoms and pain control fail, "abnormal illness behavior" may develop, which includes physical changes in sleep, appetite, and social activity. Somatic symptom preoccupation can occur with associated depression and anxiety. Marked prolonged disability may result particularly if disease control and pain management have not been successful (13). The distinction between acute cancer pain and chronic pain may become blurred (15).

Nociceptive Pain: Somatic and Visceral

When a tissue is traumatized by injury, invasion, or inflammation, local peripheral nerves are stimulated in the skin or organs producing nociceptive pain. Opioids and anti-inflammatories are useful in the management of this pain, which is subdivided into somatic, myofascial, and visceral types.

Somatic pain is well localized and is commonly described as throbbing, sharp, aching, and (rarely) burning. Examples include bone metastasis, incisional pain, and arthritic joint pain. *Myofascial* pain arises from similar mechanisms. The hallmark is "trigger points," which are focal points, and when stimulated generate an explosive regional pain response. At rest, symptoms include tightness, pulling, and spasms (such as in head and neck strains). NSAIDs, heat/ice, stretching, physical therapy, trigger point release by dry needling, the use of Tens (transcutaneous electrical nerve stimulation), and occasionally local botox (botulinum toxin A) injections are employed for the relief of these symptoms.

Visceral pain similarly results from tissue damage to organs, with associated irritation or inflammation to local nerves. Painful perceptions are often deeper and less focal than somatic pain. Reports of pressure, tightening, and cramping are noted. Radiation occurs (such as cardiac or pleural pain) to more distant sites. (An explicit example would be celiac pain with origins in the epigastrium that radiates through the back.) Colicky spasms (biliary, intestinal, and renal colic) are common and are often associated with symptoms of nausea, vomiting, and diaphoresis like other visceral pains. Treatments include opiates, NSAIDs, steroids, and occasionally procedures such as nerve blocks.

Neuropathic pain occurs with central or peripheral nerve tissue inflammation (chemotherapy, HSV, Hepatitis C, HIV infections, or metabolic toxicities) injury, tumor invasion, or surgical intervention and results in aberrant neurotransmission (16). Characteristic paroxysmal sensations, such as lancinating, burning, and prickling, may be accompanied by heightened painful sensitivity to light touch (allodynia). Anatomic localization combined with the above descriptors aid in this diagnosis. Examples include "shingles," phantom pain, diabetic neuropathy, and complex regional pain syndromes (formerly called reflex sympathetic dystrophy and causalgia). Management includes opioids, steroids, antidepressants, anticonvulsants, and local anesthetic or topical agents (17).

Recognizing early weakness, sensory, or motor function losses on exam assist in the prevention of progressive neurological dysfunction. Changes such as solitary sensory loss or focal pain, a "red Flag", may warn the clinician of an evolving neurologic emergency. A "band-like" squeezing sensation around the trunk or new onset back pain may herald ensuing cord involvement or compression in cancer patients (18). Likewise, new headache, vision changes, or sudden onset of dizziness may be a harbinger of quiescent CNS metastasis, which if undetected can prove catastrophic.

Breakthrough pain is a transient exacerbation of pain occurring in patients with otherwise stable, persistent pain. An estimate of 19% to 95% of all patients with pain may experience this based on the definition used (1). Depending on the author, subtypes include incident (related to movement or activity) and idiopathic pain. Persistent existence of breakthrough pain can portend poor outcomes, lower patient satisfaction, and increase healthcare utilization (1). Higher pain intensity has been associated with breakthrough pain, somatic pain, younger age, and lower performance status (14).

A separate type of pain is *end of dose failure pain,* which occurs when medication dosing is inadequate in strength or length of action.

Existential pain is synonymous with suffering or psychic pain. The experience of pain is profoundly affected by mortal angst, which in turn is influenced by premorbid personality, coping mechanisms, as well as psychosocial-spiritual support systems. Pain of this nature is not responsive to opioid manipulations, is just as "real," and is therefore more difficult to manage. Unfinished business in life (goals unmet), financial strains, fear (such as that of dying), and leaving behind loved ones are common concerns that contribute to marked suffering. If this very significant part of a patient's experience is avoided, the soul-searching questions (and possible resolutions) that arise when an individual faces mortality are neglected. Questions must be addressed, tasks at hand (such as family issues) need to be dealt with, and personal opportunities to grow (for both the physician and the patient) should be recognized.

The recognition and management of suffering requires the attention of an interdisciplinary team in conjunction with the patient's support system. Utilizing counseling, spiritual ministry, or religious support, in conjunction with creative modalities of art, music, recreational therapies, and even healing touch, may greatly assist an individual who is preparing for the reality of the struggle ahead, whatever it may be. Honest communication is essential; it aids both the individual and family to make progressive steps in coping with illness and mortality. Practitioners who have recognized issues of their own mortality are better prepared to help with existential pain of patients.

Total pain is the aggregate of all types of pain that an individual experiences. In order to obtain relief, one must treat *all* natures of pain and suffering. Most individuals will commonly present with a mixed picture of pain. Treatment needs to be directed to each type of distress to be successfully ameliorated (Fig. 1).

PAIN ASSESSMENT

For a complete evaluation of pain to occur, an evaluation starts with a thorough history and physical exam. The history includes, but is not limited to, a focus on primary complaint, other distressing symptoms, medications, herbal treatments, and folk remedies in use. Details of pain should include sites and distribution (local or multiple sites? radiating?) onset, duration (acute or chronic), and temporal variations in experience. The quality of distress (pain types noted above), associated symptoms (sensory, motor, autonomic changes), the impact on sleep, mood (QOL), function (activities of daily living or ADL, and work), as well as exacerbating and alleviating factors, all require documentation. Visual inspection to evaluate body posture and habitus (bracing, crying, moaning, sweating, restlessness, wincing, or gasping) should be recorded as well. To quantify the individual's experience, notation must be made of the severity of pain experienced.

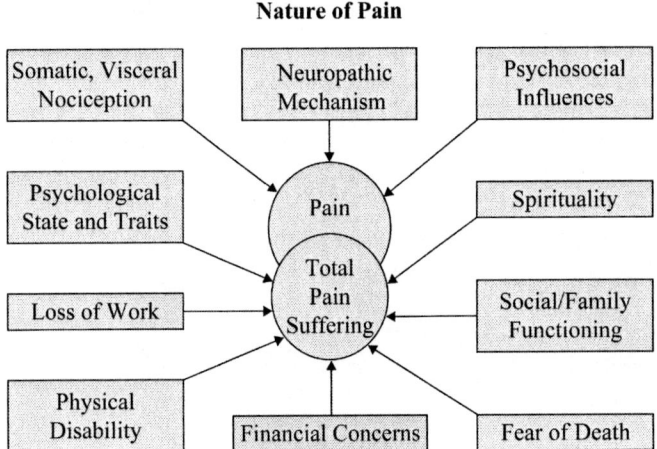

Figure 1 Total pain diagram.

"Documentation of pain intensity within the medical records of hospitals and cancer centers has been considered a requirement for excellence in the quality improvement process for health care providers." (19,20).

SCALES FOR PAIN MEASUREMENT

Since pain perception is inherently subjective, the gold standard of assessing pain is simply to ask the patient (21). In order to facilitate details on the quantity of pain, several scales have been developed. A review of instruments, such as NRS (numeric rating scale) VRS (verbal rating score), and VAS (visual analog scale), suggest that these are all valid ways to assess pain severity (22). The NRS describes pain on an 11-point scale, with 0 being no pain and 10 the worst pain imaginable (23). It may be used alone or in conjunction with the VAS. The VAS is a horizontal line with dividing marks 0 to 10 at 1 cm intervals, and is used for ages 9 and older (Fig. 2).

The VRS is a simple pain description, with ratings of no pain, mild, moderate, or severe (the worst pain ever had or could be imagined). It may also be used in conjunction with a simplified VAS. The Wong-Baker Faces Pain Rating Scale is used alternately in both adults and children over the age of three. Instructions are available in many languages (26).

PSYCHOSOCIAL HISTORY ASSESSMENT

To understand a person, one must delve into his psychological experience in addition to physical symptoms. An individual's coping mechanism, support systems (vs. isolation), home situation, finances, religion, spiritual and cultural preferences

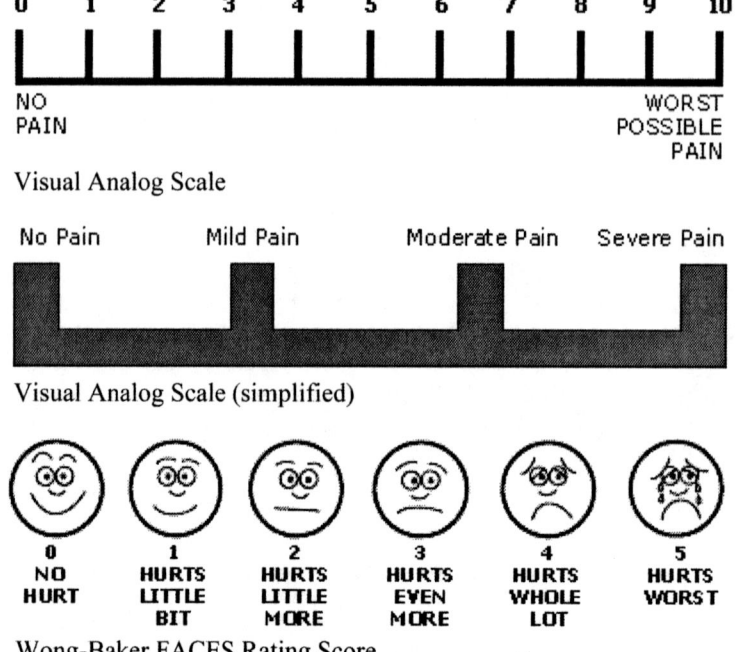

Figure 2 The scales. *Source*: Refs. 23–25.

are just the beginning of insights into ways to provide support. Other valuable data include present functionality, past or present mood disorders, drug/alcohol problems, and significant losses/grief. It is important to appreciate the current meaning of the illness (a challenge or punishment?) and the goals of care (cure or pain relief?). If these issues are not addressed during the initial history and physical exam, details may be obtained through later encounters with the clinician or interdisciplinary members' interactions.

TREATING PAIN: PRINCIPLES OF PAIN CONTROL AND ANALGESIC THERAPY

1. Analgesic interventions should be integrated into a comprehensive patient evaluation and management plan.
2. The emotional and cognitive aspects of pain must be recognized and treated.
3. Pain is most often under treated, not over treated.
4. Pain control must be individualized.
5. Identify and treat the source of the pain.

6. Consider a multimodality approach that applies both pharmacologic and nonpharmacologic therapies.
7. If drug therapy is used, select the appropriate drug and route and optimize administration.
8. Anticipate and manage side effects.
9. Address patient concerns if opioids are indicated; understand and communicate the difference between physical and psychological dependence (below), and proactively address the risk of misuse or abuse and addiction.
10. Avoid using placebos to treat pain (27).

APPLYING ANALGESIC PRINCIPLES: THE WORLD HEALTH ORGANIZATION ANALGESIC LADDER

To assist in the development of a clinically consistent approach to pain management, the WHO, in 1986, designed this three-step analgesic ladder (Fig. 3) (28). Through an individualized application of analgesics (choice of medication, dose, and adjuvant medication) based on the nature and severity, pain can be relieved in 70% to 90% of the patients (29). The WHO pain management ladder categorizes the level of pain intensity by steps, with the milder symptoms occurring on the first rung. Ascending the steps accommodates increasing

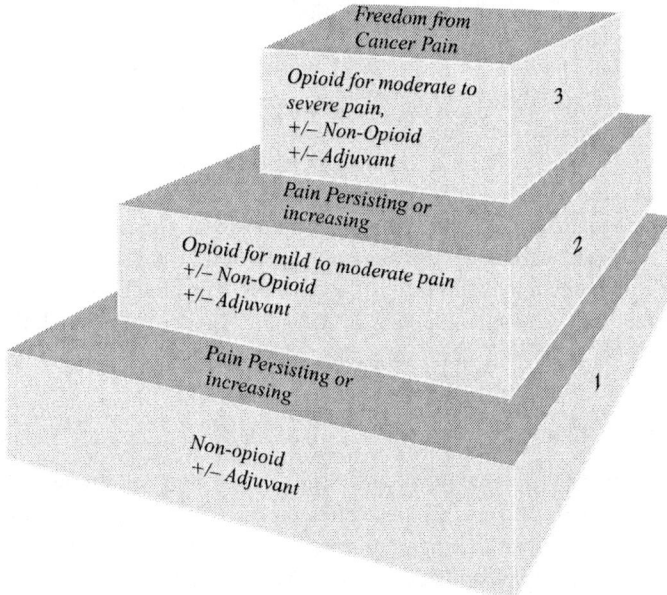

Figure 3 World Health Organization analgesic ladder. *Source*: From Ref: 28.

severities of pain, as well as negotiating differing types of pain through the addition of adjuvant medications and therapies.

Step 1, mild 0–3/10 pain starts with nonopioid analgesia and adds an adjuvant as clinically indicated by the nature of the pain. This group of drugs includes acetaminophen, aspirin, and NSAIDs. When used alone, the anti-inflammatories are best for mild pain. They are also often used as co-analgesic (steps 2 and 3) with opioids to maximize pain control. Inflammatory pain such as with acute injury (dental, postoperative) and bone pain are examples that are most frequently aided by these medications. This group exhibits a "ceiling" effect for analgesia, beyond which there is no further analgesic benefit; however, it does not produce tolerance or physical dependence (29).

Step 2, moderate 4–6/10 pain uses the analgesics that have previously been referred to as "weak opioids." Often, these are the same opioids used in step 3, but in smaller doses and in combined formulations with first-rung medications, acetaminophen, and aspirin as co-analgesics. In fact, these same opioids such as oxycodone are either the same or stronger than the standard of morphine in comparable doses (Table 1). Moderate pain can be well managed with these medications, which include codeine (usually in combination with acetaminophen), percocet (oxycodone and acetaminophen), vicodan (hydrocodone and acetaminophen), percodan (oxycodone and aspirin), and tramadol. Combination analgesics (such as vicodan, percocet) are dose limited by ceiling effects of the co-analgesic agent (from step 1 below). For example, in vicodan, the acetaminophen component limits the dosing to eight tablets a day (with 500 mg acetaminophen/5 mg of hydrocodone formulation). At all steps, adjuvant medications are added as appropriate for the nature of pain. A recent Cochrane review did not substantiate the addition of a "weak opioid" to the first rung of the WHO ladder, but instead, recommended maximizing doses of the NSAID before the addition of or replacement with an opioid (30).

Step 3, severe 7–10/10 pain is a crisis level of pain and deserves acute attention and management with the class previously called "strong opioids" for adequate relief. The gold standard of opioid pain management is morphine. This and similar morphine-like agonists make up the preponderance of this step, used alone and in combination with medications from steps 1 and 2, plus appropriate adjuvants. "Plain opioids" (those without acetaminophen or aspirin), also previously called step 3, are said to exhibit no ceiling effect in analgesia.

MEDICATION OVERVIEW

Acetaminophen is an antipyretic analgesic with little, if any, anti-inflammatory effect. Used by itself or with opiates, it is less efficacious in inflammatory pain than the NSAIDs. *Caution:* dose ceilings are important for this drug whether used alone (step 1) or in combination (step 2) and must be limited to 4 g or less (2 g with liver dysfunction or chronic alcohol use, and under 3 g in the elderly) due to risk of potential hepatotoxicity (31).

Table 1 Equianalgesic Conversion (Daily Oral Morphine Equivalents or DOME)

Drug	Oral (mg)		IV (mg)	PO:IV ratio
Morphine	30		10	3:1
Codeine	200		130	1:5
Hydrocodone	30–60		None	—
Oxycodone	20		None	—
Hydromorphone	7.5		1.5	5:01
Oxymorphone	10–15		1	10 to 15:1
Propoxyphene	100		50	2:1
Levophanol	4		2	2:1
Meperidine	300		100	3 or 4:1
Methadone: convert from daily oral morphine equivalents (noted in mg) × % = calculated methadone dose	DOME <90 mg 90–300 mg 300–600 mg 600–1000 mg >1000 mg	Methadone use 20–30% 10–20% 8–12% 5–10% <5%	1–3	Variable
Fentanyl	none		100 µg	
Different equianalgesia for each of the following fentanyl products				
Fentanyl transdermal	100 µg/hr = approximately 3 mg/hr IV morphine see package insert for DOME equivalents		n/a	Do not start in opioid-naive patients (taking less than 45 DOME)
OTFC Oral transmucosal fentanyl citrate (Actiq)	200 µg = 6–12 mg oral MS (or 2–4 IV MS) 400 µg = 12–24 mg oral MS (or 4–8 mg IV MS)		n/a	Slower absorption than fentanyl buccal tablet
Fentanyl buccal tablet (Fentora)	100 µg = 200–400 µg OTFC 200 µg = 600 µg OTFC 400 µg = 1200 µg OTFC		n/a	Fentanyl products are not interchangeable

Source: From Refs. 29, 35–39.

Nonsteroidal anti-inflammatories as a class are "useful in a broad range of pain syndromes of diverse mechanisms," but there are no data to support its therapeutic superiority to alternative options in any particular setting other than inflammation (29,32). Unlike opioids, NSAIDs have a ceiling effect beyond which there is no beneficial analgesia; they do not develop tolerance, dependence, and are not associated with abuse and addiction. NSAIDs, like aspirin, are antipyretic and their primary action is inhibition of prostaglandin formation

(33). "Although the efficacy and mechanism of action are well known, nonsteroidal anti-inflammatories remain underused medication for pain management, especially where opioids are being administered" (34). If a nonsteroidal from one class is ineffective, it is useful to sequentially try alternate classes to obtain a therapeutic response. *Caution:* significant renal dysfunction and GI bleeding are among the risks. Cox-2 selective inhibitors may increase the risk of serious or potentially fatal cardiovascular events (MI, CVA) in proportion to duration of use.

NSAID classes (31): It is useful to become familiar with one or two from each class as well as their specific side effects. The derivatives of each class are listed below.

Salicylates: Aspirin, diflunisal
Acetic acid: Indomethacin, sulindac, etodolac, mefanamic acid, meclofenamate, tolmentin, ketorolac, diclofenac
Proprionic acid: Ibuprofen, naproxen, fenoprofen, ketoprofen, flurbiprofen, oxaprozin
Enolic acid: Piroxicam, meloxicam, nalbumetone
COX-2 selective inhibitor: celecoxib

Opioids are all measured against morphine as the "gold standard of pain control." Morphine and its related compounds are used in the management of cancer pain. With similar analgesic and side effect profiles, the choice is largely based on the clinician's preference rather than evidence-based studies. Structural modifications have produced morphine derivatives, many of which are more potent than the parent drug (availability varies by country). Pharmacologic properties are similar, though individual responses may vary greatly. These individual differences are poorly understood (31), but are presumed to be based on genetic differences as well as pharmacologic receptor site preferences for each medication (29). When a poor response or intolerable side effects occur, the patient should be rotated to another opioid. When rotation occurs, it is important to recognize the marked strength differences between the opiates (Table 1) and the need to reduce dose due to limited cross-tolerance. As a class, the opioids are well absorbed from the entire GI tract. Some have lipophilic properties (fentanyl), which allow for absorption through the buccal mucosa, skin, SC, IM, epidural, and intrathecal routes. First-pass metabolism occurs with oral administration of opioids (through the liver), yielding an effective lower analgesic response than a comparable parenteral dose. The analgesic difference varies by opioid and is a basis for conversion tables (Table 1). Opioids can be agonist, agonist-antagonist, and antagonist based on interactions with receptor subtypes. In the management of cancer pain, pure agonists are most commonly used (29) and will be reviewed below.

SIGNIFICANT OPIOID FACTS

Morphine, a naturally occurring alkaloid of the opium poppy, is the "gold standard" (reference standard) analgesic by which other opioids are compared in terms of efficacy and side effects. For reasons of historical use (nearly 200 years), clinical familiarity, world-wide availability, and low cost, it is often considered the drug of choice in cancer management. Morphine is well absorbed orally, has extensive liver metabolism (first pass), and may have some extrahepatic metabolism in the small bowel and proximal tubule, which could be important with liver dysfunction (31). *Caution:* metabolites of morphine include inert morphine-3-glucuronide (M-3-G, which may contribute to excitatory effects) and morphine-6-glucuronide, which is believed to be twice as potent as the parent compound. The latter metabolite, like morphine, is excreted in kidney in proportion to the creatinine clearance. With diminishing renal function, M-3-G accumulates in both blood and CSF, and is associated with toxicity including myoclonus and seizure activity. Use morphine with care in impaired renal function. If renal dysfunction is sudden in onset, symptoms of opioid toxicity may develop, necessitating withdrawal, dose reduction, or interval lengthening (31). Formulations include oral (both long- and short-acting), rectal, parenteral, and intraspinal.

Codeine, another naturally occurring analgesic, is used for its antitussive and antidiarrheal properties. Most commonly, it is administered with acetaminophen to improve its effectiveness. *Caution:* Cytochrome P450 (CYP2D6) is *required* to actively metabolize it to morphine (the only active metabolite). Genetic variation may leave individuals with minimal, if any, activity, hence little or no pain relief (approximately 10% of the Caucasian population) (31). Like other opiates, it is well absorbed from GI tract, but there can be considerable variation (12–84%) (40). When used in conjunction with acetaminophen, the same cautions for ceiling effects apply (available formulations: oral and parenteral routes).

Hydrocodone, another synthetic codeine analog, is roughly equivalent with similar uses. *Caution:* there is a narrower therapeutic index than codeine with higher incidence of adverse effects, especially in impaired renal function. Severe toxicity has been reported, presumable through metabolic accumulations similar to morphine of the glucuronide moieties (oral) (40).

Oxycodone, a synthetic morphine derivative, is frequently used in low-dose combination with nonopioids for step 2, or alone as immediate or sustained release for step 3. Metabolites are *not* thought to contribute to pharmacologic effects (oral as immediate-release and long-acting formulations are available).

Oxymorphone is also a synthetic derivative of morphine and has been recently re-released. Stronger than the parent compound, it accumulates similarly in renal failure, requiring dose-interval lengthening. It appears more closely related to hydromorphone in structure and strength (41). *Caution:* respiratory depression has been reported with parenteral administration of oxymorphone, and requires judicious and slow titration starting at one-third to half the dose, especially in the face of existing pulmonary disease, CNS depression, debilitation, or with any other sedatives (42). Nausea and vomiting are more common than morphine when used by Patient Controlled Analgesia (PCA), though less sedation occurs (oral with immediate-release and long-acting formulations, parenteral and rectal formulations exist).

Hydromorphone is another synthetic morphine derivative that is more potent (Table 1) and largely excreted by kidneys. *Caution:* hydromorphone also has a metabolite, hydromorphone-3-glucuronide which is renally excreted, and may contribute to morphine-like side effects in patients with renal disease (oral and parenteral routes available) (31,35).

Fentanyl is similar in action to morphine but 100 times more potent. A synthetic opioid with rapid onset or action, which has less histamine release, and hence less pruritus. Higher lipid solubility allows for transdermal use as well as administration through the buccal mucosa. *Caution:* fevers, diaphoresis, increased metabolic rate, or heat exposure can cause marked increases fentanyl transdermal absorption resulting in toxicity. Muscular rigidity occurs with fentanyl, more commonly with bolus dosing (parenteral, transdermal, buccal application, epidural, and intrathecal routes are available).

Methadone is a synthetic opioid with a long half-life ranging from 12 to 150 hours (averaging 24 hr). There is an associated slow rise in drug concentrations as well as onset of analgesia and side effects (steady state occurs at about one week). It is inexpensive, but often not readily available. It has additional N-methyl-D-aspartate (NMDA) properties (discussed under adjuvant medications), which can reduce opioid tolerance, and may also provide use for neuropathic pain. *Caution:* its use should be limited to clinicians who are familiar with the pharmacologic properties and prescribe it frequently. There are numerous drug interactions (including antiretrovirals, antibiotics, tricyclic antidepressants, etc.) that should be carefully evaluated. Qt intervals require monitoring, especially in the face of preexisting cardiac disease or concomitant use of medications, which interfere with cardiac conduction or cause electrolyte disturbances (43). Equianalgesic dosing is controversial (oral, IV) (31,40).

Tramadol is a synthetic codeine derivative with similar weak mu receptor binding and effects like morphine. It may have less constipation and respiratory depression at equianalgesic doses. Analgesia is produced by central inhibition of uptake of norepinephrine and serotonin. Reportedly, it is as effective as morphine or meperidine for mild to moderate pain (even in cancer), but not as useful in severe pain. Maximum dose is 400 mg/day (oral, rectal, parenteral routes are included in availability) (31).

NOT RECOMMENDED FOR ANALGESIA

Propoxyphene is structurally related to methadone (with similar pharmacologic properties) and has extensive first-pass metabolism. Potency is thought to be half to two-third as strong as codeine (31) *Caution:* the weaker active opioid metabolite norpropoxyphene can penetrate the CNS, accumulate, and yield excitatory effects (tremulousness and seizures) as well as respiratory depression at more toxic doses. Other rare toxicities include hepatotoxic reaction, cardiac conduction disorders, and dangerous interactions with carbamazepine, warfarin, and alcohol (31,40).

Meperidine is a synthetic opioid agonist no longer recommended for the treatment of chronic pain due to concerns of toxicity. Despite long-held beliefs by clinicians, its effects on smooth muscle are similar to other opioids. It *does* appear to be effective in the treatment of post-anesthetic shivering (31). *Caution:* the active metabolite norpethidine, a potent convulsant, is less potent as an analgesic and accumulates readily in renal failure, (may also with normal renal function) causing hyperexcitability and seizures, which cannot be blocked by naloxone. It is a dangerous drug if used in conjunction with MAOI and may produce fatal toxicities (thought to be from excess serotonin yielding hyperpyrexia, muscle rigidity, and seizures) (40).

Mixed agonists-antagonists (penazocine, butorphanol, and nabuphine) are not recommended in chronic pain since they can block uptake of the agonist drugs often needed for analgesia.

DOSE ESCALATION FOR PAIN CONTROL

Increases in analgesia by less than 25% to 30% of a given medication dose are unlikely to be noted by a patient. In severe pain, 50% to 100% increases are recommended, which may need to be administered parenterally every 15 to 20 minutes until pain is relieved (29). Mild to moderate pain often does not need loading doses, but rather regular dose titration upward by 25% to 50% (regardless of starting dose) to achieve relief. Basal dose infusions or long-acting opioids should not be increased by more than 100% at a time (with normal renal function) regardless of how many bolus or breakthrough doses have been used. Individuals who are aged, have renal impairment or hepatic impairment will need a reduction in the escalation. Immediate release opioids (without acetaminophen) can be increased safely, if needed, in two-hour increments. Long-acting opiate doses can be changed every 24 hours, fentanyl patch (duragesic) every 48 to 72 hours (29), or methadone no less then every 72 hours (44,29).

ADJUVANT MEDICATIONS

Commonly used for treating conditions other than pain, these medications enhance pain relief through nonopioid mechanisms (34). They are used at all levels of the WHO ladder. Cherny has helpfully divided these into four main groups (29) and has been adapted below.

1. Neuropathic adjuvant agents: These are often needed to maximize analgesia since there may be a diminished responsiveness of this type of pain to opioids (29).

Antidepressants (oral, transdermal), for many years, have been used to manage neuropathic pain, and are often the first choice of treatment (45). Tricyclics are the best studied of this class, are well absorbed orally, and have a long half-life. Low doses are initiated and slowly titrated up for response. Presynaptic CNS membrane blockade of serotonin or norepinephrine is thought to be the mechanisms of action. Tricyclics stabilize nerve membranes acting like local anesthesia (34), and enhance morphine-like analgesia reducing dose requirements.

Unique preparations have been used to reduce pain with electrotherapy in DM neuropathy (31). Transdermal preparations have been used for severe inflammatory bowel disease (when unable to take oral doses) (34). And newer studies suggest oral topical application may be useful for mucositis pain (46). Tricyclics provide analgesia within 24 hours of administrations, indicating that the effects are not related to antidepressant action (which takes 1 week) (34). *Caution:* side effects of dry mouth, urinary retention, constipation, sedation, orthostatic hypotension, and cardiac arrhythmia require monitoring. The secondary amines (desipramine, nortriptiline, clomipramine) show less anticholinergic effect and less sedation than the tertiary amines (e.g., amitriptiline). Amitriptiline has the best evidence for neuropathic effectiveness, but apparently has no influence on HIV-related neuropathies (45). Select serotonin reuptake inhibitors (SSRIs) have been minimally effective (34,47). Serotoninnorepinephrine reuptake inhibitors (SNRIs) in particular duloxetine (FDA approved) has been useful in diabetic neuropathy, but venlafaxine is less consistent in response.

Anticonvulsants block sodium channels reducing neuron excitability, and may work in neuropathic pain where opioids (have little or no efficacy) may fail. The best evidence has been for carbamazepine, especially in trigeminal neuralgia (48), but the hematologic risks has limited its usefulness (29) Oxycarbazine is reported to have fewer side effects, but no controlled studies exist at present. Gabapentin (thought to work on calcium channels) is commonly used and supported by data for use in postherpetic neuralgia (PHN) and painful diabetic neuropathy. More recently, pregabalin has emerged with more stable pharmacokinetics and is cost effective in the same neuropathic states (49). Lamotrigine shows the most promise in central pain syndromes and diabetic neuropathy. Topiramate is FDA approved for the treatment of migraines. Phenytoin is limited in use due to side effects, and valproic acid is without controlled studies to support it. Clinical trials are underway for clonazepam, tiagabine, and vigabatrin for the use in neuropathic analgesia (48). *Caution:* doses and monitoring are often the same as in seizure management, and may require monitoring of hematologic values (medication specific). Side effects include mental clouding, dizziness, and sedation (as well as drug-specific side effects that require familiarity with each medication).

2. Multipurpose adjuvant medications: This category includes corticosteroids, clonidine, NMDA receptor antagonists, and local agents such as topical local anesthetics.

Corticosteroids act by decreasing prostaglandin production, thereby reducing inflammation, edema, and neuronal excitability. This provides usefulness in the treatment of acute cord compression, headache from brain metastasis, bone pain, and neuropathic back pain. Corticosteroids also increase appetite and abate nausea. Commonly used corticosteroids include betamethasone, dexamethasone, and prednisone. Intrathecal administration can produce analgesia (34). *Caution:* side effects include hypertension, hyperglycemia, GI ulceration, immunosuppression, and precipitation of psychiatric disorders. Long-term use may lead to the development of Cushing's syndrome or development of proximal myopathy, osteoporosis, and aseptic necrosis. The duration of therapy increases the risks of the later side effects.

The alpha-2 agonist clonidine has been used to improve postoperative analgesia. When given intra-articularly or intrathecally (spinal surgery) with morphine, it can decrease pain and increase analgesic duration. In other surgeries, clonidine proves less beneficial (34). Clonidine is also useful in the management of chronic cancer pain.

Local anesthetics block sodium channels, reducing neuronal hyperexcitability (34). Topical application alleviates mucosal ulcer pain as well as numbs cutaneous areas before procedures (lumbar puncture, venipuncture). The benefit is seen in neuropathic states, such as distal symmetrical polyneuropathy of HIV disease, DM, complex regional pain syndromes, postmastectomy (18) and postthoracotomy pain as well as with postherpetic neuralgia. *Caution:* systemic absorption can cause seizures.

Antiarrythmics (systemic anesthetics) have not proved useful in neuropathic pain (34).

Another topical agent is capsaicin, which has been shown to be helpful in post-mastectomy pain, chronic neuropathic pain, and diabetic neuropathy through the depletion of substance P from local terminals, decreasing nerve transmission in C fibers and producing analgesia (34).

NMDA receptor antagonists facilitate peripheral hyperalgesia (windup central sensitization), antagonism may prevent or counteract opioid tolerance. Reports of pain reduction with ketamine and dextromethorphan support a decrease in opioid need. In fact, ketamine as an adjunct to opioids, increased pain relief by 20% to 30% and allowed a reduction in opioids dose by 25% to 50% (18,34).

3. Adjuvant analgesics for bone pain: There is surprisingly limited data found for efficacy of NSAIDs in bone pain (2,29), yet some patients appear to benefit greatly. Corticosteroids are used in difficult situations (29). Bisphosponates, according to a Cochrane review, show modest effectiveness that should be used only if analgesia and radiation are inadequate. Similarly, limited evidence was found for calcitonin (22). Radiolabeled agents such as strontium are often effective (2) as first-line agents and localizes to all involved bone area with selective absorption; however, data is conflicting as to its use as an adjuvant to external beam radiotherapy. Radiopharmaceuticals (samarium, rhenium) are also showing promising results (29).

4. Adjuncts for visceral pain: There is limited supportive evidence for these agents for bladder spasm, colicky abdominal pain, and tenesmic pain. Oxybutynin has been used for bladder spasms with some success, and NSAIDs may also be helpful. There is no pharmacologic relief for rectal spasm, though a recent report shows nebulized salbutamol may reduce the

severity of symptoms (29). Other reports of calcium blocker, clonidine, chlorpromazine, and benzodiazepines have anecdotally been successful (29). Benzodiazepines, in addition to relaxation, cause some analgesia separate from anxiolysis, thought to be from a direct effect on opioid receptors (34). Colic has been treated with scopolamine (IV, sublinqual) as well as octreotide (29). Belladonna and Opium (B&O) suppositories (50,51), as well as tincture of opium, are also used for smooth muscle spasm.

INVASIVE STRATEGIES

Other consultative services should be added to the armamentarium of analgesia. These include judicious referral to anesthesiology and pain services for botox injections (botulinum toxin type A) for myofascial pain, epidural, intrathecal, and other blocks specific to the nature of pain (celiac plexus for epigastric and pancreatic pain). Often blocks are done in conjunction with interventional radiology. Radiologic procedures also include radiation for symptomatic treatment of lesions (mass effect and bone pain). Rehabilitation may use "dry needling" for myofascial pain as well as the application of Tens (transcutaneous nerves stimulation). GI referrals may be made for implants (such as stents for pancreatic cancer and obstructive tumors). Consultation for palliative surgery (catheters, ureteral stents, surgery for bone disease, and amputation) may be beneficial when relief can not be otherwise obtained (22).

NONPHARMACOLOGIC STRATEGIES

Nonpharmacologic strategies include psychological support (chaplaincy, counseling, psychiatry, and social work), rehabilitative medicine (occupational and physical therapy), and CAM (complementary and alternative medical therapies). CAM includes the healing techniques of acupuncture, hypnosis, Reiki (energy medicine), healing and therapeutic touch, the use of the labyrinth, as well as other diversional therapies of massage, music, art, recreational and pet therapies, as well as biofeedback, imagery, and relaxation techniques.

MISCONCEPTIONS AND BARRIERS TO GOOD PAIN MANAGEMENT

Pain Myths

1. Pain is proportionate to the injury (just check a local emergency room). If no cause of pain is identified, then the complaint is (thought) due to psychological causes (examples, headaches, neuropathic and phantom pain, causalgia).

2. A patient who describes a pain as severe or rates it high on numerical or VASs, and does not look ill, writhe, or grimace, is exaggerating his/her pain (note, some individuals guard for comfort, others feel they will be disbelieved).
3. Patients who do not take analgesics, but continue to complain of pain are not cooperating with treatment (not all pain responds to given medications or there may be intolerable side effects) (52).

DEFINITIONS IN PAIN MANAGEMENT

Tolerance is a state of adaptation in which exposure to a drug induces changes that result in the diminution of one or more of the drugs effects over time (53).

Individuals on medications for prolonged periods may have reduction in beneficial as well as adverse effects, each occurring at different rates. Such occurrences are common with many classes of drugs including alpha adrenergic agents, antidepressants, beta blockers, corticosteroids, and opiates (alcohol also develops tolerance). This often occurs with progressive disease.

Physical dependence is a state of adaptation that is manifested by a drug-class-specific withdrawal syndrome that can be produced by abrupt cessation, rapid dose reduction, decreasing blood level of the drug, and/or administration of an antagonist (53).

Like tolerance, this is a normal response that may occur after persistent use of a given class of medication, including opioids. With opioids, this is thought to occur after a week or longer on consistent doses. This adaptation results in a new level of homeostasis, which accommodates the medication dose. If opioids are withdrawn abruptly, this *will* precipitate withdrawal symptoms. Thus, patients may continue to use opioids after pain has subsided to prevent withdrawal symptoms. Clinicians often mistake this for addiction; this is *not* the same. When the need for analgesia resolves, an individual can safely be tapered over time to prevent symptoms of opiate withdrawal. Recognize that this dependency is a temporary condition, which occurred after the body adapted to opioids and can be reversed. This is seen with many medications including coffee.

"*Addiction* is a primary, chronic, neurobiologic disease with genetic, psychosocial, and environmental factors influencing its development and manifestations. It is characterized by behaviors that include one of more of the following; impaired control over drug use, compulsive use, continued use despite harm, and craving." (53).

Abnormal behaviors include extremes such as theft and prostitution in order to access the desire drug. This occurs most commonly in individuals who seek out opioids for reason other than pain. Those who are treated for pain reportedly have a lower incidence of addiction. An idiosyncratic adverse reaction to exposure in a biologically and psychosocially vulnerable person may result in addiction; it cannot be predicted, but occurs at an estimated low frequency. In a recent review, cancer patients on long-term opioids were estimated to have an addiction rate of 0% to

7.7%; however, reservations must be applied to these figures since some studies (mistakenly) included individuals with tolerance and dependence in their definition of addiction (54). Noncancer populations are estimated higher (54). Clinicians fear this situation when prescribing opiates, often resulting in underprescribing.

Pseudoaddiction is a term that describes a patient's behavior when he is under treated. Patients with unrelieved pain may become focused on obtaining medications, may clock watch, and may otherwise seem inappropriately "drug seeking." Even behaviors such as illicit drug use and deception can occur as the patient attempts to obtain relief. Pseudoaddiction can be distinguished from true addiction in that the behaviors resolve when pain is effectively treated (53). Patients may become desperate and go to more than one provider in an effort to get adequate pain relief. This behavior is the iatrogenic result when a well-meaning practitioner under-prescribes (oligo-opioid or little opioid) for fear of "causing addiction," in an individual who has unmet pain control needs.

CONCLUSION

Total pain is made up of more than just physical pain. Total pain can involve a physical component as well as a suffering component. Suffering involves psychological and coping factors, social support, loss issues, fear of death, financial concerns, and spiritual concerns. It is not unusual for individuals with cancer to have suffering issues as well as physical pain. To help relieve total pain, in particular suffering, the entire healthcare team should be involved; most notably, those on the team who work with nonpharmacologic approaches to relieving pain including social service workers; spiritual care counselors; recreation, art, massage and reiki, music, pet therapists; and volunteers. We as health professionals may not always be able to cure the cancer or totally relieve pain; however, we can help patients find meaning in their pain. The goal is to heal by helping the patient find a sense of wholeness in life.

REFERENCES

1. Burton AW. Outpatient management of breakthrough pain. Medscape Neurology and Neurosurgery; 2005. www.medscape.com/viewarticle/506124
2. Carr DB, Goudas LC, Balk EM, et al. Evidence report on the treatment of pain in cancer patients. J Natl Cancer Inst Monogr 2004(32):23–31.
3. Parkin DM, Bray F, Ferlay J, et al. Global cancer statistics, 2002. CA Cancer J Clin 2005; 55(2):74–108.
4. Levin DN, Cleeland CS, Dar R. Public attitudes toward cancer pain. Cancer 1985; 56(9):2337–2339.
5. Fine PG. Principles of effective pain management at the end of life (CME/CE). Medscape from WebMD; 2006.

6. Ng K, von Gunten CF. Symptoms and attitudes of 100 consecutive patients admitted to an acute hospice/palliative care unit. J Pain Symptom Manag 1998; 16(5):307–316.
7. Portenoy RK, Lesage P. Management of cancer pain. Lancet 1999; 353(9165): 1695–700.
8. Miaskowski C. The next step to improving cancer pain management. Pain Manag Nurs 2005; 6(1):1–2.
9. International Association for the Study of Pain. Pain terms: a list with definitions and notes on usage. Recommended by the IASP Subcommittee on Taxonomy. Pain 1979; 6(3):249.
10. Anand KJ, Craig KD. New perspectives on the definition of pain. Pain 1996; 67(1): 3–6; discussion 209–211.
11. King TL, McCool WF. The definition and assessment of pain. J Midwifery Womens Health 2004; 49(6):471–472.
12. Marco CA, Plewa MC, Buderer N, et al. Self-reported pain scores in the emergency department: lack of association with vital signs. Acad Emerg Med 2006; 13(9):974–979.
13. Jay SM, Elliott C, Varni JW. Acute and chronic pain in adults and children with cancer. J Consult Clin Psychol 1986; 54(5):601–607.
14. Portenoy RK, Payne D, Jacobsen P. Breakthrough pain: characteristics and impact in patients with cancer pain. Pain 1999; 81(1-2):129–134.
15. Burton AW, Fanciullo GJ, Beasley RD, et al. Chronic pain in the cancer survivor: a new frontier. Pain Med 2007; 8(2):189–198.
16. Caraceni A, Portenoy RK. An international survey of cancer pain characteristics and syndromes. IASP Task Force on Cancer Pain. International Association for the Study of Pain. Pain 1999; 82(3):263–274.
17. Collins SD, Chessell IP. Emerging therapies for neuropathic pain. Expert Opin Emerg Drugs 2005; 10(1):95–108.
18. Shaiova L. Difficult pain syndromes: bone pain, visceral pain, and neuropathic pain. Cancer J 2006; 12(5):330–340.
19. Phillips DM. JCAHO pain management standards are unveiled. Joint Commission on Accreditation of Healthcare Organizations. JAMA 2000; 284(4):428–429.
20. Caraceni A, Brunelli C, Martini C, et al. Cancer pain assessment in clinical trials. A review of the literature (1999–2002). J Pain Symptom Manag 2005; 29(5):507–519.
21. Thomas JR, von Gunten CF. Pain in terminally ill patients: guidelines for pharmacological management. CNS Drugs 2003; 17(9):621–631.
22. Chang VT, Janjan N, Jain S, et al. Update in cancer pain syndromes. J Palliat Med 2006; 9(6):1414–1434.
23. McCaffery M, McCaffery M, Pasero CL. Pain Clinical Manual. 2nd ed. St. Louis, MO: Mosby; 1999.
24. Graham RB. The Purpose of Pain Scales, 2006 (http://wwwintelihealthcom/IH/ihtPrint/WSIHW000/29721/32087html?hide=t&k=basePrint).
25. Wong DL, Hockenberry MJ, Wilson D, et al. Wong's Essentials of Pediatric Nursing, 7th ed. St. Louis, MO: Elsevier Mosby; 2005.
26. Wong DL, Whaley LF, Kasprisin CA. Clinical Handbook of Pediatric Nursing, 2nd ed. St. Louis, MO: Mosby; 1986.
27. Ducharme J. Acute pain and pain control: state of the art. Ann Emerg Med 2000; 35(6):592–603.
28. WHO. WHO Analgesic Ladder 1996.

29. Cherny NI. The pharmacologic management of cancer pain. Oncology 2004; 18(12): 1499–1515; discussion 1516, 1520–1521, 1522, 1524.
30. McNicol E, Strassels SA, Goudas L, et al. NSAIDS or paracetamol, alone or combined with opioids, for cancer pain. Cochrane Database Syst Rev 2005(1): CD005180.
31. Goodman LS, Gilman A, Brunton LL, et al. Goodman & Gilman's the Pharmacological Basis of Therapeutics, 11th ed. New York: McGraw-Hill, 2006.
32. McNicol E, Strassels S, Goudas L, et al. Nonsteroidal anti-inflammatory drugs, alone or combined with opioids, for cancer pain: a systematic review. J Clin Oncol 2004; 22(10):1975–1992.
33. American Pain Society. Principles of Analgesic Use in the Treatment of Acute Pain and Cancer Pain, 4th ed. Glenview, IL: American Pain Society, 1999.
34. Goldstein FJ. Adjuncts to opioid therapy. J Am Osteopath Assoc 2002; 102(9 suppl 3): S15–S21.
35. Fine PG. Principles of Effective Pain Management at the End of Life CME/CE, 2006.
36. Cephalon CL. FENTORATM CII (fentanyl buccal tablet), 2006.
37. Wolters Kluwer Health Inc. Pharmacy and Therapeutics Review: Oxymorphone Hydrochloride, 2006.
38. Aronoff GM, Brennan MJ, Pritchard DD, et al. Evidence-based oral transmucosal fentanyl citrate (OTFC) dosing guidelines. Pain Med Malden 2005; 6(4):305–314.
39. McCarter GC, Strykowski JM. ASHP 2006: Highlights of the 2006 American Society of Health-System Pharmacists Midyear Clinical Meeting. In: WebMD; 2006.
40. Doyle D. Oxford Textbook of Palliative Medicine, 3rd ed. New York: Oxford University Press, 2004.
41. Prommer E. Oxymorphone: a review. Support Care Cancer 2006; 14(2):109–115.
42. Waknine Y. FDA Safety Changes: Opana and Sodium Chloride Saline Irrigation Solution CME. Medscape Medical News, 2006.
43. Waknine Y. FDA Safety Changes: Dolophine CME. Medscape Medical News, 2007.
44. Weissman DE. Fast Fact and Concept 020; Opioid Dose Escalation. End-of-Life Palliative Education Resource Center, 2005.
45. Saarto T, Wiffen PJ. Antidepressants for neuropathic pain. Cochrane Database Syst Rev 2005(3):CD005454.
46. Epstein JB, Epstein JD, Epstein MS, et al. Management of pain in cancer patients with oral mucositis: follow-up of multiple doses of doxepin oral rinse. J Pain Symptom Manag 2007; 33(2):111–114.
47. Argoff CE. The coexistence of neuropathic pain, sleep, and psychiatric disorders: a novel treatment approach. Clin J Pain 2007; 23(1):15–22.
48. Jensen TS. Anticonvulsants in neuropathic pain: rationale and clinical evidence. European J Pain 2002; (6 suppl A):61–68.
49. Tarride JE, Gordon A, Vera-Llonch M, et al. Cost-effectiveness of pregabalin for the management of neuropathic pain associated with diabetic peripheral neuropathy and postherpetic neuralgia: a Canadian perspective. Clin Therapeutics 2006; 28(11): 1922–1934.
50. Emanuel LL, VonGunten C. Education for Physicians on End-of-Life Care Participants Handbook, 1999:MT7.
51. Ferrell BR, ed. Textbook of Palliative Care Nursing. 1st ed. Oxford: Oxford University Press, Inc., 2001.

52. Archard G, Collett, B. The Practical Guide to the Provision of Chronic Pain Services for Adults in Primary Care. Royal College of General Practitioners and the British Pain Society, 2004.
53. Savage S, Covington EC, Heit H, et al. Definitions Related to the Use of Opioids for the Treatment of Pain. American Academy of Pain Medicine, 2007.
54. Hojsted J, Sjogren P. Addiction to opioids in chronic pain patients: a literature review. Eur J Pain 2007; 11(5):490–518.
55. Kehlet H. Multimodal approach to control postoperative pathophysiology and rehabilitation. British j Anaesth 1997; 78(5):606–617.

18

Management of Anxiety and Depressive Symptoms

Jimmie C. Holland, Talia R. Weiss, and Maria Rueda-Lara
Department of Psychiatry and Behavioral Sciences, Memorial Sloan-Kettering Cancer Center, New York, New York, U.S.A.

INTRODUCTION

"We are not ourselves when nature, being oppressed, commands the mind to suffer with the body." King Lear, Act II.

Supportive care in cancer has evolved rapidly in recent years to improve the control of patients' symptoms even in the face of treatment that is not curative. Laudatory as this is, the attention has focused largely on physical symptoms, and particularly pain. The focus on the "psychic suffering" has been considerably less. Yet, Shakespeare's observation relates well to the patients with cancer, when "the mind is commanded to suffer with the body." It is this "suffering of the mind" that psycho-oncology addresses to reduce distress and improve the quality of life (1). It is reassuring that supportive care is increasingly giving attention to the psychological or "human" side of care (2). This chapter outlines the recognition, diagnosis, and management of the most common forms of distress that the oncologist confronts—anxiety and depressive symptoms.

For an oncologist in a busy practice, faced with a distressed patient, the issue is to quickly determine "Is this patient's level of distress 'normal' or 'not normal' and should it be treated?" A large survey of almost 5000 patients with cancer showed that, overall, 35% of the patients were experiencing significant distress (3). The percentage was even greater in patients with brain, pancreas, and lung cancer.

To assist the oncologist in routinely taking these common symptoms into account and treating the "whole patient," The National Cancer Centers Network (NCCN) established a multidisciplinary Panel on Management of Distress in Cancer in 1997 (4). This panel has developed consensus- and evidence-based clinical practice guidelines, which are updated annually. The American Psychosocial Oncology Society adopted these guidelines to provide the basis for its Handbook "Quick Reference for Oncology Clinicians: The Psychiatric and Psychological Dimensions of Cancer Symptom Management" (5). The handbook provides a rapid "psych curbside consult" in a small handbook suitable for the use in the clinic and while on hospital rounds (5). It may be ordered online at www.apos-society.org.

The guidelines were developed to provide a rapid way to screen for level of distress in the busy oncology clinics, thereby assuring that the psychological domain is included in routine care, with guidelines for management by the oncologist and recommendations for triage of the patient to the appropriate discipline when more extensive evaluation and treatment are needed.

The NCCN panel first determined that the terms "psychological" and "psychiatric" are strongly disliked by patients who fear being "labeled" as "psychiatric." The word "distress" was chosen as an acceptable, normal, and non-stigmatizing term that covers the range of psychological, social, and spiritual problems patients experience with life-threatening illness. The primary oncology team, particularly the oncologist and clinic nurse, are the "front line" of psychological care for all patients; the cornerstone of good psychosocial care. To do this, the oncologist must be able to identify the common symptoms of distress, and provide information about illness and treatment in the context of a trusting relationship. Figure 1 (NCCN DIS-5) outlines the common and expected distress symptoms and the evaluations and interventions that the team should utilize in care, recognizing the patient to be reevaluated at the next visit and referred to social work or mental health if not improved (6). Figure 1A (NCCN DIS-B) outlines patients who are at increased risk for distress and the points in illness when they are most vulnerable (7).

The NCCN guidelines strongly endorse the screening of all new patients for level of distress, using the same successful paradigm that has improved pain management in the United States. The common tool used now for asking about pain is, "How is your pain on a scale of 0–10?" Patients understand this, and can accurately report their subjective pain level. Similarly, NCCN distress guidelines recommend using the Distress Thermometer, which is a graphic "thermometer" of a 0 to 10 scale, asking "What is the level of your distress, 0–10?" It can be presented to the patient in the waiting room on a touch screen or paper and pencil (Fig. 2, DIS-A, NCCN Distress Thermometer) (8). This single-item scale serves as a "broad-stroke" approach to be followed by more specific questions, usually by the nurse, if patients score 4 or above on the scale. The oncology nurse is often the person who asks the additional psychosocial questions. There are currently free online lectures for nurses about screening for distress on the APOS website at www.apos-society.org.

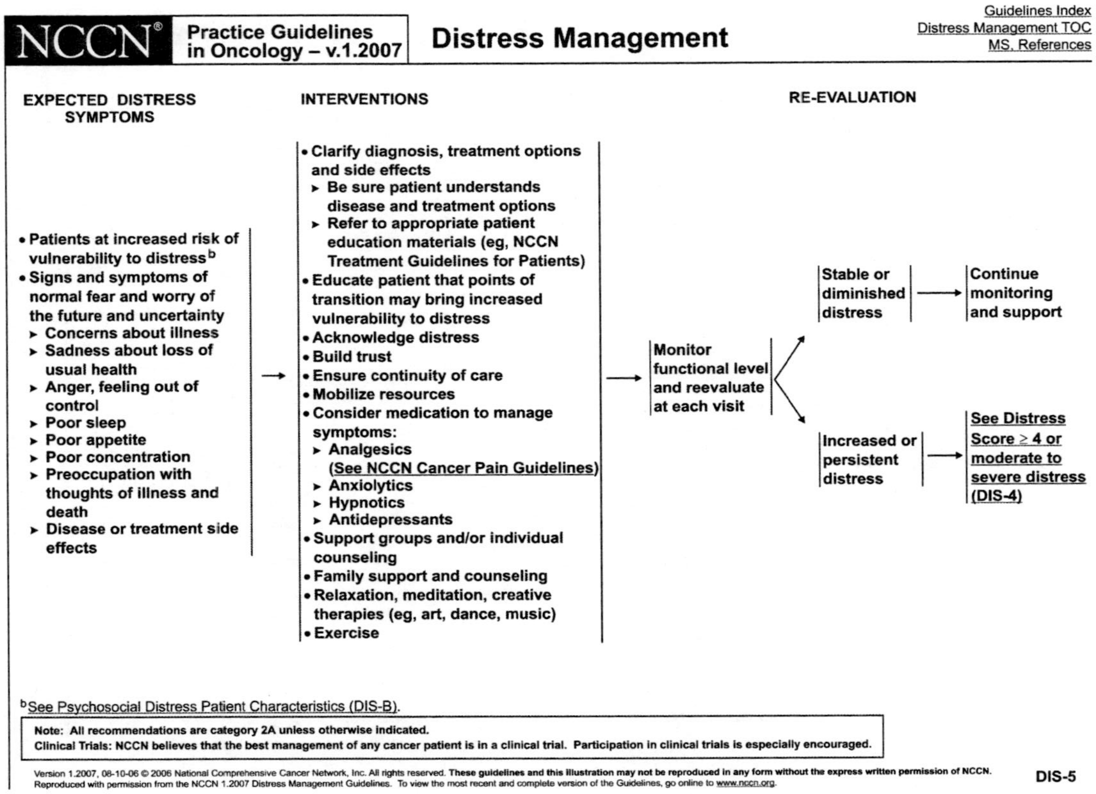

Management of Anxiety and Depressive Symptoms

Figure 1 Distress management: expected distress symptoms, interventions, re-evaluation.

NCCN Practice Guidelines in Oncology – v.1.2007 | **Distress Management**

Guidelines Index
Distress Management TOC
MS, References

PSYCHOSOCIAL DISTRESS PATIENT CHARACTERISTICS[c]

PATIENTS AT INCREASED RISK FOR DISTRESS[d]

- History of psychiatric disorder/substance abuse
- History of depression/suicide attempt
- Cognitive impairment
- Communication barriers[e]
- Severe comorbid illnesses
- Social problems
  - Family/caregiver conflicts
  - Inadequate social support
  - Living alone
  - Financial problems
  - Limited access to medical care
  - Young or dependent children
  - Younger age; woman
  - Other stressors

PERIODS OF INCREASED VULNERABILITY

- Finding a suspicious symptom
- During workup
- Finding out the diagnosis
- Awaiting treatment
- Change in treatment modality
- End of treatment
- Discharge from hospital following treatment
- Stresses of survivorship
- Medical follow-up and surveillance
- Treatment failure
- Recurrence/progression
- Advanced cancer
- End of life

[c]For site-specific symptoms with major psychosocial consequences, see Holland, JC, Greenberg, DB, Hughes, MD, et al. Quick Reference for Oncology Clinicians: The Psychiatric and Psychological Dimensions of Cancer Symptom Management. (Based on NCCN Distress Management Guidelines). IPOS Press, 2006. Available at www.apos-society.org.
[d]From the NCCN Palliative Care Clinical Practice Guidelines in Oncology. Available at www.nccn.org.
[e]Communication barriers include language, literacy, and physical barriers.

Note: All recommendations are category 2A unless otherwise indicated.
Clinical Trials: NCCN believes that the best management of any cancer patient is in a clinical trial. Participation in clinical trials is especially encouraged.

Version 1.2007, 05-10-06 © 2006 National Comprehensive Cancer Network, Inc. All rights reserved. These guidelines and this illustration may not be reproduced in any form without the express written permission of NCCN. Reproduced with permission from the NCCN 1.2007 Distress Management Guidelines. To view the most recent and complete version of the Guidelines, go online to www.nccn.org.

DIS-B

Figure 1A Distress management: patient characteristics.

Management of Anxiety and Depressive Symptoms

NCCN® Practice Guidelines in Oncology – v.1.2007

Distress Management

Guidelines Index
Distress Management TOC
MS, References

SCREENING TOOLS FOR MEASURING DISTRESS

Instructions: First please circle the number (0-10) that best describes how much distress you have been experiencing in the past week including today.

```
      10  Extreme distress
       9
       8
       7
       6
       5
       4
       3
       2
       1
       0  No distress
```

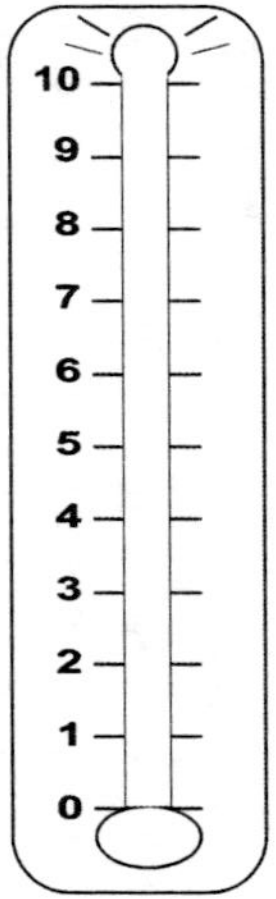

Second, please indicate if any of the following has been a problem for you in the past week including today. Be sure to check YES or NO for each.

YES NO Practical Problems
- ☐ ☐ Child care
- ☐ ☐ Housing
- ☐ ☐ Insurance/financial
- ☐ ☐ Transportation
- ☐ ☐ Work/school

Family Problems
- ☐ ☐ Dealing with children
- ☐ ☐ Dealing with partner

Emotional Problems
- ☐ ☐ Depression
- ☐ ☐ Fears
- ☐ ☐ Nervousness
- ☐ ☐ Sadness
- ☐ ☐ Worry
- ☐ ☐ Loss of interest in usual activities

- ☐ ☐ Spiritual/religious concerns

YES NO Physical Problems
- ☐ ☐ Appearance
- ☐ ☐ Bathing/dressing
- ☐ ☐ Breathing
- ☐ ☐ Changes in urination
- ☐ ☐ Constipation
- ☐ ☐ Diarrhea
- ☐ ☐ Eating
- ☐ ☐ Fatigue
- ☐ ☐ Feeling Swollen
- ☐ ☐ Fevers
- ☐ ☐ Getting around
- ☐ ☐ Indigestion
- ☐ ☐ Memory/concentration
- ☐ ☐ Mouth sores
- ☐ ☐ Nausea
- ☐ ☐ Nose dry/congested
- ☐ ☐ Pain
- ☐ ☐ Sexual
- ☐ ☐ Skin dry/itchy
- ☐ ☐ Sleep
- ☐ ☐ Tingling in hands/feet

Other Problems: _____

DIS-A

Version 1.2007, 08-10-06 © 2006 National Comprehensive Cancer Network, Inc. All rights reserved. These guidelines and this illustration may not be reproduced in any form without the express written permission of NCCN. Reproduced with permission from the NCCN 1.2007 Distress Management Guidelines. To view the most recent and complete version of the Guidelines, go online to www.NCCN.org.

Figure 2 Screening tool for measuring distress: distress thermometer.

The largest routine screening study of new patients at Johns Hopkins found that 35% had significantly elevated levels of distress (3). Early validation studies showed 5 to be the clinically appropriate cut off, compared to the score for clinical "caseness" on the Hospital Anxiety Depression Scale; however, later studies have identified 4 as best (9–12). The Problem List, which is on the same page with the Distress Thermometer, asks the patient to check the reasons for their distress. The problems checked determine whether referral should be to social work (for practical and psychosocial needs), mental health (for a psychiatric disorder in which medication may be needed), or clergy (when a spiritual crisis is present). Figure 3 (NCCN DIS-4) (13) gives an algorithm for the use of the brief screening tool, noting how the cut-off score (≥ 4) for distress assists in determining patients who should be referred for more extensive psychological evaluation and those who should continue to be managed by the primary team and community resources (13).

These guidelines assure that the psychosocial aspects are a part of total care, from initial visit when baseline screening should be done and repeated as clinically appropriate. The most common symptoms of distress encountered by the oncologist are anxiety and depression. Their management is outlined below.

ANXIETY DISORDERS

Anxiety is the commonest form of distress seen in patients at all stages of disease. It is often mild and managed by reassurance by the oncologist; however, more significant levels require evaluation to identify the etiology and treatment. The NCCN guidelines for management of anxiety disorder provide a useful framework for recognition, differential diagnosis, and treatment (Fig. 4, NCCN DIS-14) (14). It outlines the common signs of anxiety that may be occurring due to the fear of illness, but may also have a medical or medication etiology.

Symptoms may be largely physical (tachycardia, diaphoresis, restlessness, pacing, tremor, insomnia, dry mouth) or psychological (fears, worry about specific problems of illness or treatment), or of an impending procedure. When the basis is response to illness, it is usually situationally related and is referred to as an Adjustment Disorder with Anxiety. However, in presence of more significant anxiety, a workup must be done to rule out medically related causes. Pain is the most common cause of anxiety. It diminishes with adequate pain control measures. Table 1 outlines the range of frequent medical problems and medications that may produce anxiety. Also, an early symptom of alcohol or opioid withdrawal may be acute anxiety and tremulousness. One should also take a history as to the presence of a pre-existing anxiety disorder: Generalized Anxiety Disorder, Panic or Phobic Disorder, PTSD, chemotherapy-conditioned disorder (response nausea and vomiting with anxiety), and obsessive compulsive disorder (OCD).

The treatment of anxiety is psychopharmacologic and psychological. The medications ordinarily used are benzodiazepines, selective serotonin reuptake inhibitors (SSRIs), and low-dose antipsychotics. Benzodiazepines are useful

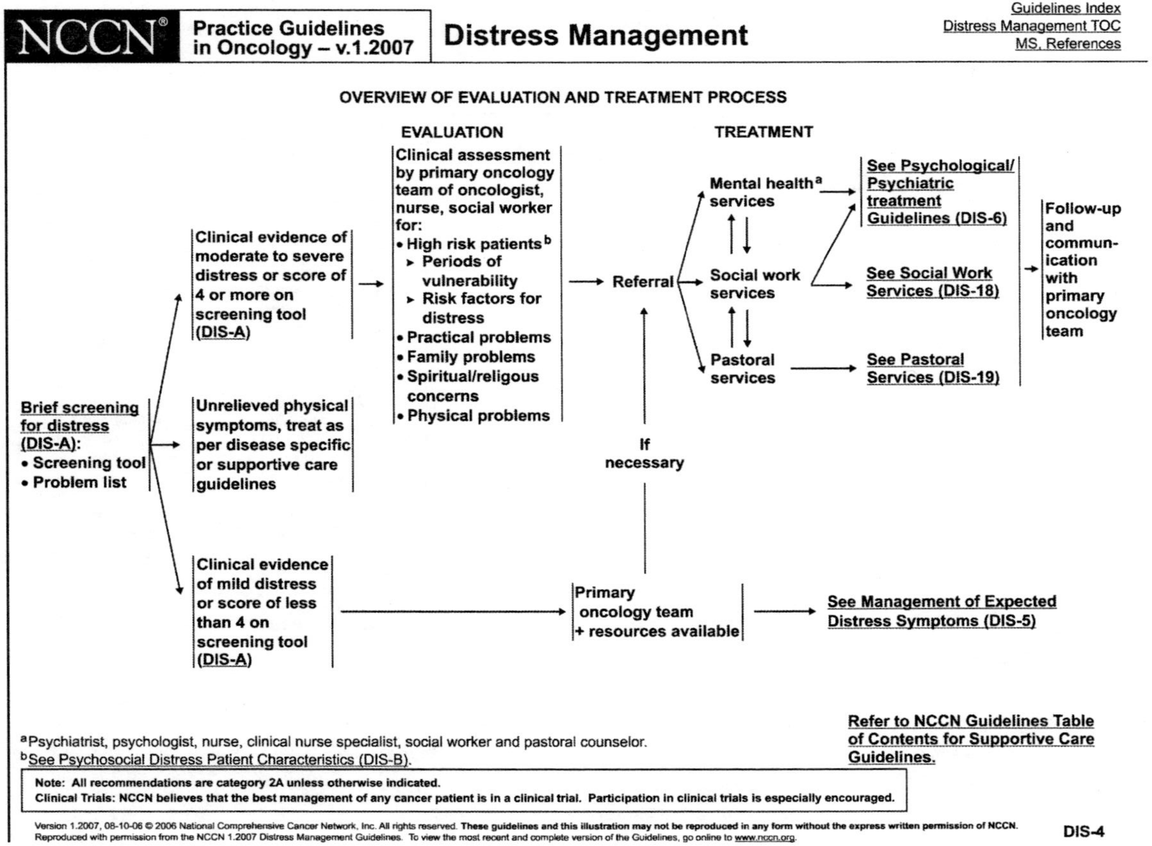

Management of Anxiety and Depressive Symptoms 325

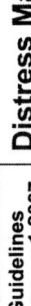

Figure 3 Distress management: overview of evaluation and treatment process.

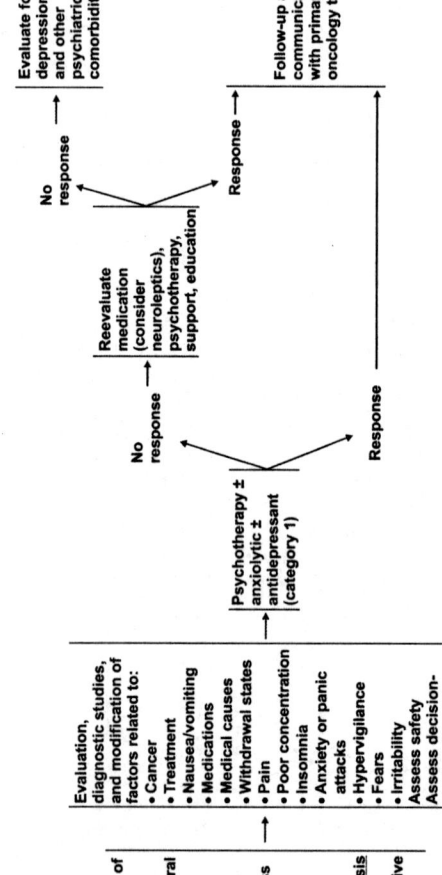

Figure 4 Anxiety disorder: signs, symptoms, evaluation/treatment/follow-up plan.

Table 1 Medical and Medication-Related Anxiety

Metabolic	Hyperkalemia
	Hyperthermia
	Hypoglycemia
	Hyponatremia
Tumor-related	Delirium (restlessness, agitation)
	Pain
	CNS neoplasms
	Carcinoid syndrome
	Para neoplastic disorders
Endocrine	Adrenal
	Thyroid
	Parathyroid
	Pituitary
	Pheocromocytoma
Cardiovascular	Arrhythmia
	Congestive heart failure
	Myocardial infarction
	Angina pectoris
	Valvular disease
Pulmonary	Pulmonary embolism
	Asthma
	Chronic obstructive pulmonary disease
	Peumothorax
	Pulmonary edema
Medications	Corticosteroids
	Neuroleptics used as antiemetics (akathesias)
	Sympathotomimetic agents
	Antibiotics (cephalosporins, acyclovir, isoniazid)
Withdrawal states	Alcohol, opioids, sedatives hypnotics, caffeine

because of the immediate relief they produce and are often given initially with an SSRI, which is slow to produce an anti-anxiety effect. Table 2 outlines the commonly used drugs and their dosage. Patients are often fearful of addiction to benzodiazepines and must be encouraged to use them and reassured that they will be monitored.

In terms of non-pharmacologic interventions, several forms of psychotherapy and counseling are useful:

1. Support from the primary oncology team with attention to control troublesome symptoms (e.g., insomnia).
2. Referral to social work or mental health for supportive psychotherapy, given either one on one or in groups.

Table 2 Medications Commonly Used to Treat Anxiety

Drug	Brand name	Starting dose (mg)	Maintenance dose (mg)
SSRIs: selective serotonin reuptake inhibitors			
Escitalopram[a]	Lexapro®	10–20	10–20
Fluoxetine[a]	Prozac®	10–20 (qAM)	20–60
Paroxetine[a]	Paxil®	20 (qAM)	20–60
Sertraline[a]	Zoloft®	20–25 (qAM)	50–150
Benzodiazepines			
Alprazolam	Xanax®	0.25–1.0	PO q 6–24 hr
Clonazepam	Klonopin®	1.5–2.0	PO q 6–24 hr
Diazepam	Valium®	2–10	PO/IV q 6–24 hr
Lorazepam	Ativan®	0.5–2.0	PO/IM/IVP/IVPB q 4–12 hr

Source: From Ref. 5. APOS quick reference for oncology clinicians, Charlottesville, VA, 2006.
Abbreviations: IM, intramuscular; IVP, IV push; IVPB, IV piggyback; PO, oral.
[a]Available in liquid form.

3. Cognitive behavioral therapy helps patients through cognitive reframing of symptoms, guided imagery, relaxation, and meditation.
4. The internet and virtual groups are emerging as easily accessible, but are largely unsupervised.

Supportive and behavioral interventions trials have been conducted at all stages of disease. Evidence from meta-analyses support the inclusion of psychotherapy as evidence-based in clinical practice guidelines in the United States and Australia (15,16). While the oncologist treats most situational anxiety well, when the etiology is a pre-existing anxiety disorder, referral to a mental health professional is useful. OCD and Generalized Anxiety Disorders are often resistant to treatment and both can significantly complicate the management of cancer therapy.

DEPRESSION (MOOD DISORDERS)

The challenge for the oncologist is to determine when the normal sadness that accompanies life-threatening illness has reached a level that deserves a full evaluation and treatment. Similar to anxiety, there are medical issues and medications that may cause depression. A workup must consider a wide range of potential correctable causes in the differential diagnosis. It is important that significant depressive symptoms not be dismissed as a presumption of being part of cancer. Equally difficult is the fact that physical symptoms of cancer and somatic symptoms of depression are similar (e.g., insomnia, fatigue, poor concentration). When the sadness begins to interfere with coping, by insomnia, fatigue, or distress, this represents the most common depressive disorder: situational depression, called Adjustment Disorder with Depressive Symptoms. Most of these patients are handled well by the oncology team with reassurance and medications to target their specific symptoms (e.g., insomnia, fatigue).

However, persistent and more severe symptoms require a thoughtful workup since there are many medical causes for depressive symptoms. These depressive symptoms in their moderate levels are called subsyndromal depression, indicating that they are distressing but do not reach the criteria for a Major Depressive Disorder (characterized by dysphoria, anhedonia, hopelessness, guilt, change in sleep, appetite, concentration, feeling life is not worth living, and suicidal risk). Major depression is seen less often than the subsyndromal disorders, but it causes the greatest risk of suicidal behavior. Mania is unusual in cancer patients, but is seen most often in response to medication or in a patient with pre-existing bipolar disorder.

The NCCN guidelines for recognition and management of mood disorders (Fig. 5: NCCN DIS–10, Fig. 6: NCCN DIS–11) (17,18) outline the common mood disorders and the evaluation of the symptoms and factors that may contribute to depressive symptoms. After establishing the cause, treatment includes correcting the medical problem or stopping the medication, when possible (e.g., interferon). Often, the offending agent cannot be removed and treatment must be instituted for the depression. Suicidal-risk patients should be immediately referred to a psychiatrist.

Table 3 outlines the common medical causes for depression. Most common and most likely to produce suicidal thoughts is unrelenting and unrelieved pain. Medications, chemotherapy agents, metabolic derangement, and some sites of cancer are associated with greater depression. The role of pro-inflammatory cytokines is becoming more clear in producing symptoms of depression, fatigue, anxiety, and poor concentration (19,20). This may account for the association of pancreatic cancer, for example, with greater depression.

Assessment of Suicide Risk

Any patient who is significantly depressed should be asked about suicidal ideation. Asking about it does not increase the risk. In fact, it decreases the risk. A question like "Do you ever have thoughts that life isn't worth living?" can be followed with more direct questions if that is positive. Most patients admit to "thinking about it" and express, "I would do it if things get bad enough." Of more concern (and higher risk) are patients with unrelieved pain, advanced disease, prior depression, or alcohol or substance abuse, who pose greater suicidal risk.

Management

Depression is treated by psychological and psychopharmacologic interventions. Psychological support from the primary care team is critical. Referral for

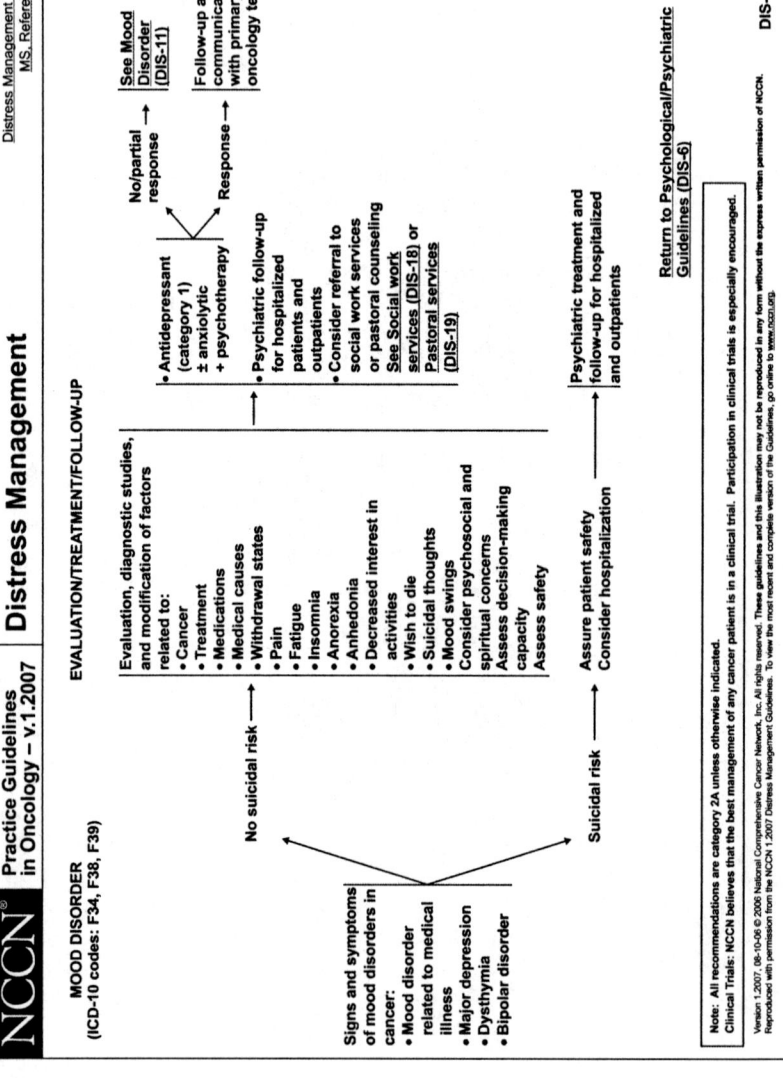

Figure 5 Mood disorder: signs, symptoms, evaluation/treatment/follow-up plan.

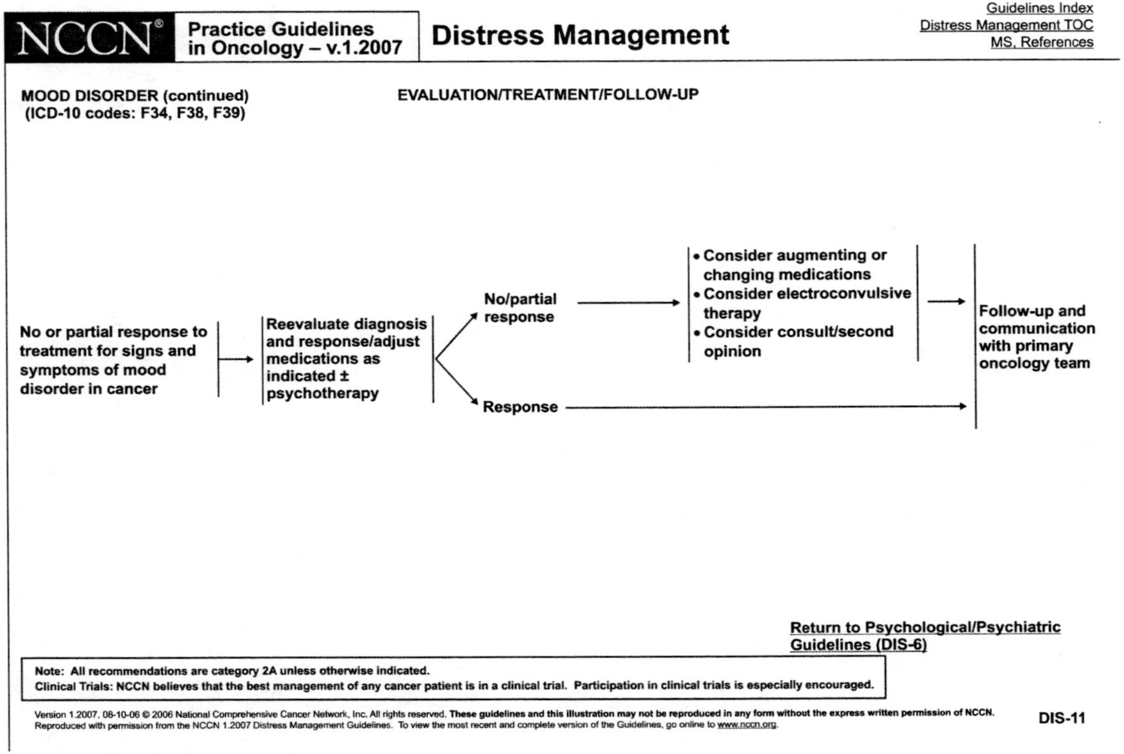

Management of Anxiety and Depressive Symptoms 331

NCCN® Practice Guidelines in Oncology – v.1.2007

Distress Management

Guidelines Index
Distress Management TOC
MS, References

MOOD DISORDER (continued)
(ICD-10 codes: F34, F38, F39)

EVALUATION/TREATMENT/FOLLOW-UP

No or partial response to treatment for signs and symptoms of mood disorder in cancer → Reevaluate diagnosis and response/adjust medications as indicated ± psychotherapy

- No/partial response → • Consider augmenting or changing medications
  • Consider electroconvulsive therapy
  • Consider consult/second opinion → Follow-up and communication with primary oncology team
- Response →

Return to Psychological/Psychiatric Guidelines (DIS-6)

Note: All recommendations are category 2A unless otherwise indicated.
Clinical Trials: NCCN believes that the best management of any cancer patient is in a clinical trial. Participation in clinical trials is especially encouraged.

Version 1.2007, 06-10-06 © 2006 National Comprehensive Cancer Network, Inc. All rights reserved. These guidelines and this illustration may not be reproduced in any form without the express written permission of NCCN. To view the most recent and complete version of the Guidelines, go online to www.nccn.org.
Reproduced with permission from the NCCN 1.2007 Distress Management Guidelines.

DIS-11

Figure 6 Mood disorder: continued.

Table 3 Medical Causes of Depressive Symptoms

Unrelieved pain	Significant cause of depression as well as fear of unrelieved pain; a major variable in physician-assisted suicide request
Medications	Corticosteroids may cause marked mood change.
	Opioids, analgesics, interferon alpha, and interleukin 2 are particularly related.
	Vinca alkaloids, L-asparaginase, procarbazine
Metabolic	Electrolyte abnormalities, particularly sodium, thyroid, and parathyroid function
Cancer	Pancreatic, occult, brain tumors, and CNS lymphomas

Source: Adopted from Ref. 5. Table 6.8. APOS quick reference for oncology clinicians, Charlottesville, VA, 2006.

supportive or cognitive behavior psychotherapy is supported by meta-analyses of clinical trials, which show a significant evidence base (21). In Australia and the United States, evidence-based clinical practice guidelines include psychotherapeutic interventions (16,21).

Psychopharmacologic Management

Patients with mood disorders are treated by antidepressants, largely, but also psychostimulants, which rapidly improve alertness and may reduce fatigue. Table 4 outlines the commonly used medications. While there are few controlled trials in cancer for psychotropic drugs, the few that have been done, when reviewed in the meta-analyses, support their efficacy and inclusion in the guidelines (16,21).

SUMMARY

In supportive care, psychiatric and psychologic aspects are being increasingly incorporated in routine care. Control of distress is often central to a patient's well-being and ability to carry on communication with others and lead a normal family life, as well as to comply with treatment. Severe and acute forms of distress (often depression and anxiety occur together) interfere with cancer treatment and can become central to overall management. The availability today of evidence-based clinical practice guidelines has been a major step forward. Indicators for quality of psychosocial care are being developed, which will permit accountability to be possible in this area that has been seen as "fuzzy" and weak in its scientific base. That can no longer be held true.

Table 4 Medications Commonly Used to Treat Depression

Medication	Brand Name	Starting Dose (mg)	Therapeutic Range	Common Adverse Effects/Comments
SSRIs: selective serotonin reuptake inhibitors				
Fluoxetine[a]	Prozac®	5–10	5–40	Varying degrees of gastrointestinal distress, nausea, headache, insomnia, increased anxiety, sexual dysfunction; sertraline, citalopram, and escitalopram produce the least P450 system interactions
Sertraline[a]	Zoloft®	25–50	25–200	
Paroxetine[a]	Paxil®	5–10	5–40	
Citalopram[a]	Celexa®	10–20	10–40	
Escitalopram[a]	Lexapro®	5–10	5–20	
Newer antidepressants				
Bupropion	Wellbutrin®, SR & XL	75	75–300	Activating, seizures if predisposed; no sexual dysfunction
Venlafaxine	Effexor®, XR	18.75	18.75–225	Activating, nausea, anxiety, sedation, sweating, hypertension
Duloxetine	Cymbalta®	20–30	20–60	Activating, nausea, anxiety
Mirtazapine	Remeron®	7.5–15	7.5–45	Sedation, weight gain; dissolvable tablet form available
Stimulants and wakefulness-promoting agents				
Dextroamphetamine	Dexedrine®	2.5	5–30	Possible cardiac complications; agitation, anxiety, nausea
Methylphenidate	Ritalin®	2.5	5–10 twice a day	
Modafinil	Provigil®	50	50–200	Activating, nausea, cardiac adverse effects; usually well-treated

Source: From Ref. 22.
[a]Available in liquid form. Holland, Evcimen, ASCO Educational Book 2007.

REFERENCES

1. Holland J. History of psycho-oncology: overcoming attitudinal and conceptual barriers. Psychosom Med 2002; 64:206–221.
2. Holland JC, Boettger S. Depression and anxiety. In: Handbook of Supportive Care in Oncology. Manhasset, NY: CMP Healthcare Media, Oncology Publishing Group, 2005.
3. Zabora J, Brintzenhofe Szoc K, Curbow B, et al. The prevalence of psychological distress by cancer site. Psycho-Oncology 2001; 10:9–28.
4. Holland JC, Anderson B, Breitbart W, et al. The NCCN Distress Management Clinical Practice Guidelines in Oncology. J NCCN 2007; 5:66–98.
5. APOS Institute for Research and Education. Quick Reference for Oncology Clinicians: The Psychiatric and Psychological Dimensions of Cancer Symptom Management. Charlottesville, VA: IPOS Press, 2006.
6. Expected Distress Symptoms, Interventions, Re-Evaluation (DIS-5). Reproduced with permission from the NCCN. v.1. 2007. The Complete Library of NCCN Clinical Practice Guidelines in Oncology, v.1.2007 Distress Management. Jenkintown, Pennsylvania: NCCN.
7. Psychosocial Distress Patient Characteristics (DIS-B). Reproduced with permission from the NCCN. v.1. 2007. The Complete Library of NCCN Clinical Practice Guidelines in Oncology, v.1.2007 Distress Management. Jenkintown, Pennsylvania: NCCN.
8. Screening Tools for Measuring Distress (DIS-A). Reproduced with permission from the NCCN. v.1. 2007. The Complete Library of NCCN Clinical Practice Guidelines in Oncology, v.1.2007 Distress Management. Jenkintown, Pennsylvania: NCCN.
9. Hoffman BM, Zevon MA, D'arrigo MC, Cecchini TB. Screening for distress in cancer patients: the NCCN rapid-screening measure. Psycho-oncology 2004; 13:792–799.
10. Akizuki N, Yamawaki S, Akechi T. et al. Development of an impact thermometer for use in combination with the distress thermometer as a brief screening tool for adjustment disorders and/or major depression in cancer patients. J Pain Symptom Manag 2005; 29(1):91–99.
11. Jacobsen P, Donovan K, Trask P, Fleishman S, et al. Screening for psychologic distress in ambulatory cancer patients. Cancer 2004; 103(7):1494–502.
12. Ransom S, Jacobsen P, Booth-Jones M. Validation of the distress thermometer with bone marrow transplant patients. Psycho-oncology 2006; 15(7):604–612.
13. Overview of Evaluation and Treatment Process (DIS-4). Reproduced with permission from the NCCN. v.1. 2007. The Complete Library of NCCN Clinical Practice Guidelines in Oncology, v.1.2007. Distress Management. Jenkintown, Pennsylvania: NCCN.
14. Anxiety Disorder (DIS-14). Reproduced with permission from the NCCN. v.1. 2007. The Complete Library of NCCN Clinical Practice Guidelines in Oncology, v.1.2007 Distress Management. Jenkintown, Pennsylvania: NCCN.
15. Fricchione G. Clinical practice. Generalized anxiety disorder. NEJM 2004; 351(7):675–682.
16. National Breast Cancer Centre and National Cancer Control Initiative. Clinical Practice Guidelines for the Psychosocial Care of Adults with Cancer. National Breast Cancer Centre, Camperdown, NSW, 2003.
17. Mood Disorder (DIS-10). Reproduced with permission from the NCCN. v.1. 2007. The Complete Library of NCCN Clinical Practice Guidelines in Oncology, v.1.2007

Distress Management. Jenkintown, Pennsylvania: National Comprehensive Cancer Network.
18. Mood Disorder (DIS-11). Reproduced with permission from the NCCN. v.1. 2007. The Complete Library of NCCN Clinical Practice Guidelines in Oncology, v.1.2007 Distress Management. Jenkintown, Pennsylvania: National Comprehensive Cancer Network.
19. Cleeland CC, Bennet, GJ, Dantzer, R. et al. Are the Symptoms of Cancer and Cancer Treatment Due to a Shared Biologic Mechanism? A Cytokine-immunologic Model of Cancer. Cancer 2003; 97:2919–2925.
20. Musselman DL, Miller, AH, Porter MR. Higher than normal plasma interleukin-6 concentrations in cancer patients with depression: preliminary findings. Am J Psychiatr 2001; 158:1252–1257.
21. Jacobsen P, Donovan K, Swaine Z, Watson I. Management of anxiety and depression in adult cancer patients: toward an evidence-based approach. Oncology: An Evidence-Based Approach. New York, NY: Springer-Verlag, 2006.
22. Holland J, Alici Evcimen, Y. Common psychiatric problems in elderly patients with cancer. American Society Clinical Oncology Educational Book 43rd Annual Meeting 2007:307–311.

19

End-of-Life Care

Amy P. Abernethy
Division of Medical Oncology, Department of Medicine, Duke University Medical Center (DUMC), Durham, North Carolina, U.S.A. and Department of Palliative and Supportive Services, Flinders University, Bedford Park, South Australia, Australia

Joshua S. Barclay
Division of General Internal Medicine, Department of Medicine, Duke University Medical Center (DUMC), Durham, North Carolina, U.S.A.

Jane L. Wheeler
Division of Medical Oncology, Department of Medicine, Duke University Medical Center (DUMC), Durham, North Carolina, U.S.A.

David C. Currow
Department of Palliative and Supportive Services, Flinders University, Bedford Park, South Australia, and Cancer Australia, Canberra, Australia

INTRODUCTION

Despite improvements in survival rates following the introduction of a host of novel therapies, end-of-life care remains an unavoidable—and a rich and important—component of the cancer clinician's practice. While end-of-life care is often a highly individualized proposition, with each patient's care tailored to address the many facets of his/her condition and circumstances, there are common threads that characterize the experiences of patients, families, and caregivers in the last two weeks of a patient's life. These shared experiences can be anticipated and, placed within a context of comprehensive care at the end of life, can be used to prepare and deliver truly supportive care for the patient, family, and caregiver, as well as for others involved in the patient's care.

PHILOSOPHY OF CARE AT END OF LIFE

Care provided at the end of life differs from other patient care in several distinct ways. First, its goal is to optimize the patient's experiences of living and dying, and to sustain best possible quality of life, rather than to extend survival or effect cure. While end-of-life care can be delivered concomitantly with disease-remitting therapies, it commonly becomes the sole focus of care as the patient approaches death. Secondly, patients and those close to them attribute emotionally charged meaning to end-of-life experiences and to the end of life itself, and these meanings are of direct relevance to the tailoring of clinical care. Death may signify release to a traditionally religious patient who has suffered a long illness, while it may signal defeat to this patient's adult children who are involved in medical decision making and end-of-life planning. Thirdly, care at this phase of life engages others, in addition to the patient, in a more intensive manner than does care at less critical or starkly transitional times. Patients at the end of life rarely present as a single unit of care; instead, end-of-life issues typically involve extensive networks of caregivers, families, and friends, each of whom bring their own care needs. Fourth, end of life entails certain unique physiological changes that shape and direct clinical care. Finally, the need to address the whole person—in mind, body, and spirit—through care that is multidimensional and comprehensive, is amplified at the end of life. Best end-of-life care addresses and coordinates three dimensions of being for the patient: physical, psychosocial, and spiritual.

PATTERNS OF EXPERIENCE AND CARE AT END OF LIFE

Because symptoms experienced at the end of life span the physical, psychosocial, and spiritual domains, a care strategy that integrates these realms will most effectively meet the needs of patient and family/caregivers. Table 1 presents common symptoms reported by end-of-life patients and their loved ones, and shows the concerns and issues encountered at this final phase of the disease trajectory. Emotional suffering and grief are common as patients, family, and friends struggle to adapt to new information regarding a terminal diagnosis. Patients often must adapt to new roles as they accept the loss of previous identities, aspirations, and hopes. Families often must take on new roles as caregivers, requiring them to modify long-held visions of their future. Clinicians

Table 1 Domains of Terminal Symptoms and Prevalence

Symptom	Prevalence at end of life
Physical	
General	
Pain	22–76%
Dry Mouth	6–70%
Altered Sleep	29–57%
Decreased Energy	83–96%
Pulmonary	
Dyspnea	23–65%
Cough	17–62%
Gastrointestinal	
Decreased Appetite	52–93%
Nausea	13–49%
Vomiting	10–26%
Diarrhea	7–22%
Constipation	39–65%
Dysphagia	28–52%
CNS alterations	
Delirium	29–48%
Confusion	44–68%
Musculoskeletal	
Myoclonus	16%
Weakness	82%
Genitourinary	
Dysuria	7%
Incontinence	34%
Psychosocial	
Disorders	
Adjustment	10–16%
Anxiety	7–79%
Depression	3–82%
Feelings	
Worried	70%
Nervous	44%
Guilt	28%
Loneliness	37%
Spiritual	
Meaninglessness	40–58%
Fear	51%
Desired Hope Resources	42%
Desired Spiritual Resources	39%

Source: From Refs. 54, 56, 100–104.

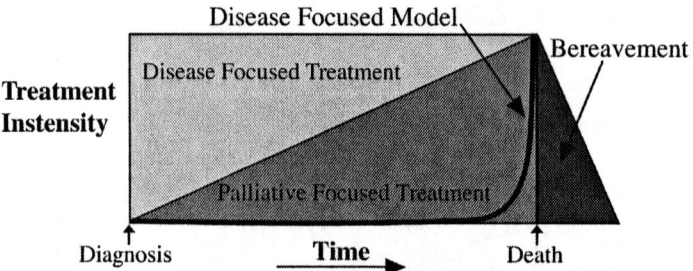

Figure 1 Integration of disease-focused and palliative treatments.

can help patients and families by providing, in addition to appropriate medical therapy, the emotional support and expert guidance that will help patients and their loved ones navigate through the late stages of disease and end of life.

Clinicians often face difficulty in determining when to begin to address end-of-life concerns and initiate symptom management. The traditional disease-oriented model of end-of-life care focused efforts on cure-directed therapies early in the course of an illness, switching to a palliative focus just prior to death. More recently, there has been a push to start palliative care earlier in the course of the disease. In this model, aggressive symptom management begins with the patient's diagnosis of a life-limiting illness, and gradually assumes a larger role in the care plans as the disease progresses (Fig. 1).

END-OF-LIFE CARE: PHYSICAL

Many of the common complaints of patients at end of life have been covered in other chapters of this book. Please see the following chapters [in brackets] for previous discussion of the following symptoms: nausea and vomiting, [Chapter 10], fatigue, [Chapter 2], diarrhea and constipation, [Chapter 12], and pain, [Chapter 17]. This section will focus on several common end-of-life symptoms not addressed in other chapters.

Dyspnea

A highly subjective symptom, dyspnea manifests as a sensation of breathlessness arising from a combination of underlying pathology, the signaling of neural pathways, and the patient's perception (1). Patients' descriptions of dyspnea vary widely and depend, at least in part, on the individual's disease, ethnic/racial background, previous experiences, and emotional state. Patients often report dyspnea that seems out of proportion to known underlying lung disease. When dyspnea does not improve despite maximal treatment for the underlying illness, it is termed "refractory dyspnea." While a host of pharmacologic and nonpharmacologic interventions have been studied for relief of dyspnea, opioids (either oral or parenteral) and oxygen are most frequently used at the end of life.

The mechanism of action of opioids in reducing dyspnea is poorly understood; these agents may act centrally, peripherally, or by reducing anxiety (2). Opioids reduce ventilatory response to carbon dioxide (3), hypoxia (4,5), inspiratory flow resistive loading (6), and exercise (7). In addition, morphine decreases oxygen consumption both at rest and while exercising in healthy individuals (7).

Jennings et al. (8), systematically reviewed all data on the use of opioids through 2001 in an attempt to evaluate the evidence. Meta-analysis of nine studies demonstrated a highly statistically significant effect of oral and parenteral opioids on the sensation of breathlessness (overall pooled effect size –0.31, 95% CI –0.50 to –0.13, $p = 0.0008$); nebulized opioids were not effective. The clinical effect size was relatively small (approximately 8 mm on a 100-mm visual analog scale (VAS) with baseline levels of dyspnea of 50 mm).

In 2003, Abernethy et al. published the results of a trial using oral morphine in opioid-naïve adults with refractory dyspnea. Despite optimal management, 48 patients with refractory dyspnea were enrolled in an adequately powered eight-day randomized, double-blind, crossover study in which they received either 20 mg oral morphine sulfate or placebo. The morphine product used was a 24-hour, sustained-release preparation. The primary outcome was the sensation of breathlessness measured on a 100 mm VAS. The mean baseline morning dyspnea score was 43 (SD = 26). Morphine improved dyspnea with mean improvements of 6.6 mm in the morning ($p = 0.011$) and 9.5 mm in the evening ($p = 0.006$). Relative improvement over baseline dyspnea was 15% to 22%. These results were similar to the estimate of efficacy for oral and parenteral opioids generated by Jennings et al. Morphine did not depress the respiratory rate, and no episodes of severe sedation or obtundation were recorded. The main side effect was constipation ($p = 0.021$), but neither treatment caused more vomiting, confusion, sedation, or appetite suppression. Those who received morphine also described better sleep at night ($p = 0.039$) despite the fact that the medication was administered each morning.

To date, the majority of evaluations for opioids in refractory dyspnea have focused on patients with underlying chronic obstructive pulmonary disease (COPD). Current data do not clarify the ideal dose of morphine, the additive effect of opioids, whether all opioids provide equal effect, or whether the effect would be as substantial in diseases other than COPD. Practically, when the patient is opioid-naive, a reasonable starting dose is 20 mg once daily of sustained-release morphine, if the drug is available and the patient does not have a contraindication to morphine. When the once-daily product is not available, then the 15-mg twice-daily, long-acting morphine product can be prescribed, which is initially administered once a day and increased to twice a day after five to seven days if the patient tolerates the medication and has residual breathlessness. When the patient has a contraindication to morphine, long-acting oxycodone can be used, starting at 10 mg once a day and increasing to twice a day after five to seven days as tolerated and needed. If an opioid-tolerant patient is already on a regular dose of morphine or another opioid, sequentially increase the opioid by 20% of the total daily dose every three to five days until the breathlessness is relieved or side effects occur (9).

Palliative oxygen is commonly prescribed for symptomatic relief in cancer patients with refractory dyspnea who do not meet funding criteria for long-term domiciliary oxygen. While it is indicated for severely hypoxemic patients, a meta-analysis of two small studies, with a total of 59 patients, found that oxygen failed to improve dyspnea in mild- or nonhypoxemic cancer patients (standardized mean difference (SMD) -0.14, 95% CI -0.29 to 0.00; $p = 0.05$). A multinational randomized controlled trial is currently underway to evaluate the benefit of palliative oxygen versus medical air in patients with refractory dyspnea; preliminary results indicate that the burden of oxygen therapy, which includes cost, tubing, confinement to a concentrator, and exaggeration of the sick role, may outweigh its benefit in many patients' perception.

Delirium

Delirium, characterized by disturbance of consciousness, cognition, and perception, occurs in 28% to 83% of patients as they approach end of life and causes considerable distress for patients, families, caregivers, and providers (10,11). Delirium usually arises as an indirect result of factors associated with the patient's underlying cancer, such as treatment side effects, metabolic disorder, nutritional deficiency, or infection; the evidence suggests that the effects of medications, particularly opioids, are the most common cause of delirium in end-of-life patients (12). Two types of delirium are observed in this population: agitated/hyperactive delirium or hypoactive delirium. In either case, the signal is an acute change in the patient's level of arousal, manifesting as disorientation, visual or auditory hallucinations, change in speech pattern, memory or language alteration, or sleep/wake cycle upset; symptoms typically wax and wane over time (13). In clinical diagnosis, delirium is assessed at the bedside using assessment scales, such as the Delirium Rating Scale (14), Confusion Assessment Method (15), Delirium Symptom Interview (16), Memorial Delirium Assessment Scale (17), or the more general and widely recognized Mini-Mental State Examination (MMSE) (18).

To manage delirium, the clinician typically discontinues all medications, especially psychoactive ones, which are not absolutely necessary; thereafter, the goal of treating delirium is, in most cases, to restore patients to a state closer to their baseline mental state, rather than to suppress agitation or sedate them (19). The presence of family and friends, familiar surroundings, consistent care staff including nurses, and a calm setting may help. In palliative care patients, intravenous or oral haloperidol, starting at 0.5 mg twice daily and titrated upward, is the drug of choice. Clinicians have additional options in other useful neuroleptic drugs, including intravenous chlorpromazine, risperidone, and transmucosal olanzapine. Benzodiazepines (lorazepam, midazolam) may help calm the patient, but are generally avoided because they may worsen delirium by further sedating and disinhibiting the patient or by causing agitation. When terminal delirium is severe, especially in an actively dying patient, the clinician may opt for an alternative strategy to sedate the patient through continuous infusion of benzodiazepine (midazolam) and barbiturate (pentobarbital) (20,21), although this strategy is usually reserved for the most severe cases that are causing great distress to the patient and family.

Death Rattles

Noisy ventilation ("death rattles" or "terminal secretions") due to oscillatory movements of accumulated bronchial mucosa and salivary secretions is common in patients who are at the end of life and unable to clear secretions by coughing or swallowing (22). Previous observational studies have estimated that death rattles occur in up to 90% of unconscious dying patients (23–25). Intervention to reduce secretions is often instituted to alleviate the distress of the attendant relatives, even when the patient seems settled (25,26).

Standard practice in cases of death rattles can include suctioning, positioning, and explaining to the patient's family; however, the mainstay of pharmacological management is the use of anticholinergic agents, also known as muscarinic receptor blockers (22,23). These include scopolamine, hyoscyamine, glycopyrrolate, and atropine. In awake and aware patients, all of these agents can cause varying degrees of blurred vision, sedation, confusion, delirium, restlessness, hallucinations, palpitations, constipation, and urinary retention. The primary difference in these drugs is whether they are tertiary amines, which cross the blood-brain barrier (scopolamine, atropine), or quaternary amines, which do not (hyoscyamine, glycopyrrolate). Drugs that cross the blood-brain barrier are apt to cause central nervous system toxicity (sedation, delirium).

The case for using antimuscarinic agents in the end-of-life setting has been extrapolated from evidence of efficacy in reducing bronchial secretions during intubation and bronchoscopy, and pharmacological studies in healthy volunteers (27). Noisy ventilation at the end of life relates to airway secretions from bronchial and salivary sources, both containing muscarinic receptors. Few clinical studies are available to ascertain the effectiveness of pharmacological interventions at the end of life, with observational studies reporting current practice in an unblinded way (22,28). The comparative studies of scopolamine (hyoscine hydrobromide) and glycopyrrolate have not been randomized; however, effectiveness ranging from 35% to 79% to reduce noisy respirations has been reported (29,30). The potentially distressing anticholinergic side effects are almost impossible to assess because patients are invariably obtunded.

In practical terms, nonpharmacological measures should be the focus of treatment for death rattles. Exceptional nursing care, positioning, suctioning, and psychological support for family members are paramount as they can alleviate concerns of patients and family without introducing additional medications. Rarely, medications can prove useful and when elected, the clinician can use scopolamine patches starting at approximately 1 mg every 3 days or glycopyrrolate injections at 0.2 mg subcutaneously, repeated if there is no response after an hour.

Nutrition and Hydration

Nutrition and hydration, both essential for life itself, often become highly charged issues for families caring for a loved one with a potentially life-limiting illness. Fearing that withdrawal of nutrition or hydration will result in a painful death by starvation, many families request nutrition and hydration support even for terminally ill patients. Consequently, nutrition and hydration are some of the last therapies to be withdrawn at the end of life (31,32).

Despite the frequency of use, the evidence does not suggest that nutritional supplementation provides patients nearing end of life with benefit in terms of prevention of aspiration, improved survival, increased activity, or alleviation of cachexia (33). A study that randomized patients with cancer to receive or not receive a nutritional intervention found no difference in survival, energy balance, or exercising capacity (34). As patients progress towards death, they eat less, and hunger is not an issue for the vast majority of patients (35). Observational studies of dying patients who are no longer receiving hydration or nutrition have not demonstrated an increase in discomfort (36,37). Therefore, nutritional supplementation at the end of life is not recommended (38), except in select scenarios such as gastrointestinal complications with limited spread of malignancies, especially involving obstruction (39).

While the data on providing nutrition at the end of life are relatively clear, data on the role of hydration are not. The prevalence of thirst in patients at the end of life has been estimated to be 25% to 83% (40,41). However, the association between thirst and dehydration at the end of life has not been established (40,42). The proponents of the use of artificial hydration argue that the use of judicious hydration may alleviate or prevent symptoms resulting from decreased clearance of metabolites and medications, such as delirium, agitation, nausea, and myoclonus (43,44). Here, the data are conflicting. In a prospective, randomized trial of hydration therapy in seemingly dehydrated patients with metastatic cancer, patients in the hydration arm showed improvement in symptoms of myoclonus and sedation (45). However, a separate multicenter study evaluating terminally ill patients found no difference in myoclonus, confusion, or agitation in hydrated versus not hydrated patients (46).

While the potential benefits of hydration have been noted, there are also arguments about the potential harms of hydration at the end of life (47). These include worsening pulmonary congestion, peripheral edema, ascites, and increased need for voiding and diuretic use (46,48). In order to maintain enteral, intravenous, or subcutaneous access, increased use of restraints is often required, thus subjecting patients to the prospect of injury or discomfort (49). Through the use of good mouth care and small offerings of water or ice chips, patients who do not receive hydration are able to achieve a comfortable death (37). While there is little evidence that hydration prolongs life in actively dying patients, opponents of terminal hydration express concerns that artificial hydration serves to artificially prolong the dying process (50,51).

In acutely dying patients, most experts do not recommend the routine use of artificial hydration. Providers should discuss prognosis, goals of care, and possible benefits and harms of hydration and nutritional therapy with both the patient and caregivers. In situations where patients or families insist on therapies that are unlikely to be beneficial, a time-limited trial with explicit, objective criteria for desired outcomes may be the best option.

END-OF-LIFE CARE: PSYCHOSOCIAL

Death is a difficult emotional process for patients, caregivers, family members, and health care providers, all of whom have a unique relationship to the individual approaching the end of life. Psychosocial issues add complexity to end-of-life care, and they can be difficult to discern or diagnose. Emotions that are normal in terminally ill patients often resemble depression; physical symptoms normally associated with end of life are part of the somatic diagnostic criteria for psychiatric illnesses. Nonetheless, because of the morbidity associated with psychiatric illness at the end of life, health care providers must be vigilant for signs and symptoms of pathology. For clinicians treating patients near the end of life, awareness of psychological concerns takes on greater importance as patients move closer to dying and psychological distress often increases (52).

It is estimated that up to 82% of the terminally ill patients experience some form of psychiatric illness (53,54), including adjustment disorder (10–16%) (55,56), depressive disorders (3–82%) (55,56), and anxiety disorders (7–79%) (54,56). Despite the high prevalence of psychiatric symptoms at the end of life, physicians often find it difficult to discuss emotions during the medical interview. Many physicians report that they feel uncomfortable with their skill in discussing emotional topics, especially bad news (57,58). The structure of the medical encounter and reimbursement restrictions also discourage clinicians from discussing psychosocial issues (59). Often physicians are afraid that discussions will take too long or elicit feelings in the patient that they will be unable to handle. The evidence should dispel this fear; studies have shown that when physicians acknowledge patients' emotional concerns, encounters are actually shorter (60).

Depression

Identifying and differentiating between preparatory grief and depression in a dying patient can be quite difficult, even for seasoned clinicians. In general, depressed patients tend to remain in a consistently sad state, have a poor view of themselves, maintain a sense of hopelessness, and show little pleasure in new situations or from memories of prior events (61,62). In contrast, patients with normal grief reactions typically experience a progression of feelings, are able to maintain a realistic view of themselves, and can adjust their goals of care to maintain hope. The importance of identifying depression at the end of life has been highlighted by several studies that have shown an increase in morbidity and reported sequelae resulting from untreated depression. Depression, hopelessness, loss of meaning in life, and loss of interest in activities are risk factors for desire of hastened death (63,64). Patients who have their psychosocial needs addressed are less likely to persist in their desire for death (65).

Several instruments have been created or adapted to help identify depression in the terminally ill. These include the Beck Depression Inventory-Short Form (BDI-SF) (66), Hospital Anxiety and Depression Scale (HADS) (67), Edmonton Symptom Assessment Scale (ESAS) (68), Edinburgh Depression Scale, and Brief Edinburg Depression Scale (BEDS) (69). A simple screening instrument was developed by Chochinov, consisting of the single question, "Are you depressed?" (66). While the initial study demonstrated a sensitivity and specificity of 100% in a North American population, subsequent work has generally demonstrated less consistent results (68,70). The addition of a second question regarding a loss of interest in activities had good sensitivity in non-palliative care patients (71), but did not meet predetermined validity standards when assessed in a palliative care population (72). Single-question screening items have been expanded to other areas of psychosocial suffering, including overall distress and spiritual distress, with good results (73,74). Ultimately, clinicians should use the method that is most applicable to their clinical setting and patient population. It is critical that clinicians assess terminally ill patients for symptoms of distress.

The treatment of depressive symptoms in the end-of-life patient may follow guidelines established for general care of psychiatric illness, with certain adjustments. The use of pharmacologic therapy must take into account the patient's prognosis. When the patient has a limited life expectancy, there may not be time to titrate and achieve an effect with selective serotonin reuptake inhibitors (SSRIs), and psychostimulants may offer a more realistic treatment strategy.

Caregiver Distress

Psychosocial problems afflict not only the patient with a terminal illness; up to 50% of caregivers of terminally ill cancer patients experience psychiatric morbidity (75,76). Many families are unprepared for the financial, emotional, and physical commitment of caring for a loved one at end of life (77). In addition, families often lack the necessary medical knowledge and skills to anticipate care needs. Because of the demands of caregiving, many family members are forced to leave their jobs or work part-time, thus adding financial strain to an already emotionally intense period. Caregivers often neglect their own health care and emotional needs because of the burden of caregiving (78).

A primary way in which physicians can help both caregivers and terminally ill patients is by providing effective symptom relief (79). Control of both pain and non-pain symptoms can help alleviate or prevent depression in patients, just as treatment of depression may improve pain control (80,81). Reductions in patients' psychosocial distress can also decrease the caregiving burden and the psychological effects of terminal illness on caregivers (82).

One of the clinician's most powerful therapeutic assets, in offering support for end-of-life patients and family members, is simply his/her presence. By being available, discussing difficult topics, and helping manage troublesome symptoms, the physician can provide significant support. Caregivers who report that physicians listen to their opinions and concerns are less likely to report depressive symptoms (83). Good communication, including anticipatory guidance and explanations of what will occur, is essential. Appropriate referrals to agencies that can provide assistance, such as hospice, can greatly support family members (84). In all cases, effective communication, listening, and availability go far toward alleviating suffering at the end of life.

Communication

Communicating bad news to patients and families is an essential but challenging component of supportive care for terminally ill patients, and is one that warrants special discussion. Providing accurate information to patients and caregivers is very important, not only because it facilitates collaborative decision-making, but also because the way in which bad news is broken can affect the subsequent emotional health of patients and their loved ones (64).

Many healthcare providers experience great difficulty in delivering an accurate prognosis. Often physicians consciously provide an overly optimistic assessment of a patient's prognosis (85,86); alternatively, they may not provide prognostic information to the patient until he/she is very close to death, if at all (87,88). For their part, patients often interpret prognostic information in a highly optimistic way, seemingly choosing to believe that they will be an exception to the rule (89). The manner in which physicians provide information to patients has been shown to influence patients' perceptions of prognosis, and therefore, their choices regarding therapy (90,91). Information provided in a positive manner, such as percent surviving, is perceived to be better than the same information phrased negatively, such as percent dying. Patients often use falsely optimistic perceptions in choosing aggressive medical therapy, despite the fact that terminally ill patients who choose aggressive care garner no survival benefit compared to those choosing palliative measures only (92).

Many physicians worry that providing an accurate prognosis will rob patients of hope (93,94). Patients and caregivers rate the support of hope very highly, and stress that they do not want doctors to diminish it, even at the end of life (95,96). In terminal illness, however, physicians can define hope in such a way that it does not imply cure. They can instead help patients develop a realistic assessment of their prognosis, and work toward realistic goals, such as reduction of pain, alleviation of distressing symptoms, and relationship closure with loved ones (64). Many people worry that accurate prognosis, coupled with depression, will cause the patient to lose his/her fighting spirit. While it is important that psychiatric illness be treated, a recent systematic review found little evidence to support the idea that a fighting spirit improves morbidity or mortality (97).

Existing guidelines for breaking bad news to patients and families, though they typically do not have empirical evidence to support their use, are based on good communication principles and consensus expert opinion, and have good face validity (98,99). The initial step in a formal discussion of bad news is preparation. Clinicians should discuss how patients would like to receive prognostic information, and whether they actually desire it, before starting any conversation about bad news. The physician should bear in mind that patients and families vary in their views of who should be involved in discussions of prognosis, what information should be conveyed, the setting in which such a discussion should occur, and who should deliver the information. Clinicians should endeavor to have accurate, up-to-date information available during any discussion, and to deliver the information themselves. Ideally, the setting should be private and free from distractions.

A discussion of bad news should begin with the clinician asking the patient or family what information they already know. This helps the clinician to evaluate the patient's and family's level of understanding and to anticipate their reactions. The level of information sought and the best way to provide that information will be guided by the patient and his/her family. The physician can then deliver the information, stopping frequently to check for understanding or questions. A good rule of thumb is to give no more than three items of information before pausing to make sure that the patient and family are following. After the discussion, the clinician should check for a sound understanding, for example, by asking the patient and family to summarize information in their own words. At the end of the discussion, a clear agenda should be established, covering what the patient and family will do, what the physician will do, and when the next contact will occur.

END-OF-LIFE CARE: SPIRITUAL

As the patient approaches the end of life, the spiritual needs of patients, families, and caregivers typically become heightened. Good care of the spirit is therefore integral to excellent end-of-life care. Care of the spirit helps the patient and loved ones address existential issues that they will almost certainly face, such as "What is the meaning of life?" "Why am I here?" "What have I achieved in my life?" "How do I fit into the universe?" and "What will happen to 'me' after my death?" The clinician should be aware that patients', families', and caregivers' religious belief systems, and/or their personal belief system regarding our spiritual nature, will influence their reactions to these large spiritual questions.

Although physicians are not typically trained to provide spiritual care, patients and families often expect that health professionals can adequately introduce and discuss the subject of care of the spirit. Many people value an expected death as an opportunity to discuss and resolve any outstanding spiritual issues, and expect to complete this work in the context of their loved one's medical care. Yet the prospect of providing spiritual care to someone at the end of life challenges many clinicians.

Cancer care at the end of life, perhaps more than in any other phase of the illness, is provided by a multidisciplinary care team. Being comfortable with exploring and discussing spiritual issues is a key competency for each member of the end-of-life care team. Because patients and their families may initiate a discussion about spiritual concerns at any time, each member of the care team needs to be able to appropriately and professionally discuss spiritual care. While certain specific issues may need to be referred to an appropriate person in the pastoral care team, many spiritual issues can be safely explored by the team member with whom they are first raised. Clinicians must have considered the important spiritual and existential questions themselves in order to be able to converse meaningfully with patients about their beliefs and concerns. In these conversations, clinicians do not seek to share their own views about such issues, but rather to understand the breadth and complexity of a person's orientation toward this potentially complex area of life, and to use this understanding to identify needs that should be addressed by other professionals (e.g., chaplain or psychotherapist), to guide the delivery of compassionate care and to incorporate insights into "whole-person" focused clinical decisions.

Many people, especially in developed countries, encounter death very infrequently and may not even face it for the first time until well into their adult lives. As a person watches someone whom they love die, especially the first time, the confrontation with mortality can be profound. Clinicians may see this personal experience manifest in a variety of emotions—anger, fear, and powerlessness—and these emotions can, at times, be directed toward clinical staff as well as toward family members, the dying person, a deity, or some other construct. Encounters with death often force individuals to confront questions that many of us, on a day-to-day basis, prefer to ignore. Principal among these are questions about the nature and purpose of suffering, the reason for suffering, and the injustice of a painful or premature death.

As people express their beliefs and interpretations about spiritual issues with family members, the emotional rawness of dying and death can become magnified. Long-ignored or contentious issues often arise in a family at this time. In these situations, clinicians can help refocus family members on the goal of this aspect of care—to support patients in exploring and expressing their spirituality at the end of life, to the extent they would wish and in the manner that is most meaningful and comfortable for them. Containing or managing family conflict is crucial to ensure that patients can approach death in a context of full support, which covers their medical, psychosocial, and spiritual needs.

Clinicians may tend to look to a patient's, family's, or caregiver's belief system to evaluate their orientation toward spirituality, life, dying, and death. Although individuals may identify a particular belief system or religion, clinicians must avoid the temptation to assume particular interpretations or beliefs based on the religion or belief system nominated. A religion may provide the clinician with a broad guide to a person's beliefs; however, it will not furnish the details required to understand the ways in which this person will respond to arising spiritual concerns, or how to best support the patient in the context of spiritual care. Belief systems may help to structure wider conversations that occur around life and death, but clinicians should remember that spirituality and religion are not one and the same thing. A patient need not adhere to any particular system of belief in order to successfully resolve existential or spiritual issues. As outlined earlier in the chapter, belief systems may either relieve or worsen anxiety and fear as death approaches. Fears of lack of faith or of losing faith in the face of the unknown can greatly exacerbate anxiety. Belief systems that are challenged either by the disease (i.e., "Only bad people get this disease, and I have been good") or by the mode of death (i.e., "No one should suffer like this") can further challenge an individual's long-held views.

Ultimately, coming to peace with God, the universe, a higher power, or a belief system is an opportunity valued by people as death approaches. Those who are dying, their families, and caregivers will appreciate the clinician's efforts to ensure that they have the space, quietness, encouragement, and support to explore important spiritual issues.

END-OF-LIFE CARE: THE LAST DAYS OF LIFE

Clinicians must be able to actively recognize the process of dying from cancer. The diagnosis is supported by a continued expected deterioration of a person's overall condition with increasing lethargy, decreasing levels of consciousness, and at times, increasing confusion, increasing time spent sleeping, less spontaneous movement, and often changes in patterns of respiratory effort. For many people, the systemic signs can include progressive hypotension, diminishing oxygenation, and progressive loss of peripheral perfusion.

Alternatively, the terminal phase of cancer may be signaled by a sudden change in condition—an intracerebral bleed, a pulmonary embolus, a perforated viscous, or an overwhelming sepsis. When this change is superimposed on the condition of someone already moribund, continued symptom control becomes the primary aim. Understanding patients' wishes—often through conversations that they have had with their families both over the course of this illness and over the course of life more broadly—will help determine the best course of action. Many people, in the event of a catastrophic change in their condition, may wish to focus on comfort, while others may wish to try to achieve improvement in functions.

Whether the end of life approaches as an expected decline or as an unexpected catastrophic deterioration where the person would want nothing further done, the issue of comfort is absolutely paramount. All clinical actions should contribute to the comfort of the person who is dying.

Physical Care

Attention to the nursing care of the cancer patient at the end of life is crucial. Mouth care, ensuring that the dying person's mouth is clean and moist, will aid comfort. Continued attention to positioning is important. Using an air mattress will help to shift the person's weight. If an air mattress is not available, repositioning the person regularly will relieve musculoskeletal pain from inertia, and maintain skin integrity in order to avoid the excruciating (and difficult to control) pain of skin tears and pressure areas. Likewise, gentle elevation of the head of the bed may help if noisy upper respiratory tract secretions are a concern.

Medications and Hydration

All medications currently being administered to the patient must be reviewed, and those that directly contribute to comfort should be continued. This list may include more medications than just those that were introduced for symptom control in the palliative phase of the illness. For example, in type I diabetes, it may be necessary to prevent hyperglycemia in order to spare the patient from unquenchable thirst. Ensure that essential medications are available in a form that can be administered to someone who may not predictably be swallowing. Alternative formulations include sublingual, subcutaneous, intravenous, transdermal, intranasal, and rectal delivery. Review any nutritional supplements and any parenteral hydration at this time. Almost always, parenteral hydration should be stopped, with appropriate advice to the family, as over-hydration will worsen respiratory symptoms and potentially secretions in the gut, which may cause vomiting.

As mentioned, moist secretions have not been shown to respond to any particular therapy. The widespread use of anticholinergics continues. If used, hyoscine butylbromide and glycopyrrolate do not cross the blood-brain barrier and would not worsen any centrally mediated agitation.

Physical agitation can occur in the patient's final days. Ensure that this agitation is not due to pain, urinary retention, or constipation. Treatment may include a regular dose of a long-acting benzodiazepine. Benzodiazepines can precipitate or worsen delirium, and they should be used with care.

Communication with the Family

Communication with the family should be a key focus for health professionals as a patient nears death. What does the family expect? A trusted clinician should clearly, but compassionately, describe the process of dying. Patients should be reassured that, in most cases, the person dying gently slips into a coma and life ebbs away with no dramatic manifestations of dying. The clinician should emphasize that the sole focus of care is the dying person's comfort.

The Person Who Is Unconscious

Even when a patient is unconscious, clinical staff should carefully assess him/her to ensure comfort. This cannot be done from the door of the person's room. An examination is required, with special attention to the face (Is it relaxed?), respiration (Is it regular, not labored?), and positioning (Is the patient positioned comfortably?). The clinician should continue to explain to the patient what is happening in the clinical examination as if he or she were conscious, and should reassure the family that symptom control medications need to continue to ensure comfort even though consciousness is lost. Especially if continued at the equivalent dose, there is no concern that these medications may hasten death. It is important to ensure that family members understand that loved ones, even when unconscious, will still recognize their voice and touch.

Many family members have a strong desire to be present at the time of death. This specific time point can be difficult to predict, even as the patient's body shuts down. The need to be present varies from family to family, and within families, from one individual to another. If family member(s) have a particular wish to be present at the patient's time of death, the clinician may want to set up a vigil roster to ensure that one member of the family is always present during the patient's last days.

REFERENCES

1. American Thoracic Society, Dyspnea. Mechanisms, assessment, and management: a consensus statement. Am J Respir Crit Care Med, 1999; 159:321–340.
2. Leach RM. Palliative medicine and non-malignant, end-stage respiratory disease. In: Doyle D, Hanks G, Cherny N, Calman K, eds. Oxford Textbook of Palliative Medicine, 3rd ed. New York: Oxford University Press, 2005.
3. Eckenhoff JE, Oech SR. The effects of narcotics and antagonists upon respiration and circulation in man. A review. Clin Pharmacol Ther 1960; 1:483–524.
4. Weil JV, McCullough RE, Kline JS, et al. Diminished ventilatory response to hypoxia and hypercapnia after morphine in normal man. NEJM 1975; 292(21): 1103–1106.
5. Santiago TV, Pugliese AC, Edelman NH. Control of breathing during methadone addiction. Am J Med 1977; 62(3):347–354.
6. Kryger MH, Yacoub O, Dosman J, et al. Effect of meperidine on occlusion pressure responses to hypercapnia and hypoxia with and without external inspiratory resistance. Am Rev Respir Dis 1976; 114(2):333–340.
7. Santiago TV, Johnson J, Riley DJ, et al. Effects of morphine on ventilatory response to exercise. J Appl Physiol 1979; 47(1):112–118.

8. Jennings AL, Davies AN, Higgins JP, et al. A systematic review of the use of opioids in the management of dyspnoea. Thorax 2002; 57(11):939–944.
9. Bruera E, MacEachern T, Ripamonti C, et al. Subcutaneous morphine for dyspnea in cancer patients. Ann Intern Med 1993; 119(9):906–907.
10. Massie M, Holland J, Glass E. Delirium in terminally ill cancer patients. Am J Psychiatry 1983; 140:1048–1050.
11. Minagawa H, Uchitomi Y, Yamawaki S, et al. Psychiatric morbidity in terminall ill cancer patients: a prospective study. Cancer 1996; 78:1131–1137.
12. Bruera E, Miller L, McCallion J, et al. Cognitive failure in patients with terminal cancer: a prospective study. J Pain Symptom Manage 1992; 7:192–195.
13. Moryl N, Carver AC, Foley KM. Holland-Frei Cancer Medicine, 6th edition. In: Kufe DW, Pollock RE, Weichselbaum RR, et al., eds. Holland-Frei Cancer Medicine, 6th ed. Amsterdam: Elsevier 2003:1113–1123.
14. Trzepacz P, Baker R, Greenhouse J. A symptom rating scale for delirium. Psychiatry Res 1988; 23:89–97.
15. Inouye S, van Dyck C, Alessi C, et al. Clarifying confusion: the confusion assessment method. A new method for detection of delirium. Ann Intern Med 1990; 113:941–948.
16. Albert M, Levkoff S, Reilly C, et al. The delirium symptom interview: an interview for the detection of delirium symptoms in hospitalized patients. J Geriatric Psychiatr Neurol 1992; 5:14–21.
17. Breitbart W, Rosenfeld B, Roth A, et al. The Memorial Delirium Assessment Scale. J Pain Symptom Manage 1997; 13:128–137.
18. Folstein M, Folstein S, McHugh P. "Mini-mental state." A practical method for grading the cognitive state of patients for the clinician. J Psychiatr Res 1975; 12:189–198.
19. Casarett DJ, Inouye SK. Diagnosis and management of delirium near the end of life. Ann Intern Med 2001; 135:32–40.
20. McNamara P, Minton P, Twycross R. The use of midazolam in palliative care. Pall Med 1991; 5:244–249.
21. Truog R, Berde C, Mitchell C, et al. Barbiturates in the care of the terminally ill. New Engl J Med 1992; 327:1678–1682.
22. Bennett M, Lucas V, Brennan M, et al. Using anti-muscarinic drugs in the management of death rattle: evidence-based guidelines for palliative care. Pall Med 2002; 16(5): 369–374.
23. Hughes AC, Wilcock A, Corcoran R. Management of "death rattle." J Pain Symptom Manage 1996; 12(5):271–272.
24. Bennett MI. Death rattle: an audit of hyoscine (scopolamine) use and review of management. J Pain Symptom Manage 1996; 12(4):229–233.
25. Power D, Kearney M. Management of the final 24 hours. Irish Med J 1992; 85(3): 93–95.
26. Watts T, Jenkins K. Palliative care nurses' feelings about death rattle. J Clin Nurs 1999; 8(5):615–616.
27. Bennett M, Lucas V, Brennan M, et al. Using anti-muscarinic drugs in the management of death rattle: evidence-based guidelines for palliative care. Pall Med 2002; 16(5):369–374.
28. Wildiers H, Menten J. Death rattle: prevalence, prevention and treatment. J Pain Symptom Manage 2002; 23(4):310–317.

29. Back IN, Jenkins K, Blower A, et al. A study comparing hyoscine hydrobromide and glycopyrrolate in the treatment of death rattle (see comment). Pall Med 2001; 15(4):329–336.
30. Hughes A, Wilcock A, Corcoran R, et al. Audit of three antimuscarinic drugs for managing retained secretions. Pall Med 2000; 14(3):221–222.
31. Mercadante S, Ferrera P, Girelli D, et al. Patients' and relatives' perceptions about intravenous and subcutaneous hydration. J Pain Symptom Manage 2005; 30(4): 354–358.
32. Asch DA, Faber-Langendoen K, Shea JA, et al. The sequence of withdrawing life-sustaining treatment from patients. Am J Med 1999; 107(2):153–156.
33. Finucane TE, Christmas C, Travis K. Tube feeding in patients with advanced dementia: a review of the evidence. JAMA 1999; 282(14):1365–1370.
34. Lundholm K, Daneryd P, Bosaeus I, et al. Palliative nutritional intervention in addition to cyclooxygenase and erythropoietin treatment for patients with malignant disease: effects on survival, metabolism, and function. Cancer 2004; 100(9): 1967–1977.
35. McCann RM, Hall WJ, Groth-Juncker A. Comfort care for terminally ill patients. The appropriate use of nutrition and hydration. JAMA 1994; 272(16):1263–1266.
36. Pasman HR, Onwuteaka-Philipsen BD, Kriegsman DM, et al. Discomfort in nursing home patients with severe dementia in whom artificial nutrition and hydration is forgone. Arch Intern Med 2005; 165(15):1729–1735.
37. Ganzini L, Goy ER, Miller LL, et al. Nurses' experiences with hospice patients who refuse food and fluids to hasten death. NEJM 2003; 349(4):359–365.
38. Casarett D, Kapo J, Caplan A. Appropriate use of artificial nutrition and hydration: fundamental principles and recommendations. NEJM 2005; 353(24):2607–2612.
39. Duerksen DR, Ting E, Thomson P, et al. Is there a role for TPN in terminally ill patients with bowel obstruction? Nutrition 2004; 20(9):760–763.
40. Burge FI. Dehydration symptoms of palliative care cancer patients. J Pain Symptom Manage 1993; 8(7):454–464.
41. Ellershaw JE, Sutcliffe JM, Saunders CM. Dehydration and the dying patient. J Pain Symptom Manage 1995; 10(3):192–197.
42. Morita T, Tei Y, Tsunoda J, et al. Determinants of the sensation of thirst in terminally ill cancer patients. Support Care Cancer 2001; 9(3):177–186.
43. Lawlor PG. Delirium and dehydration: some fluid for thought? Support Care Cancer 2002; 10(6):445–454.
44. Mercadante S, Ripamonti C, Casuccio A, et al. Comparison of octreotide and hyoscine butylbromide in controlling gastrointestinal symptoms due to malignant inoperable bowel obstruction. Support Care Cancer 2000; 8(3):188–191.
45. Bruera E, Sala R, Rico MA, et al. Effects of parenteral hydration in terminally ill cancer patients: a preliminary study. J Clin Oncol 2005; 23(10):2366–2371.
46. Morita T, Hyodo I, Yoshimi T, et al. Association between hydration volume and symptoms in terminally ill cancer patients with abdominal malignancies. Ann Oncol 2005; 16(4):640–647.
47. Morita T, Shima Y, Miyashita M, et al. Physician- and nurse-reported effects of intravenous hydration therapy on symptoms of terminally ill patients with cancer. J Palliat Med 2004; 7(5):683–693.
48. Lanuke K, Fainsinger RL, DeMoissac D. Hydration management at the end of life. J Palliat Med 2004; 7(2):257–263.

49. Ferris FD, von Gunten CF, Emanuel LL. Competency in end-of-life care: last hours of life. J Palliat Med 2003; 6(4):605–613.
50. Chiu TY, Hu WY, Chuang RB, Chen CY. Nutrition and hydration for terminal cancer patients in Taiwan. Support Care Cancer 2002; 10(8):630–636.
51. Brard L, Weitzen S, Strubel-Lagan SL, et al. The effect of total parenteral nutrition on the survival of terminally ill ovarian cancer patients. Gynecol Oncol 2006; 103(1): 176–180.
52. Butler LD, Koopman C, Cordova MJ, et al. Psychological distress and pain significantly increase before death in metastatic breast cancer patients. Psychosom Med 2003; 65(3):416–426.
53. Wilson KG, Chochinov HM, Skirko MG, et al. Depression and anxiety disorders in palliative cancer care. J Pain Symptom Manage 2007; 33(2):118–129.
54. Solano JP, Gomes B, Higginson IJ. A comparison of symptom prevalence in far advanced cancer, AIDS, heart disease, chronic obstructive pulmonary disease and renal disease. J Pain Symptom Manage 2006; 31(1):58–69.
55. Akechi T, Okuyama T, Sugawara Y, et al. Screening for depression in terminally ill cancer patients in Japan. J Pain Symptom Manage 2006; 31(1):5–12.
56. Maguire P, Walsh S, Jeacock J, et al. Physical and psychological needs of patients dying from colo-rectal cancer. Palliat Med 1999; 13(1):45–50.
57. Baile WF, Glober GA, Lenzi R, et al. Discussing disease progression and end-of-life decisions. Oncology 1999; 13(7):1021-1031; discussion 31–36, 38.
58. Sise MJ, Sise CB, Sack DI, et al. Surgeons' attitudes about communicating with patients and their families. Curr Surg 2006; 63(3):213–218.
59. Chibnall JT, Bennett ML, Videen SD, et al. Identifying barriers to psychosocial spiritual care at the end of life: a physician group study. Am J Hosp Palliat Care 2004; 21(6):419–426.
60. Levinson W, Gorawara-Bhat R, Lamb J. A study of patient clues and physician responses in primary care and surgical settings. JAMA 2000; 284(8):1021–1027.
61. Periyakoil VS, Hallenbeck J. Identifying and managing preparatory grief and depression at the end of life. Am Fam Physician 2002; 65(5):883–890.
62. Noorani NH, Montagnini M. Recognizing depression in palliative care patients. J Palliat Med 2007; 10(2):458–464.
63. Breitbart W, Rosenfeld B, Pessin H, et al. Depression, hopelessness, and desire for hastened death in terminally ill patients with cancer. JAMA 2000; 284(22): 2907–2911.
64. Schroepfer TA. Critical events in the dying process: the potential for physical and psychosocial suffering. J Palliat Med 2007; 10(1):136–147.
65. Ganzini L, Nelson HD, Schmidt TA, et al. Physicians' experiences with the Oregon Death with Dignity Act. NEJM 2000; 342(8):557–563.
66. Chochinov HM, Wilson KG, Enns M, et al. "Are you depressed?"; Screening for depression in the terminally ill. Am J Psychiatr 1997; 154(5):674–676.
67. Lloyd-Williams M, Friedman T, Rudd N. An analysis of the validity of the Hospital Anxiety and Depression scale as a screening tool in patients with advanced metastatic cancer. J Pain Symptom Manage 2001; 22(6):990–996.
68. Lloyd-Williams M, Dennis M, Taylor F. A prospective study to compare three depression screening tools in patients who are terminally ill. Gen Hosp Psychiatry 2004; 26(5):384–389.

69. Lloyd-Williams M, Shiels C, Dowrick C. The development of the Brief Edinburgh Depression Scale (BEDS) to screen for depression in patients with advanced cancer. J Affect Disord 2007; 99(1-3):259-264.
70. McKenzie N, Marks I. Quick rating of depressed mood in patients with anxiety disorders. Br J Psychiatry 1999; 174:266-269.
71. Whooley MA, Avins AL, Miranda J, et al. Case-finding instruments for depression. Two questions are as good as many. J Gen Intern Med 1997; 12(7):439-445.
72. Robinson JA, Crawford GB. Identifying palliative care patients with symptoms of depression: an algorithm. Palliat Med 2005; 19(4):278-287.
73. Kelly B, McClement S, Chochinov HM. Measurement of psychological distress in palliative care. Pall Med 2006; 20(8):779-789.
74. Steinhauser KE, Voils CI, Clipp EC, et al. "Are you at peace?": one item to probe spiritual concerns at the end of life. Arch Intern Med 2006; 166(1):101-105.
75. Pitceathly C, Maguire P. The psychological impact of cancer on patients' partners and other key relatives: a review. Eur J Cancer 2003; 39(11):1517-1524.
76. Haley WE, LaMonde LA, Han B, et al. Family caregiving in hospice: effects on psychological and health functioning among spousal caregivers of hospice patients with lung cancer or dementia. Hosp J 2001; 15(4):1-18.
77. Rabow MW, Hauser JM, Adams J. Supporting family caregivers at the end of life: "they don't know what they don't know." JAMA 2004; 291(4):483-491.
78. Stein MD, Crystal S, Cunningham WE, et al. Delays in seeking HIV care due to competing caregiver responsibilities. Am J Public Health 2000; 90(7):1138-1140.
79. Rose K. How informal carers cope with terminal cancer. Nurs Stand 1997; 11(30):39-42.
80. Lin EH, Katon W, Von Korff M, et al. Effect of improving depression care on pain and functional outcomes among older adults with arthritis: a randomized controlled trial. JAMA 2003; 290(18):2428-2429.
81. Bair MJ, Robinson RL, Katon W, et al. Depression and pain comorbidity: a literature review. Arch Intern Med 2003; 163(20):2433-2445.
82. Redinbaugh EM, Baum A, Tarbell S, et al. End-of-life caregiving: what helps family caregivers cope? J Palliat Med 2003; 6(6):901-909.
83. Emanuel EJ, Fairclough DL, Slutsman J, et al. Understanding economic and other burdens of terminal illness: the experience of patients and their caregivers. Ann Intern Med 2000; 132(6):451-459.
84. Christakis NA, Iwashyna TJ. The health impact of health care on families: a matched cohort study of hospice use by decedents and mortality outcomes in surviving, widowed spouses. Soc Sci Med 2003; 57(3):465-475.
85. Glare P, Virik K, Jones M, et al. A systematic review of physicians' survival predictions in terminally ill cancer patients. BMJ 2003; 327(7408):195.
86. Lamont EB, Christakis NA. Prognostic disclosure to patients with cancer near the end of life. Ann Intern Med 2001; 134(12):1096-1105.
87. Anselm AH, Palda V, Guest CB, et al. Barriers to communication regarding end-of-life care: perspectives of care providers. J Crit Care 2005; 20(3):214-223.
88. Clayton JM, Butow PN, Tattersall MH. When and how to initiate discussion about prognosis and end-of-life issues with terminally ill patients. J Pain Symptom Manage 2005; 30(2):132-144.

89. Thorne S, Hislop TG, Kuo M, et al. Hope and probability: patient perspectives of the meaning of numerical information in cancer communication. Qual Health Res 2006; 16(3):318–336.
90. Moxey A, O'Connell D, McGettigan P, et al. Describing treatment effects to patients. J Gen Intern Med 2003; 18(11):948–959.
91. Young JM, Davey C, Ward JE. Influence of "framing effect" on women's support for government funding of breast cancer screening. Aust N Z J Public Health 2003; 27(3):287–290.
92. Weeks JC, Cook EF, O'Day SJ, et al. Relationship between cancer patients' predictions of prognosis and their treatment preferences. JAMA 1998; 279(21):1709–1714.
93. Curtis JR, Patrick DL, Caldwell ES, et al. Why don't patients and physicians talk about end-of-life care? Barriers to communication for patients with acquired immunodeficiency syndrome and their primary care clinicians. Arch Intern Med 2000; 160(11):1690–1696.
94. Knauft E, Nielsen EL, Engelberg RA, et al. Barriers and facilitators to end-of-life care communication for patients with COPD. Chest 2005; 127(6):2188–2196.
95. Heyland DK, Dodek P, Rocker G, et al. What matters most in end-of-life care: perceptions of seriously ill patients and their family members. CMAJ 2006; 174(5): 627–633.
96. Wenrich MD, Curtis JR, Ambrozy DA, et al. Dying patients' need for emotional support and personalized care from physicians: perspectives of patients with terminal illness, families, and health care providers. J Pain Symptom Manage 2003; 25(3): 236–246.
97. Petticrew M, Bell R, Hunter D. Influence of psychological coping on survival and recurrence in people with cancer: systematic review. BMJ 2002; 325(7372):1066.
98. Vaidya VU, Greenberg LW, Patel KM, et al. Teaching physicians how to break bad news: a 1-day workshop using standardized parents. Arch Pediatr Adolesc Med 1999; 153(4):419–422.
99. Baile WF, Buckman R, Lenzi R, et al. SPIKES-A six-step protocol for delivering bad news: application to the patient with cancer. Oncologist 2000; 5(4):302–311.
100. Brandt HE, Ooms ME, Deliens L, et al. The last two days of life of nursing home patients: a nationwide study on causes of death and burdensome symptoms in the Netherlands. Pall Med 2006; 20(5):533–540.
101. Conill C, Verger E, Henriquez I, et al. Symptom prevalence in the last week of life. J Pain Symptom Manage 1997; 14(6):328–331.
102. Hall P, Schroder C, Weaver L. The last 48 hours of life in long-term care: a focused chart audit. J Am Geriatrics Soc 2002; 50(3):501–506.
103. Tranmer JE, Heyland D, Dudgeon D, et al. Measuring the symptom experience of seriously ill cancer and noncancer hospitalized patients near the end of life with the memorial symptom assessment scale. J Pain Symptom Manage 2003; 25(5):420–429.
104. von Gunten CF. Interventions to manage symptoms at the end of life. J Pall Med 2005; 8(suppl 1):S88–S94.

20

Risk Prediction of Chemotherapy-Associated Toxicity in Patients Receiving Cancer Chemotherapy

Gary H. Lyman and Nicole M. Kuderer

Department of Medicine, Duke University School of Medicine and the Duke Comprehensive Cancer Center, Durham, North Carolina, U.S.A.

INTRODUCTION

Prognostic or risk models evaluate the association between an outcome (dependent variable)—such as disease, response, and survival—and one or more predictive or prognostic factors (independent variables). Such models are used for a number of purposes, including to (1) improve our understanding of a disease process, (2) improve the design and analysis of clinical trials, (3) generate risk stratification, (4) assist in comparison of outcome between treatment groups in nonrandomized studies by allowing adjustment for case mix, (5) define risk groups based on prognosis, (6) predict disease outcome more accurately or parsimoniously, and (7) act as a guide for clinical decision making including treatment selection and patient counseling (1). In general, there are two major types of models depending upon the purpose of the study: 1. explanatory models and 2. predictive models.

EXPLANATORY MODELS

Explanatory models are often used to identify risk factors that are associated with the outcome of interest in an exploratory study. In other cases, the primary focus is on the relationship of the outcome with a specific risk factor when there is concern that the relationship between the risk factor and outcome may either be confounded by other factors or the strength of the relationship may be modified by an interaction term. Clinical experience and expertise are of considerable importance in the modeling process, particularly in identifying potential confounding factors and effect modifiers in advance of the study.

Confounding

Confounding occurs when an apparent association between a risk factor and an outcome is altered by the relationship of each to a third factor (Fig. 1). Therefore, confounding may results in a treatment effect being falsely obscured or falsely observed due to an association of a variable with both treatment (or exposure) and the outcome of interest, i.e., confounding factors may obscure a true relationship between variables or create an apparent relationship that does not actually exist. Figure 2A illustrates the potential impact of ignoring confounding of the relationship between treatment intensity and survival in a situation where younger patients do better than older patients, but where the treatment effect (slope) is similar. If the impact of age is ignored, the observed treatment effect illustrated by the flat line is observed, which does not reflect the true treatment effect in either older or younger patients. If the treatment effect is adjusted for age, the average treatment effect illustrated by the intermediate dashed line has the same slope as that found for both older and younger patients. Confounding is sometimes simply addressed in a stratified analysis where the relationship between the risk factor and the outcome is assessed separately for different levels

Confounding

Confounding: treatment effect is either falsely obscured or falsely observed due to an association with both treatment and outcome

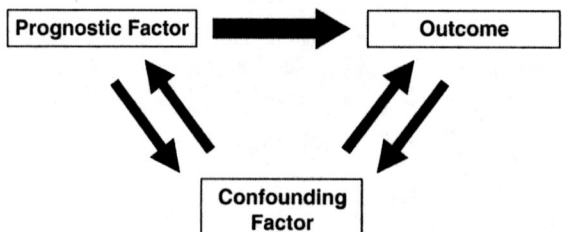

Figure 1 Schematic of the relationship between a prognostic factor and a clinical outcome, which may become confounded by another factor if such a factor is associated with both the prognostic factor of interest as well as the clinical outcome of interest.

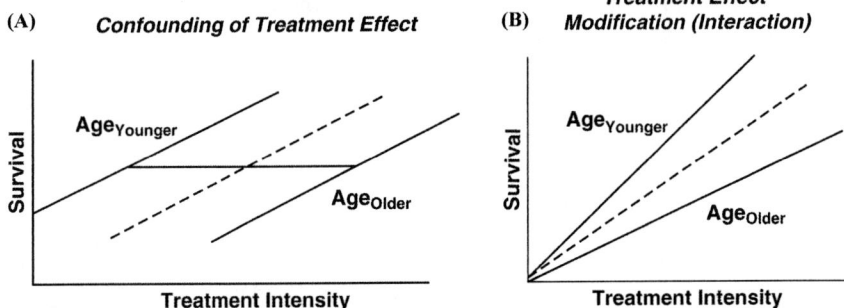

Figure 2 Hypothetical illustration of the relationship between treatment and survival when another factor, such as age, functions as a confounding factor (2A), or an effect modifier (2B). If a confounding factor is ignored, a significant relationship between treatment and outcome may be falsely observed or falsely obscured (flat line). If an effective modifier or interaction term is ignored, the resulting estimate of the overall treatment effect (slope) may be incorrect and not be an accurate estimate of the treatment effect in any group of subjects.

of the confounding factor. For instance, if age is confounding a relationship between treatment and survival, that relationship may be assessed separately in younger and older patients to adjust for confounding. The limitation of this approach primarily relates to small numbers when multiple categories within a confounding factor or multiple factors need to be considered. Alternatively, multivariate methods permit study of the relationship between risk factors and outcome simultaneously adjusting for known or suspected confounding factors. Multivariate models have the capability of addressing multiple potential confounding factors, simultaneously incorporating most, if not all, of the subjects. Clearly, such analyses can only adjust for potential confounding factors that are actually considered, measured, and included in the analysis. Confounding of the relationship between dependent and independent variables may still exist with factors that are unknown, unmeasured, or otherwise not included in the model. When the focus is on the identification or evaluation of specific risk factors, the model permits the study of the independent contribution of each to the outcome of interest. When the analysis is focused on one main predictor, its relationship with the primary outcome can be estimated while being adjusted for all of the potential confounding factors considered in the model.

Interaction

Dealing with potential interaction can be one of the most challenging aspects of developing risk models. Interaction or effect modification represents the situation in which an interacting variable alters the level of association between a risk factor and an outcome. For instance, age would represent an effect modifier if the relationship between treatment and survival (treatment effect) were different for younger and older patients. Interaction is sometimes referred to as synergism or antagonism depending upon whether the effect is increased or decreased by the interacting term. Figure 2B illustrates the potential impact of ignoring interaction upon the relationship between treatment intensity and survival in a situation where the outcome without treatment is essentially the same, but the treatment effect (slope) is greater in younger patients than older patients. If the impact of age is ignored, the observed treatment effect illustrated by the dashed line does not reflect the true treatment effect in either older or younger patients but something in between. One would want to preserve in some way the true treatment effect of both younger and older patients. It is very important that any potential effect modifiers or interaction terms be considered *a priori* as the evaluation for interaction involves subgroup analyses and multiple testing issues. While an interaction term may also be a confounding factor, confounding and interaction are different and must be dealt with differently. As discussed above, confounding can often be adequately dealt with by including the variable in a multivariate risk model that automatically adjusts for its effect. Interaction, on the other hand, cannot be addressed in such a straightforward manner. Nevertheless, it is important to explore and identify interactions and consider them in the analysis. Effect modification or interaction can be identified either by stratified analysis of the treatment effect for different levels of the candidate interaction term or by incorporating a variable consisting of the product of the effect modifier and the risk factor into the model. If either approach does not demonstrate significant interaction, the interaction term can essentially be ignored. Such a variable could still represent a confounding variable and should be evaluated. On the other hand, where there is significant interaction, such as with age in the example above, it should not be ignored since a multivariate model without the interaction term will provide only an "average" treatment effect that may not be accurate for either men or women.

There are two options in dealing with interaction in risk models. The investigator may choose to present separate models for different levels of the interaction term, e.g., different models for younger and older patients. Outcome differences between subgroups should be assessed by testing for interaction between the risk factor and the interaction term, rather than by separate analyses within subgroups, which may have limited power due to smaller sample size. Alternatively, a single model can be presented by including as variables in the model, both the variables in question, e.g., treatment and age, as well as an interaction variable generally created as a product term of the two variables. Again, if the interaction variable is found to be nonsignificant, it should be deleted from the final model. If it is significant, all three terms must be retained which, unfortunately, results in a model that is complex and difficult to explain. The relative risk estimates, such as odds ratios or hazard ratios, are no longer simply single fixed numbers based on a single regression coefficient, but rather represent an equation where the relative risk is a function of the other variable term and will change as the value of that variable changes. In the example above, the relative risk for survival with treatment is not a discrete number but a function of age, and it will be different for younger and older patients. Likewise, of course, the relative risk for survival with age is not a discrete number but a function of treatment in a similar way. Such results are understandably difficult to understand and perhaps even more difficult to explain.

Risk Factors

The selection of risk factors for inclusion in a model represents arguably the most challenging issue with regard to risk modeling. Ideally, such models should include all relevant and important risk factors and potential confounding factors. Variable selection should be guided by the knowledge and experience of the clinician and often appears to be more of an art rather than a science. Often, however, risk factors are identified through the use of a statistical model using exploratory techniques such as forward or backward stepwise variable selection methods. Since such an approach selects variables to fit the specific set of data, it is fraught with many potential problems including model instability and exaggeration of relative risk estimates and their associated level of significance. A more valid approach is the selection of risk factors based on a fundamental understanding of the pathophysiology of the disease and pharmacology of treatment, prior knowledge, and experience. Evaluation of a model based on risk factors identified *a priori* is less likely to lead the investigator astray. In addition, multiple comparison issues must be considered when selecting many risk factors or cutpoints. Stepwise procedures, on the other hand, are useful exploratory approaches assuming that the results will be thoroughly investigated in confirmatory studies.

Statistical Models

The specific model or mathematical relationship between risk factors and outcome chosen depends upon the type of outcome being studied and the anticipation that the data will approximately follow the relationship defined by the model. In multivariate regression analyses, a coefficient or "slope" is estimated for each independent variable by fitting a specified model to the data while adjusting for all the other variables. Commonly used models include (1) linear regression modeling of linear function of independent variables on the mean of a normally distributed continuous outcome measure, (2) logistic regression modeling of the multiplicative product of individual predictors on a dichotomous (yes/no) outcome, and (3) proportional hazards regression modeling of the product of individual predictors on the instantaneous risk or hazard of a discrete event over time (survival).

Like a slope when there is only one independent variable, the risk factor coefficient reflects the rate of change in the outcome variable for every unit change in the predictor variable adjusted for other variables in the model. It can be shown that in logistic regression models, the exponential function (antilogarithm) of the coefficient is equivalent to the odds ratio. Likewise, it can be demonstrated that for proportional hazards regression models, the exponential function of the coefficient is equivalent to the "hazard ratio" representing the "instantaneous" risk of an event. Generally, the coefficients or the derived ratios are reported as a point estimate along with a measure of variability such as the standard error or 95% confidence limits on the estimate. Like variable coefficients, the derived estimates of relative risk are adjusted for other variables included in the model.

All models are based on specific assumptions, which must be satisfied for the results to be valid. For instance, all models assume that the observations are independent of one another such as those derived from separate patients. When a significant correlation exists between two or more variables preventing reliable estimation of the individual regression coefficients, collinearity is said to exist. Collinearity may reduce the power of the model and complicate the interpretation of the contributions of the correlated variables. Including a variable twice or one variable representing a surrogate for another variable represent examples of extreme collinearity. For lesser degrees of collinearity, investigators may choose to run the risk of ignoring it, include only the most relevant of the two correlated factors, create a composite variable, or use another type of analysis or regression, although none of these choices is ideal.

Multiple regression is the most widely used method for examining several prognostic variables simultaneously; other methods have been developed and applied, which simultaneously explore multiple factors. Regression trees, e.g., CART, work by simultaneously selecting the variable and cutpoint, which best split patients into high- and low-risk groups. The same procedure is repeated within each subgroup thus formed successively, until it reaches a stopping rule. The resulting classification of variables represents a tree. Multiple testing is a highly relevant issue here as well. Multiple testing clearly must be considered and the method is highly data dependent, yielding overly optimistic results. Likewise, neural networks are occasionally utilized, but are even more controversial suffering from less explicit variable selection methods. While these methods have gained increasing attention, they have not been shown to provide better predictions than regression methods and are often poorly applied and reported in the oncology setting.

RISK MODELS

Often, the primary purpose of a model is the overall prediction or estimation of the risk of an outcome of interest, rather than the contribution of individual risk factors. "Prognostic models" of disease outcome such as survival are often distinguished from "predictive models" of treatment outcome such as response.

Table 1 Considerations in the Design of Risk Model Studies

1. The primary and secondary hypotheses should be clearly stated, including any subgroup analyses planned in advance.
2. Consider prognostic factors for which there is sufficient evidence to warrant further investigation based on
    (i) previous studies,
    (ii) biological and clinical plausibility, and
    (iii) relevance and importance to the understanding or treatment of the disease.
3. The study population should be defined with specified inclusion and exclusion criteria and methods to judge evaluability.
4. Patient treatment should be either standardized or assigned by randomization.
5. Assays should be reproducible and performed without knowledge of the clinical data and patient outcome.
6. Estimate the sample size keeping in mind the following:
    (i) The desired power to detect meaningful differences in outcome for the major endpoints, and to reject such differences with reasonable confidence if they are not found.
    (ii) The relationship of sample size to the number of outcome events, bearing in mind that these will be less frequent in favorable prognostic groups.
    (iii) The desirability of large prospective studies of a single prognostic factor.
7. Specify the planned analysis including any cutpoints for continuous variables, proposed hypothesis testing on subgroups, and anticipated interactions in advance of the study.
8. Key study features, including the above information, should be fully detailed in a formal written protocol.

Such models may be used to group or classify subjects into discrete risk categories. Factors to consider in both the design and analysis of risk model studies are summarized in Tables 1 and 2. The simplest risk model classifies patients into "high" risk and "low" risk. The development and evaluation of such risk models may be considered analogous to that of clinical tests.

In its simplest form, a risk model predicts a single dichotomous (yes/no) outcome from a single dichotomous risk factor. For instance, one may wish to predict the risk of febrile neutropenia from a single factor such as gender. As with any test, perfect prediction of the actual outcome, such as a true positive or true negative result, is seldom achieved. Some subjects predicted to be low risk actually may experience the event (false negative), while some at high risk may fail to do so (false positive). Model predictive performance, as with clinical test performance, can be assessed in a variety of ways including sensitivity, specificity, and predictive value. The sensitivity of a model is the probability of being correctly classified if an event occurred, and the specificity is the probability of being correctly classified if an event does not occur. In clinical and risk modeling, however, the primary focus is on the probability of an event occurring based on the result predicted by the model (predictive value).

Table 2 Considerations in the Analysis of Risk Model Studies

1. Base analysis, including any hypothesis testing, on the primary and major secondary outcomes specified prior to the study.
2. Consider possible bias due to missing data.
3. Consider the issue of multiple comparisons when evaluating many prognostic factors or cutpoints and adjust tests of significance accordingly.
4. Be aware of the problems associated with the interpretation of stepwise multiple regression models, including model instability and likely exaggeration of coefficient estimates and their associated p-values.
5. Adjust the effect of new prognostic factors for existing prognostic factors of recognized and accepted importance.
6. Outcome differences between subgroups should be assessed by testing the interaction between the prognostic factor and the variable defining the subgroups rather than by separate analyses within subgroups.
7. Interpret with caution the apparent outcome or prognostic marker differences between subgroups (many such differences arise from multiple testing or small sample size within subgroups).
8. Analysis of subgroups defined only during or after completion of the study should be acknowledged as exploratory.
9. In reporting the results of a prognostic factor study
    (i) Clearly state the study design: exploratory/confirmatory, prospective/retrospective, treatment (e.g., randomized or standardized), blinding, main outcomes, etc.
    (ii) Report the number of patients excluded because of missing data.
    (iii) Specify study duration including criteria for study termination (if relevant).
    (iv) Report methods of measurement of prognostic markers, if possible, with information about reproducibility.
    (v) Define clearly all study endpoints.
    (vi) Summarize outcomes as quantitative estimates and confidence intervals.
    (vii) Emphasize the outcome differences observed for all patients more than those found among subgroups.
    (viii) Discuss any weaknesses of the study, especially related to subgroup analyses and multiple comparisons.

MODEL ACCURACY

Model predictive performance or accuracy is based on (1) discrimination, (2) calibration, and (3) power. The accuracy of a model is often summarized on the basis of the likelihood ratio representing the likelihood or odds of the event based on the predicted outcome divided by the likelihood of the event in the overall population. In the context of a prognostic model, sensitivity represents the probability of individuals experiencing events being correctly predicted to be high risk by the model. Similarly, specificity represents the probability of individuals not experiencing events being correctly predicted to be low risk by the model (Fig. 3).

The overall model discrimination is reflected in the test performance over the full range of possible criteria for defining high versus low risk, i.e., all pairs

Risk Prediction of Chemotherapy-Associated Toxicity

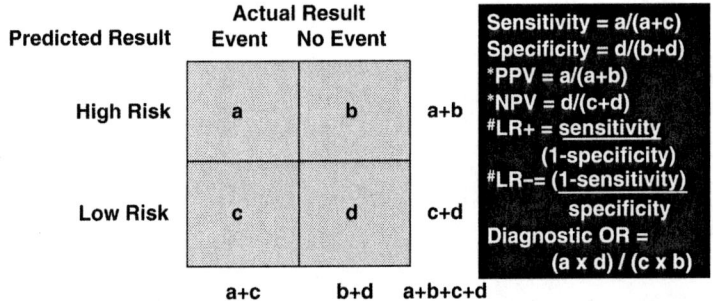

*P(N)PV = Positive (Negative) Predictive Value
#LR + (−) = Likelihood Ratio + (−)

Figure 3 Summary of estimates of risk model accuracy based on a simplified scenario of a dichotomous (yes/no) outcome and risk model classification into high-risk and low-risk patients. Possible results among a population of patients are illustrated along with the equations for estimating model performance characteristics including sensitivity, specificity, positive predictive value (PPV), negative predictive value (NPV), likelihood ratio (LR) positive (+) or negative (−) and the diagnostic odds ratio (OR).

of values for the true positive rate (sensitivity) and the false positive rate (1-specificity). The graph defined by these pair of points is termed a receiver operating characteristic (ROC) curve (Fig. 4). For dichotomous outcomes such as in logistic regression analysis, the area under the ROC curve (AUC) is equivalent to the *c index* or c statistic as a measure of concordance (2). For useful models, the AUC or c statistic varies between 0.5 and 1.0, with the best models approaching 1. The diagonal line defining the pairs of points where the true positive and false positive rates are equal represents the curve expected if the model has no discriminating capability and, therefore, conveys no information. The more the ROC curve extends into the opposing corners of the graph, the greater is the model discrimination. The overall model discrimination performance can be estimated on the basis of the model (diagnostic) odds ratio. In the simple dichotomous situation, this represents the ratio of the post-test odds in the high-risk group to the post-test odds in the low risk-group, or the likelihood ratio positive divided by the likelihood ratio negative (Fig. 3). The ratio becomes greater as the likelihood ratio positive becomes larger and the likelihood ratio negative becomes smaller. Importantly, the model odds ratio often remains relatively constant over the range of possible cutpoints.

The evaluation of model calibration or its fit to the data is generally based on the agreement between predicted risk score probabilities based on the model and the actual observed probabilities. This error in estimation, or residual analysis, can be evaluated using residual plots. For risk models, a weighted averaged global score can be generated and the accuracy of the scoring system assessed by plotting the observed versus predictive outcomes. The prediction rules can then be

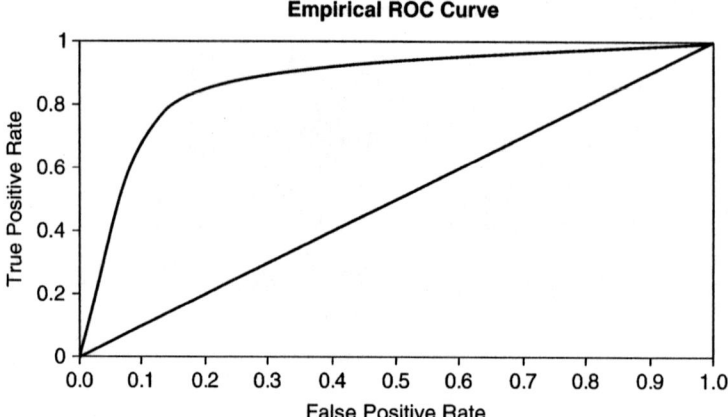

Figure 4 Graphical display of the relationship between the true positive rate and the false positive rate for a hypothetical risk model defining a receiver operating characteristic (ROC) curve. The straight line illustrates the relationship when no information is conveyed by the risk model, while the closer the ROC curve is to the corners of the graph, the better the discrimination of risk based on the model. For dichotomous outcomes, the area under the ROC curve is referred to as the c statistic.

generated based on the most accurate scoring system. Sensitivity, specificity, predictive value, and likelihood ratio can be estimated for each model and prediction rule. Calibration can be quantified on the basis of the slope of the prognostic index (3). The slope of the prognostic index or calibration slope represents the regression coefficient of the prognostic index as the only covariate in a logistic regression model. If observed and predicted probabilities agreed perfectly, the calibration slope would equal one.

The overall power of a model to predict the outcome of interest can be based on a variety of measures including the average prediction error or Brier score ranging from 0 (perfect) to 0.25 (worthless), the D statistic representing a scaled version of the model χ^2 statistic (model $\chi^2 - 1)/n$, where n is the number of subjects, and the model R^2 representing the proportion of the variation in outcome that is accounted for by the independent variables in the model (4). R^2 increases as the number of predictive variables in the model increases, while the predictive factors in a model with an R^2 close to 1 or –1 accurately predict the outcome. Another way to view R^2 is the potential to further improve outcome prediction with consideration of other variables.

MODEL VALIDATION

Model validation is ideally an external validation using an independent population of individuals not included in the original developmental sample. Internal validation can be assessed utilizing an intensive resampling technique or bootstrapping that permits one to draw inferences about the underlying population from which the sample originated by drawing samples with replacement from the original sample (5). The procedure recommended by Steyergerg includes (1) drawing a random bootstrap sample of the same size with replacement from the original, (2) selecting the same covariates and estimate the logistic regression coefficients and performance indices as described above, and (3) evaluating the model by comparing the performance in the bootstrap sample with that in the original sample, which is an unbiased estimate of the overoptimism expected for the model based on the original sample (6).

MISSING DATA

Complete data are critical to the powerful and unbiased risk estimation in multivariate models. Most modeling methods remove subjects, who are missing any of the variables included in the model potentially biasing the model results, from the calculations. All reasonable efforts should be taken to minimize missing data in a study. Any missing data, despite these efforts, should be evaluated for any relationship to the various outcomes and covariates. Imputation of missing values may be a reasonable approach if the proportion of missing values is less than 10%. Imputation methods range from simple use of the variable mean from existing values or the use of the last value carried forward in the setting of repeated measures. Regression methods based on the association of a variable with other measured variables can provide a more accurate estimate of missing values, although all of the above methods underestimate the variability of the measure. More sophisticated random sampling methods are available, which may preserve the covariance structure. None of these methods, however, is a substitute for complete and accurate data capture as a basis for modeling.

EXAMPLE

Introduction

Neutropenia and its complications, including febrile neutropenia, are major dose-limiting toxicities of systemic cancer chemotherapy. Several studies have tried to identify risk factors for neutropenic events to develop predictive models capable of identifying patients at increased risk for such complications and to guide more effective and cost-effective application of the colony-stimulating factors (7–8). A systematic review of the literature has demonstrated that age, performance status, nutritional status, chemotherapy dose intensity, and low-baseline blood cell counts were associated with the risk of severe and febrile neutropenia or reduced chemotherapy dose intensity in multivariate analysis (9). Age, diagnosis of leukemia or lymphoma, high temperature or low blood pressure at admission, and intravenous site infection along with low blood cell counts and organ dysfunction were also associated with serious medical complications of febrile neutropenia, including bacteremia and death. Available risk model studies, however, have been associated with several limitations, including retrospective analyses of small study populations, lack of independent validation, frequent missing values, and differences in the predictive factors considered. To overcome the limitations of previous studies, a prospective population study of patients with breast, lung, colorectal, and ovarian cancers, as well as malignant lymphoma initiating a new chemotherapy regimen, was undertaken (10). Primary outcomes included febrile neutropenia, severe neutropenia without fever or infection, and relative dose intensity (RDI). Despite frequent planned reductions from standard RDI, the incidence of febrile neutropenia remained, suggesting that improved methods of pretreatment assessment of patient risk factors for neutropenia are needed, including the development and validation of neutropenia risk models. Preliminary results of a risk model developed using patients in this prospective study have been presented to the Multinational Association of Supportive Care of Cancer (Table 3) (11). Based on an individual patient's calculated risk score, the model permits an estimation of the individual risk of febrile neutropenia or severe or febrile neutropenia in the first cycle of chemotherapy when most events occur (Fig. 5). While further validation of this and similar models is still needed, it is anticipated that these models will aid oncologists in clinical decision making and the selection of patients at increased risk for life threatening complications. Such patients may be candidates for the prophylactic administration of a myeloid growth factor at the start of systemic cancer chemotherapy. Similar models are under development for other hematologic complications of cancer therapy (anemia, thrombocytopenia) as well as nonhematologic complications (mucositis, nausea and vomiting, and neurotoxicity among others).

The Development and Validation of a Neutropenia Risk Model

Patient Population

The population to be utilized as the developmental data set must be fully characterized in terms of patient demographics including age, gender, and race; the cancer type and stage of disease; the treatment given including dose and schedule; and patient comorbidities and concomitant medications. The source of the population must be fully defined as well as any criteria for inclusion or exclusion. Patients, rather than encounters or cycles, must be the primary units of analysis. Important variables and cutpoints should be defined in advance.

Dependent Variables

The primary outcome variable should include various measures of myelosuppression, such as the incidence, severity, and duration of neutropenia; various infectious complications including febrile neutropenia, documented infections, or infection-related mortality; and the impact on dose reduction, treatment delay, or overall dose intensity. The secondary outcome variables may include the quality-of-life assessment and economic measures most notably related to

Table 3 Risk Model Calculator: Cycle 1 Severe or Febrile Neutropenia

	[check all that apply]		
Patient Name: _____		Date: _____	
Cancer Diagnosis: _____		DOB: _____	
History:		Points	Score
1. History of recent surgery (within six months):		2 ____	☐
2. History of prior chemotherapy:		6 ____	☐
Subtotal _____			
Concomitant Medications:			
3. Currently receiving immunosuppressives:		4 ____	☐
4. Currently receiving diuretics:		4 ____	☐
5. Currently receiving phenothiazines:		4 ____	☐
Subtotal _____			
Abnormal Baseline Laboratory Results:			
6. Elevated glucose:		2 ____	☐
7. Elevated alkaline phosphatase:		3 ____	☐
8. Elevated bilirubin:		7 ____	☐
9. Glomerular Filtration Rate < 30 ul/min		7 ____	☐
10. Absolute neutrophil count < 2000/mm^3		6 ____	☐
Subtotal _____			
Type of Cancer: (choose only one under treatment)			
11. Small cell lung cancer		23 ____	☐
12. Non-small cell lung cancer		7 ____	☐
13. Ovarian cancer		8 ____	☐
14. Non-Hodgkin's lymphoma		10 ____	☐
15. Breast cancer		8 ____	☐
16. Hodgkin's disease		2 ____	☐
Subtotal _____			
Chemotherapy:			
17. Anthracycline-based regimen:		18 ____	☐
18. Number of myelosuppressive agents: 2		5 ____	☐
>2		10 ____	☐
19. Planned relative dose intensity: >85% of standard		6 ____	☐
Unknown		3 ____	☐
20. No primary CSF prophylaxis:		20 ____	☐
		Subtotal _____	
GRAND TOTAL (Cumulative Risk Score) _____		(0-122)	

CSF = colony-stimulating factor.

resource utilization. Outcomes should be assessed separately, for each cycle of therapy, as well as cumulatively across the entire regimen.

Independent Variables

Predictive and prognostic variables should include patient and practice demographics, medical history, comorbidities concomitant medications, and common

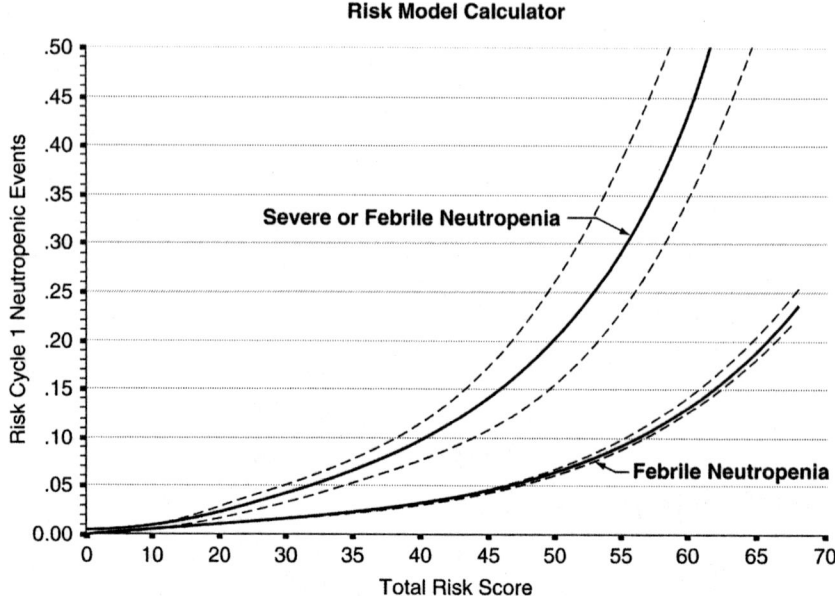

Figure 5 This represents the resulting risk model relationship between the summary score derived from Table 3 and a theoretical patient's individual risk for cycle 1 febrile neutropenia (lower curve) or severe or febrile neutropenia (upper curve) when receiving cancer chemotherapy. This is based on a large U.S. prospective study of patients initiating a new chemotherapy regimen for cancers of the lung, breast, colorectum, or ovary as well as malignant lymphoma (11). Also illustrated for each curve are the 95% confidence limits on the risk estimates derived from the risk score. This early model is undergoing additional validation studies in prospective studies.

prognostic measures including disease status, baseline blood counts, and treatment-related factors including drugs, regimen, schedule, dose intensity as well as any supportive care measures utilized. Where measures have been recorded as continuous variables or multiple categories, the analysis should initially be based on actual measures rather than arbitrarily imposed cutpoints. When incorporated, cutpoints should be based on standard and referenced parameters rather than convenience, arbitrary, or data-driven cutpoints. Possible dependent and independent variables for analysis are listed in Table 4.

Data Analysis

Descriptive

Each study measure should be assessed individually for completeness (missing data), consistency, and quality. Missing data must also be evaluated for any relationship with the primary outcomes or any of the prognostic/predictive

Table 4 Dependent and Independent Variables of Interest in Neutropenia Risk Modeling

Dependent Variables—Outcomes
A. Primary outcomes (Cycle 1: overall cycles; initial occurrence)
Neutropenic events
- Severe or febrile neutropenia;
- Febrile neutropenia hospitalization;
- Documented infection

Mortality
- Infection-related mortality;
- All deaths

Reduced dose intensity
- Dose reductions;
- Treatment delays;
- Relative dose intensity

B. Secondary outcomes
Quality of life
- Summary health profile measures
- Quality adjusted life years

Economic
- Direct costs;
  - Cost of hospitalization, length of stay, diagnostic tests, medications (antibiotics, growth factors), transfusions
  - Ambulatory costs of treating or preventing febrile neutropenia
- Indirect costs
  - Indirect, out of pocket expenses, lost wages

Independent variables—Prognostic/predictive factors
    Demographic factors: age, gender, race
    Comorbidities,
    Prior treatment
    Body surface area
    Performance status
    Treatment information:
      drugs and regimen
      dosage and schedule,
      supportive care (CSFs, erythropoietin, antibiotics)

variables. If any variable to be used in further analysis has more than 5% missing data, consideration should be given to using one of the available imputation techniques. Multiple techniques exist, which can provide unbiased estimates of missing values as well as reasonably preserve the variance structure. Summary measures should be generated for each variable including estimates of central tendency (mean, median, proportion, etc.) and of variability (standard error, confidence limits, etc.).

Analytic

The relationship between each outcome and each covariate should then be studied using both univariate and multivariate methods. Formal hypothesis testing should be limited to relationships considered *a priori* based on the literature or clinical knowledge and experience.

Modeling

Clinical outcomes are commonly represented and measured as either dichotomous variables, such as mortality, or time to event measures such as survival. Modeling of categorical or composite outcomes, which can be expressed dichotomously, may be studied using multivariate logistic regression analysis. Alternatively, outcomes representing time to an event or duration of events may be studied using the proportional hazards regression method of Cox. Covariates to be considered in the models should be specified *a priori* based on previous models generated on smaller retrospective data sets or with a firmly established biological or clinical rationale. Models should include as covariates those elements mentioned in Table 4 including the specific treatment and possible interactions as well as any other factor of known prognostic significance. Models based on the initial (derivation) population should subsequently be validated ideally on an independent population (validation).

The predictive performance of each model including discrimination, calibration, and power should be evaluated. If useful and appropriate, construction of a prognostic index or score in which the regression coefficients are used as weights may be considered. Formal tests for interaction should be applied rather than hypothesis testing between subgroups, which may have limited power. Additional issues that should be addressed during the modeling process include (1) bias due to missing data, (2) the potential impact of multiple comparisons when evaluating multiple prognostic factors or data cutpoints, and (3) the limitations of stepwise regression models including model instability and the exaggeration of coefficient estimates. Modeling ideally should be based upon fixed models incorporating variables of accepted importance and others with underlying biological or clinical rationale identified a priori, and differences in subgroups should be evaluated by testing for interaction.

While the development and validation of the model constitute critical steps in the risk model process, several additional factors must be considered, including the target user, framework within which the model will be implemented, and the planned use of the model. Likewise, the ease of implementation and compliance as well as the ultimate evaluation of the impact of the model on patient care and clinical outcomes should be considered. Properly developed and validated risk models have the potential for not only providing clinicians with a better understanding of important disease processes, but also facilitating the selection of patients for the targeted application of toxic or costly interventions in a more effective and cost-effective manner.

REFERENCES

1. Altman DG, LYMAN GH. Methodological challenges in the evaluation of prognostic factors in breast cancer. Breast Cancer Res Treatment 1998; 52:289–303.
2. Harrell FE, Califf RM, Pryor DB, et al. Evaluating the yield of medical tests. JAMA 1982; 247:2543–2546.
3. Cox DR. Two further applications of a model for binary regression. Biometrika 1958; 45:562–565.
4. Steyerberg EW, Harrell FE, Borsboom GJJM, et al: J Clin Epi 2001; 54:774–781.
5. Efron B, Tibshirani R. An Introduction to the bootstrap. Monographs on statistics and applied probability. New York. Chapman & Hall, 1993.
6. Steyerberg EW, Eijkemans MJC, Harrell FE, et al. Prognostic modeling with logistic regression analysis: in search of a sensible strategy in small data sets. Med Decision Making 2001; 21:45–56.
7. Crawford J, Dale D, Lyman GH. Chemotherapy-induced neutropenia: risks, consequences, and new directions for its management. Cancer 2004; 100:228–237.
8. Lyman GH. A predictive model for neutropenia associated with cancer chemotherapy. Pharmacotherapy 2000; 20:104S–111S.
9. Lyman GH, Lyman CH, Agboola, O. Risk models for predicting chemotherapy-induced neutropenia. Oncologist 2005; 10:427–437.
10. Crawford J, Dale DC, Kuderer NM, et al. Risk and timing of neutropenic events in adult cancer patients receiving chemotherapy: the results of a prospective nationwide study of oncology practice. J Natl Comp Canc Netw 2008 (in press).
11. Lyman G, Kuderer N, Crawford J, et al. Validation of a risk model for early neutropenic complications in patients receiving cancer chemotherapy. Supp Care Cancer 2006; 14:607.

Index

Abdominal infections in neutropenic patients, 77
Acetaminophen, 138, 261, 304, 307, 309
Acetic acid, 306
Activities of daily living (ADL) scales, 258, 271, 300
Acupuncture for fatigue management, 24
Acute leukemia patients, 92, 93, 97, 98, 99, 124, 131, 284
Acute lymphoid leukemia (ALL) patients, 92, 93
Acute myeloid leukemia (AML) patients, 92, 93, 94, 143
AML/MDS patients, 93, 98, 99
Acyclovir, 200
Addiction in pain management, 313–314
Adjuncts for visceral pain, 311–312
Adjustment disorder
  with anxiety, 324
  with depressive symptoms, 329
Adjuvants
  agents, 260, 261–262
  analgesics for bone pain, 311
  medications, 309–312
Adjuvant Zoledronic Acid to Reduce Recurrence in Patients With High-Risk Localized Breast Cancer (AZURE) trial, 251
Adriamycin, 140, 268

AES-14, 268
AIDS patients, controlled trials in, 107
Alemtuzumab, 93
Alkaloids, 270
Alpha-2 agonist, 311
American Psychosocial Oncology Society (APOS) guidelines, 320
American Society of Clinical Oncology (ASCO) guidelines, 64, 117, 120, 123, 129, 130, 131, 169, 173, 174, 175, 178, 179, 182, 196, 247, 269, 270, 284, 287
AMG 531, 143, 144
Amgen. *See* Denosumab
Amifostine, 200
Amines, 195, 310, 343
Amitriptyline, 261, 310
Amphotericin B, 98, 99, 108
  breakpoint values for, 95
  conventional, 101
  deoxycholate, 103, 104, 105, 106, 107
  lipid formulations of, 105, 107
  liposomal, 100, 101, 102
  meta-analysis involving, 97
  studies comparing azoles, itraconazole, and fluconazole with, 98–99, 104
Analgesic drugs, 260–262. *See also* Adjuvants, agents; Non-opioids; Opioids

Analgesic ladder of World Health Organization, 260, 303–304, 309
Anal sphincter
 paradoxical contraction during defecation, 209
 pressure, 212
 tone, 211
Androgen deprivation therapy (ADT), 289
Anemia in oncology
 ESA treatment, 23
  during chemotherapy, 32–38
  safety of, 39–46
  without chemotherapy, 38
 pathophysiology of, 31–32, 33
 prevalence of, 31–32
Anorectal manometry, 212
Anorexia, supportive care in, 263–264
Anthracycline, 63
 induced cardiomyopathy, 270
Anthracycline/cyclophosphamide-based emetogenic chemotherapy, 175
Antiangiogenic agents, 149, 150
Antiangiogenic therapy, 150
Antiarrythmics, 311
Antibiotics, 62, 64, 68, 69, 119, 123, 127
 broad-spectrum, 77, 101
 exposure, 92
 meta-analysis of prophylactic, 122, 124, 125
 therapy, 82, 83
  broad-spectrum, 78
  outpatient, 78, 81
Antibodies, monoclonal, 93
Anticancer therapies, 151, 152, 156, 157, 161
Anticholinergic agents, 176, 208, 209, 219, 261, 310, 343, 351. See also Antimuscarinic agents
Anticoagulation
 duration, 161
 initial, 157–158
 long-term, 158–161
Anticonvulsants, 261, 299, 310
Antidepressants, 299, 308, 309, 310, 313
Antiemetics
 agents, 169
 antihistamines, 177
 atypical neuroleptics, 177

[Antiemetics]
 benzodiazepines, 177
 cannabinoids, 176–177
 dexamethasone, 174–175
 dose of, 173
 guidelines. See American Society of Clinical Oncology (ASCO) guidelines; Mucositis Study Group of the Multinational Association for Supportive Care in Cancer and the International Society of Oral Oncology (MASCC/ISOO) guidelines; National Comprehensive Cancer Network (NCCN) guidelines
 herbs as, 178
 5-HT$_3$ receptor antagonists (5-HT$_3$-RA), 169, 172–174, 175, 178, 179, 182
 metoclopramide (MCP), 176
 metopimazine, 176
 neurokinin-1 receptor antagonist, 169, 175
 prevention based on emesis risk category, 180–181
 suggested, prophylaxis, 179
 therapy, goal of, 169
Anti-erythropoietin autoantibodies, 39
Antifungals
 broad-spectrum, 96
 classes of, 89, 90–91
 susceptibility trends, 94–95
Antihistamines, 177. See also Histamines
Anti-inflammatory agents, 299, 304
 nonsteroidal, 305, 306
 for oral mucositis, 200
Antimicrobial agents, 75, 76, 78, 83
 for oral mucositis, 200
Antimuscarinic agents, 343
Antineoplastic agents, 263, 266, 270, 271
Antioxidants for oral mucositis, 200
Antipsychotics, low-dose, 324
Anti-TNF antibodies, 93
Anxiety disorders, 324–328
Aprepitant, 169, 175
Arimidex®, 228
Arixtra for Thromboembolism Prevention in a Medical Indications Study (ARTEMIS), 154, 155

Index

Aromasin®, 228
Aromatase inhibitors, 228
  therapy, 152, 289
ASCO. *See* American Society of Clinical Oncology (ASCO) guidelines
Aspergillus species in patients with hematological malignancies, 92
Aspirin, 261, 304, 305, 306
ATAC (Arimidex®, Tamoxifen Alone or in Combination) trial, 228
Atrasentan, 230–231
Atropine, 343
Atypical neuroleptics, 177
Azoles, 92, 97, 98, 105
AZURE trial. *See* Adjuvant Zoledronic Acid to Reduce Recurrence in Patients With High-Risk Localized Breast Cancer (AZURE) trial

Bacteremia, 74, 75, 77
Bacterial infections. *See also* Polymicrobial infections
  associated with defects in host defense mechanisms, 74
  deficiencies associated with, 74
  diagnosis of, 73, 74
  nature and spectrum of, 76
  neutropenic patients. *See* Neutropenic patients, bacterial infections
  prevention of, 82–83
  signs and symptoms of, 73
  spectrum of, 74–76
  with substantial tissue involvement, 76
B2 agonists, 138
Balloon expulsion test, 211
BALP. *See* Bone-specific alkaline phosphatase (BALP)
Barbiturate, 343
Barium enema, 211
Beck depression inventory- short form (BDI-SF), 346
Benzodiazepines, 177, 312, 324, 327, 343, 351
Benzydamine hydrochloride, 200
Betamethasone, 310
Bevacizumab, 152
BFI. *See* Brief Fatigue Inventory (BFI)

Biofeedback therapy for constipation patients, 212–216
Bisacodyl, 266
Bisphosphonates, 245–251, 287, 311
  for bone loss, 228
  comparative trial of intravenous, 247–250
  meta-analyses of efficacy, 250–251
  role in reduction of skeletal morbidity, 247
BMT. *See* Bone marrow transplant (BMT)
Bone
  homeostasis, normal, 224–225.
    See also Bone metastases
  loss. *See* Osteoporosis
  markers, 227, 229, 244
  metabolism, signaling, 251
  microenvironment, 243
  mineral density, 229, 231, 287
  morphogenetic proteins, 231
  pain, adjuvant analgesic for, 311
  remodeling, 224
  resorption, 224
    biochemical markers of, 244, 251
Bone lesions. *See also* Bone metastases
  bisphosphonates trial for malignant, 247
  osteolytic and osteoblastic, 244
  plain radiograph of, 245
Bone marrow microenvironment, 225, 226
Bone marrow transplant (BMT), 14, 283, 284
Bone metastases, 243–244
  bisphosphonates for, 228, 245–251
  and breast cancer, 244–245
  cathepsin K inhibition, 231
  denosumab in, 228–229
  endothelin-1 inhibition, 230–231
  investigational indications and adjuvant therapy for, 251–252
  mechanisms of, 225–228
  osteoblastic, 226–228
  osteolytic, 225–226
  p38 mitogen-activated protein kinase inhibition, 232
  proteosome inhibitors, 231–232
  radiation therapy for, 232–233
  role of PTHrP, 229

[Bone metastases]
  surgical interventions for, 233
  Tgf-β inhibition, 231
  and treatment-related bone loss, 228
  tyrosine kinase inhibition, 230
Bone-specific alkaline phosphatase (BALP), 229
Bortezomib, 231, 270
Botox injections. *See* Botulinum toxin A injections
Botulinum toxin A injections, 299, 312
Bradycardia, 219
Breakthrough pain, 299. *See also* Pain
Breast cancer, 225
  bisphosphonates for, 245–251
  and bone metastases, 244–245
  cells, 243, 244
    and osteolytic bone metastases, 225, 226
  chemotherapy for, 138, 139, 142, 269, 284
  postmenopausal, 152, 228
  and pregnancy, 287–288
  randomized trials of, 126, 131, 283
  tamoxifen therapy in, 152, 287
Brief Edinburg Depression Scale (BEDS), 346
Brief Fatigue Inventory (BFI), 17, 20
Burst-forming unit erythroid (BFU-E), 135
Busulfan, 63
Butorphanol, 309

Cachexia, supportive care in, 264–265
Cajal, 209
Calcitonin, 311
Cancer-related fatigue (CRF). *See* Fatigue
Cancer screening, 281, 283, 291
Candida albicans, 264
Candida species
  non-albicans, 96, 97
  in solid tumor patients, 92
Candidemia treatment, 103, 104
Cannabinoids, 176–177
Capecitabine, 267
Capsaicin, 311

Carbamazepine, 308, 310
Carbapenem, 80
Carboplatin, 270
Carboxymethylcellulose, 266
Carcino-embryonic antigen (CEA), 283
Cardiomyopathy management, 270
Cardiovascular disease, 284
Caregiver distress. *See* Distress, caregiver
CART, 364
Caspofungin, 95, 98, 101, 104, 105
Cathepsin K inhibition, 231
Cbfa1. *See* Core binding factor alpha 1 (Cbfa1)
Center for Epidemiologic Studies-Depression Scale (CES-D), 263
Central venous catheters (CVC), 75
  associated thrombosis, 156–157
Cephalosporins, 80
CFU-E, 135
Chemobrain, 290
Chemoprevention, 281, 291
Chemoreceptor trigger zone (CTZ), 172, 175, 176
Chemotherapeutic agents, 196, 216, 217
  cytotoxic, 267
  emetic risk of oral, 172
  emetogenicity of
    antiemetics. *See* Antiemetics
  emetogenic risk of intravenous, 171
Chemotherapy, 97, 98, 149, 150, 169, 257, 268, 269, 280. *See also* Chemotherapeutic agents
  advances in, 169
  antitumor effects of, 174
  for breast cancer, 43, 126, 127, 138, 139, 142, 152, 156, 200, 269, 271, 284, 370
  bisphosphonates. *See* Bisphosphonates
  cisplatin-based, 174
  combination of tamoxifen and, 152
  conditioned disorder, 324
  doxorubicin-containing, 152
  emetogenic
    anthracycline/cyclophosphamide-based, 175
    high, 170, 174, 175, 176, 178
    low, 174, 182

[Chemotherapy
  emetogenic]
    minimal, 182
    moderate, 174, 175, 177, 178, 182
  fatigue prevalence in, 14
  -induced
    CNS toxicity, 271
    diarrhea, 219, 220, 266
    fibrosis, 267
    neuropathy, 271
    pneumonitis, 267
    thalidomide, 156
    thrombocytopenia, 138, 139
  -induced neutropenia, 60, 63–64, 269, 270
    cascade of, 62
    clinical trials of myeloid growth factors to prevent, 123–125
    dose escalation clinical trials, 121
    febrile. *See* Neutropenia, febrile
    prevention strategies for, 120–123
    reduction of, 129
    treatment strategies for, 119–120
  multiple-day, 182
  myelosuppressive, 60, 61, 117, 136, 137, 138, 140
  toxicity of, 123
  myelotoxic, 115
  for ovarian cancer, 287
Chemotherapy-induced nausea and vomiting (CINV), 169, 268
  antiemetics for. *See* Antiemetics
  categories of, 170, 178
  management of breakthrough and refractory, 182
  patient-related risk factors effect on, 170–171
  prevention of, 179–182
Children's Oncology Group, 285
Chlorpromazine, 312, 343
Chronic obstructive pulmonary disease (COPD), 341
C index. *See* C statistic
Cisplatin, 270
Cisplatin-based chemotherapy, 174
Clinic-based symptom assessment, 8. *See also* Symptom management
Clinician-administered psychosocial interventions, 22

Clodronate, 251
Clomid. *See* Ovarian stimulation
Clomipramine, 310
Clonidine, 310, 311, 312
Clostridium difficile, 266
CLOT trial, 159
C-Mpl receptors, 136
Cochrane system database, 250
Codeine, 304, 307, 308
Cognitive-behavioral model of cancer-related fatigue, 14–15. *See also* Fatigue
Cognitive behavioral psychotherapy, 328, 332
Colchicine, 212
Colon cancer detection, using carcino-embryonic antigen (CEA), 283
Colonic inertia, 209
Colonic transit time testing, 211
Colonoscopy, 211
Colony stimulating factors. *See* Granulocyte colony-stimulating factor (G-CSF); Granulocyte macrophage colony-stimulating factor (GM-CSF)
Colostomy bags, patients with, 217
Combination antifungal therapy, 105, 106
Communication
  at end-of-life, 347–348
  with family, 351–352
Comorbid conditions, 153
Complementary and alternative medical therapies (CAM), 312
Complementary therapies for fatigue management, 23–24. *See also* Fatigue
Comprehensive geriatric assessment (CGA), 258
Computerized adaptive testing (CAT)-administered assessments, 6
Confounding, 360–361, 362, 363
Confusion assessment method, 342
Congestive heart failure, 286, 291
Constipation
  causes of, 208
  classification of, 208–209
  criteria to define, 207–208
  diagnosis of, 209–212

[Constipation]
  management, supportive care in, 260, 261, 265–266
  medications for, 212, 213–215
  treatment of, 212–216
Coping skills training, 22
Core binding factor alpha 1 (Cbfa1), 225
Coronary artery disease after radiation therapy, 285
Corticosteroids, 169, 261, 262, 264, 268, 310–311, 313
  adrenal, 73
COX-2 selective inhibitor, 306
CRF. See Fatigue
Crohn's disease, 219
Cryotherapy, 196
  oral, 267
Cryptococcal infections, 107
Cryptococcosis neoformans, 92, 94
Cryptococcus species, 93
C statistic, 367
Cushing's syndrome, 311
CXC chemokine receptor 4 (CXCR4), 225
CXCR4. See CXC chemokine receptor 4 (CXCR4)
Cyclophosphamide, 63, 66
Cytarabine, high-dose, 271
Cytokines, 117, 118, 119, 135
  inflammatory, 265
  multifunctional, 136
    with thrombopoietic activity, 137–139
  pro-inflammatory, 329

$1,25D_3$. See 1,25-dihydroxyvitaminD_3 ($1,25D_3$)
Daily oral morphine equivalents (DOME), 305
Dalteparin, 153, 156
  trial of, 154, 159
Darbepoetin, 152
  alfa, 33, 34, 38
Dasatinib, 230
Data analysis in neutropenia risk modeling, 372–374
Death rattles at end-of-life, 343–344
Deep vein thrombosis (DVT), 149
  asymptomatic, 154

[Deep vein thrombosis (DVT)]
  CLOT trial in, 159
  complications of recurrent, 161
  rates of, 153
Defecography, 211
Delirium
  agitated/hyperactive, 342
  at end-of-life, 342–343
  rating scale, 342
  symptom interview, 342
Denosumab, 228–229, 251
Depression (mood disorders), 328–332
  at end-of-life, 345–346
  management, supportive care in, 263
Desipramine, 261, 310
Desrazoxane, antidote, 270
Dexamethasone, 152, 174–175, 264, 310
Dextroamphetamine, 262
Dextromethorphan, 311
Diarrhea
  causes of, 217
  and chemotherapeutic agents, 216–217
  chemotherapy-induced, 219, 220
  diagnosis of, 217–218
  histopathology, 216
  management, supportive care in, 266
  role of health care practitioners, 218
  treatment of, 218–220
DIC, 136
Digital rectal examination, 211
1,25-dihydroxyvitaminD_3 ($1,25D_3$), 224
Dilatation. See Vaginal dilatation
Diphenhydramine, 268
Diphenoxylate, 266
Disease-focused and palliative treatments, 340
Disease-oriented model of end-of-life care, 340
Distress. See also Anxiety disorders; Depression (mood disorders)
  caregivers at end-of-life, 346–347
  management, 321
    overview of evaluation and treatment process of, 325
    patient characteristics, 322
  NCCN's panel on management of, 320
  patient's level of, 319, 320, 324
  screening tools for measuring, 323
  thermometer, 320, 323, 324

Index

Docetaxel, 189
Dolasetron, 173
Dose
 of antiemetics, 173
 limiting toxicity of cancer
   chemotherapy, 189
 recommendations
   for aprepitant, 175
   for dexamethasone, 174
   for 5-HT$_3$-RA, 173
   for metoclopramide (MCP), 176
Doxorubicin, 267, 270
Duloxetine, 310
Dyspnea
 at end-of-life, 340–342
 management, supportive care in, 266–267

Echinocandins, 95
Edinburgh depression scale, 346
Edmonton symptom assessment scale (ESAS), 346
Edmonton symptom assessment score, 258
Egg donation. *See* In vitro fertilization (IVF)
Electroejaculation, 288
Eltrombopag, 144
ELVIS trial, 122
Emetogenic chemotherapy. *See* Chemotherapy, emetogenic
Empiric (E) antifungal therapy, 89, 92. *See also* Antibiotics
 outcome of, 101
 overall success of, 100
 versus preemptive antifungal therapy, 103
 trials in neutropenic patients, 100, 101
 Walsh's trials in, 101, 102
EN3285, 200
Endocrine therapy, 287
End-of-life care, 338–340
 last days of life, 350–352
 versus other patient care, 338
 patterns of experience and, 338–340
 philosophy of, 338
 symptoms, 339
   phychosocial, 345–348

[End-of-life care
 symptoms]
   physical, 340–345
   spiritual, 348–350
Endometrial cancer, 288
 tamoxifen in treatment of, 284
Endothelin-1, 226
 inhibition, 230–231
Enolic acid, 306
Enoxaparin, 154, 160
Epirubicin, 270
REPO. *See* Recombinant erythropoietin (rEPO)
Epoetin, 152
 alfa, 33, 34
EPO-R proteins, 41, 44
Erectile dysfunction, 288, 289
Ergosterol, 105
Erythron, 36
Erythropoiesis, 31
 iron-restricted, 36
Erythropoiesis stimulating agents (ESA), 23, 32–35
 challenges in the use of, 36–38
 safety of, 39–46
 time for intervention, 35–36
Erythropoietin, 31, 32, 41
 endogenous response of, 32, 33
 recombinant, 152
ESA. *See* Erythropoiesis stimulating agents (ESA)
Escherichia coli, 82, 117, 118, 266
Esophagitis, 200
Estrogen, 224
 therapy, intravaginal, 289
European Conference of Infections in Leukemia (ECIL), recommendations, 98, 99
European Organization for Research and Treatment of Cancer (EORTC) guidelines, 35–36, 64, 117, 129, 269, 270
Existential pain, 300
Explanatory models for chemotherapy-associated toxicity, 359
 confounding in, 360–361, 362, 363
 interactions in, 361–363
 risk factors in, 363

FACIT. *See* Functional Assessment of Chronic Illness Therapy (FACIT)
FACT-F. *See* Functional Assessment of Cancer Therapy-Fatigue (FACT-F)
FACT-G. *See* Functional Assessment of Cancer Therapy-General scale (FACT-G)
Fatigue, 33, 289–290
 assessment of, 15–20
  multidimensional measures for, 17–18, 20
  single-dimensional measures for, 16–17, 19
 cognitive-behavioral model of, 14–15
 definition, 13–14
 management of, 21–24
  supportive care in, 262
 prevalence of, 14
Fatigue symptom inventory (FSI), 17, 20, 262
FDA. *See* Food and Drug Administration (FDA)
Febrile neutropenia. *See also* Neutropenia
 risk factors of, 365
 risk models of, 369–374
Fecom, 216
Femara®, 228
Fentanyl, 306, 308, 309
Ferritin, 37
Ferroportin, 32
Fibroblast growth factor, 225
Fibroblast growth factor-20, 199
Fibrosis, 143, 267
Field cancerization, 282
Filgrastim, 117, 124
 clearance of, 125
 registration trails for, 123
First-line therapy, 104
 of IA, 105
Fluconazole, 92
 in HSCT patients, 96
 resistance rate of, 95
Flucytosine, 106, 107, 108
Fludarabine, 271
Fluoroquinolones, 122
Fluorouracil, 267, 271
5-fluorouracil (5-FU), 189, 196

Fluoxetine, 263
Fms-related tyrosine kinase 3 (FLT3), inhibitor, 230
Follow-up care, 281, 291, 292
Fondaparinux, 153, 154, 155
Food and Drug Administration (FDA), 152, 159, 188, 200, 230, 310
 approved indications for myeloid growth factors, 116, 123, 139
 draft guidance on PRO, 3
 warning against ESA, 23
Fragmin Advanced Malignancy Outcome Study (FAMOUS) study, 156
5-FU. *See* 5-fluorouracil (5-FU)
Functional Assessment of Cancer Therapy-Fatigue (FACT-F), 16, 19
Functional Assessment of Cancer Therapy-General scale (FACT-G), 19
Functional Assessment of Chronic Illness Therapy (FACIT), 3–4
Functional iron deficiency (FID), 36
Fungi
 antifungal susceptibility testing in filamentous, 94, 95
 dematiaceous, 93
 detected in blood cultures, 94
Fusariosis, 107
Fusarium species, 92

Gabapentin, 261, 289, 310
Gag reflex, 195
Galactomannan immunoassay, 94
Gastrointestinal (GI) mucositis, 201
 MASCC/ISOO clinical practice guidelines for, 198–199
Gastrostomy tube, 189, 195
GATA-1, transcription factor, 135
G-CSF, 138, 142
GEMVEN trial, 122
Generalized anxiety disorder, 324, 328
Genetic testing, 291
Geriatric depression scale (GDS), 263
German Hodgkin's Study Group trials, 121
Ginger as antiemetics, 178
Gleevec®, 230
Glutamine, 199–200

Index

Glycogen, 60
Glycoprotein, 117, 118
Glycopyrrolate, 343, 344, 351
Glycosylation, 117
GM-CSF. *See* Granulocyte macrophage colony-stimulating factor (GM-CSF)
GnRH. *See* Gonadotropin-releasing hormones (GnRH)
Gonadotropin-releasing hormones (GnRH), 228
Graduated compression stockings, 153, 155
Graft *versus* host disease (GVHD), 92, 93, 284
Gram-negative bacilli, 75
Gram-positive organisms in infections, 74, 75
Granisetron, 173
Granulocyte colony-stimulating factor (G-CSF), 59, 153, 269
  biology of, 117–118
  chemotherapy-induced neutropenia
    clinical trials to prevent, 123–125
    in treatment of, 120
  clinical
    activity of GM-CSF *versus*, 129–130
    indications similar to GM-CSF, 116, 117
    uses of, 117, 130–131
  cost effectiveness of, 269–270
  deficiencies of, 60
  FDA-approved indications for, 116
  filgrastim. *See* Filgrastim
  lenograstim. *See* Lenograstim
  meta-analysis of primary prophylaxis with, 127–129
  pegfilgrastim. *See* Pegfilgrastim
  recombinant forms of. *See* Filgrastim; Lenograstim; Pegfilgrastim
Granulocyte macrophage colony-stimulating factor (GM-CSF), 59, 153, 192, 269
  biology of, 118–119
  chemotherapy-induced neutropenia
    clinical trials to prevent, 123–125
    in treatment of, 120

[Granulocyte macrophage colony-stimulating factor (GM-CSF)]
  clinical
    activity of G-CSF *versus*, 129–130
    indications similar to G-CSF, 116, 117
    uses of, 117, 130–131
  cost effectiveness of, 269–270
  FDA-approved indications for, 115, 116
  molgramostim, 116, 118
  sargramostim, 117, 118
Granulocytopenia. *See* Neutropenia

Haloperidol, 342
HbA1c, monitoring of, 291
HCM. *See* Hypercalcemia of malignancy (HCM)
HCT. *See* Hematopoietic cell transplant (HCT)
Head and neck cancer, 189, 190, 200, 282, 286
Health-related quality of life (HRQL), 283
  assessment, 5–9
    item response theory (IRT) scores, 6–7
    minimally important difference scores, 5
    real-time symptom monitoring, 7–9
  conceptual model of, 2–3
  FACIT and NCCN experience, 3–4
  generic and targeted instruments of, 4–5
Hematology patients
  causes of IFI in, 92
  management of fungal infections in, 94
  primary antifungal prophylaxis in, 96
  prolonged neutropenica, 94
Hematopoietic cell transplant (HCT), 189–190
  clinical course of oral mucositis, 192
Hematopoietic stem cells, 59, 60, 61
Hematopoietic stem cell transplants (HSCT) patients, 92
  allogeneic, 93, 94, 96, 97, 98, 99
  studies in, 92
  use of fluconazole in, 96
Hemoglobin levels, optimal, 42–43
Hepcidin, 32, 33
Herbs as antiemetics, 178

Hereditary non-polyposis colorectal cancer (HNPCC) syndrome, 282
Herpes viruses, 200
Hirschsprung's disease, 211
Histamines, 138. *See also* Antihistamines
HLA, 93
Hodgkin's lymphoma, 121–122
Hormone replacement therapy (HRT), 288–289
Hospital anxiety depression scale, 324
Hospital-based parenteral therapy, 80
Hot flashes, 289. *See also* Menopause
HRQL. *See* Health-related quality of life (HRQL)
HRT. *See* Hormone replacement therapy (HRT)
HSCT. *See* Hematopoietic stem cell transplants (HSCT) patients
5-HT$_3$-RA. *See* 5-HT$_3$ receptor antagonists (5-HT$_3$-RA)
5-HT$_3$ receptor antagonists (5-HT$_3$-RA), 169, 172–174, 175, 178, 179, 182, 268
Hydrocodone, 304, 307
Hydromorphone, 307, 308
Hyoscyamine, 343
Hypercalcemia of malignancy (HCM), 241
Hyper-gycosylated rEPO, 33
Hyperplasia, megakaryocytic, 143
Hypothyroidism, 284, 286. *See also* Thyroid hormone
Hypoxia, tumor cell, 42–43

IA. *See* Invasive aspergillosis (IA)
Iatrogenic cancers, 284
IBS. *See* Irritable bowel syndrome (IBS)
Ice chips administration, 196
IFI. *See* Invasive fungal infections (IFI)
Ifosfamide, 140
Imantinib mesylate, 230
Immunizations, 291
Immunocompromised patients, 89
  inflammatory response in, 93, 94
Immunosuppression, 93
Immunosuppressive mechanisms, 174
Infections, bacterial. *See* Bacterial infections

Infectious Diseases Society of America (IDSA) guidelines, 82, 83
Infertility, 287, 288
Inflammatory bowel disease, 210
Inflammatory cytokines, 265
Infliximab, 93
INR levels, 157, 159
Insomnia, 15, 23
Institute of Medicine (IOM), cancer report of, 280
Instrumental activity of daily living (IADL) scales, 258, 271
Interaction in risk models, 361–363
Interleukin-1 (IL-1), 136, 137, 138
Interleukin- 3 (IL-3), 137, 138
Interleukin- 6 (IL-6), 136, 137, 138
Interleukin-11 (IL-11), 136, 137, 139
Interleukin-3 (multi-CSF), 135, 136
Intermittent pneumatic compression devices, 153
Intracytoplasmic sperm injection (ICSI), 288
Invasive aspergillosis (IA), 93, 104–106
  $(1 \to 3)$-β-D-glucan test for, 94
  first-line therapy of, 105
  galactomannan immunoassay for diagnosis of, 94
  incidence of, 92
  salvage therapy, 105
Invasive candidiasis (IC), 103–104
  $(1 \to 3)$-β-D-glucan test for, 94
  comparative trials of antifungal agents in, 104
  incidence of, 92
Invasive fungal infections (IFI). *See also* Invasive apergillosis (IA); Invasive candidiasis (IC)
  diagnosis of, 93–94
  epidemiology of, 92–93
  management of
    empiric approach in. *See* Empiric (E) antifungal therapy
    preemptive in. *See* Preemptive (PE) antifungal therapy
    prophylaxis in. *See* Prophylaxis, antifungal
  risk factors for development of, 93
  treatment of established, 103–108
In vitro fertilization (IVF), 287

Index

IOM. *See* Institute of Medicine (IOM)
Iron-restricted erythropoiesis, 36, 38
Irritable bowel syndrome (IBS), 207
IRT. *See* Item response theory (IRT)
Item banks, 6, 7
Item response theory (IRT), 6–7
ITP, 136, 137, 144
Itraconazole, 95, 97, 98, 99, 103, 104, 106, 108

Kallikrein serine protease, 227
Keratinocyte growth factors, 220, 267
  keratinocyte growth factor-1.
    See Palifermin
  keratinocyte growth factor-2, 199
Ketamine, 311
Ketoconazole, 97
Knock-out models
  of Cbfa1, 225
  of mice, 119
  of RANKL, 224
Kyphoplasty, 233

Lactate dehydrogenase (LDH), 283
Lamotrigine, 310
LASA. *See* Linear analog scale assessment (LASA)
Laser therapy, 201
Laxatives, 212
  osmotic, 266
  simulant, 265, 266
Lenalidomide, 152
Lenograstim, 116, 117
Lesions
  bone. *See* Bone lesions
  in radiation-induced oral mucositis, 192–193
Leukemia, 283, 285. *See also* Acute lymphoid leukemia (ALL); Acute myeloid leukemia (AML)
  acute, 92, 93, 97, 98, 99, 284
Leukopenia, 61
Levofloxacin prophylaxis, studies of, 82
L-glutamine, 199–200
Lidocaine, 268
Lifestyle modification factors, 287, 291

Ligand receptor interaction, G-CSF, 118
Likert scales, 19, 20
Linear analog scale assessment (LASA), 17, 19
Linear regression models, 363, 364
Liposomal amphotericin B, 100, 101, 102
LITE study, 159
Lithium carbonate, oral, 64
Logistic regression models, 363, 364
Loperamide, 219, 266
Lorazepam, 343
  trials with, 177
Low-molecular-weight heparin (LMWH), 153, 157
  advantages over long-term warfarin therapy, 159, 160
  pharmacologic prophylaxis with, 154
  trials of prophylactic, 156
  versus UFH, 155, 157, 158
Lozenges, microbial, 200
Lung cancer, 282
  non–small cell, 122, 123, 124
Lymphedema, 286
Lymph nodes, swelling. *See* Lymphedema
Lymphomas, 189, 190, 283

Maalox, 268
Mammograms, for breast cancer, 282
Mania, 329
Manometry, anorectal, 212
MASCC/ISOO guidelines. *See* Mucositis Study Group of the Multinational Association for Supportive Care in Cancer and the International Society of Oral (MASCC/ISOO) guidelines
Maximum tolerated dose (MTD), 121
McGill pain questionnaire (MPQ), 259
MCID. *See* Minimal clinically important difference (MCID)
Medical-related anxiety, 327
Medications and hydration at end-of-life, 351
Megakaryocyte (MK) erythroid progenitor (MEP), 135, 136
  role of multifunctional cytokines in, 137–139

Megakaryocytic hyperplasia, 143
Megakaryocytopoiesis, 135, 136
  role of multifunctional cytokines in, 137–139
Megestrol acetate, 264
Memorial Delirium Assessment Scale, 342
Menopause. *See also* Postmenopausal women
  and bone loss, 228
  premature, 285, 288
  treatment-induced, 289
Mentha X piperita Lamiaceae. *See* Peppermint as antiemetics
Meperidine, 308–309
Methadone, 308, 309
Methionine, 117
Methotrexate, 267
Methylcellulose, 266
Methylnaltrexone, 212
Methylphenidate, 23, 262
Metoclopramide (MCP), 176
Metopimazine, 176
MFSI. *See* Multidimensional Fatigue Scale (MFSI)
MIC, 95, 106
Micafungin, 95, 98, 99
Mice, knock-out models, 119
Microflora, oral, 191, 192
MID. *See* Minimally important difference (MID)
Midazolam, 177, 343
MILES trial, 122
Minimal clinically important difference (MCID) on HRQL scores, 5
Minimally important difference (MID) scores, 5
Mini-mental state examination (MMSE), 342
Mini-nutritional assessment (MNA), 264
Misoprostol, 212
Mixed agonists-antagonists, 309
Modafinil, 290
Model accuracy. *See* Model predictive performance
Model predictive performance, 365, 366–368

Molgramostim, 116, 118
Monocytes, 59, 60
Monotherapy, 79, 80
Morbidity of mucositis, 190
Morphine, 195, 260, 267, 304, 306, 307, 308, 309, 311, 341, 342
Mucositis
  gastrointestinal (GI), 201
  management, supportive care in, 267–268
  morbidity of, 190
  oral. *See* Oral mucositis
  pain, 310
Mucositis Study Group of the Multinational Association for Supportive Care in Cancer and the International Society of Oral Oncology (MASCC/ISOO) guidelines, 196–201
Multidimensional Fatigue Scale (MFSI), 18, 20
Multinational Association of Supportive Care in Cancer (MASCC)
  guidelines, 78, 79, 169, 173, 174, 175, 178, 179, 182
Multipurpose adjuvant medications, 310–311
Multivariate models, 361, 362, 369
Multivariate regression analysis, 363, 364, 369, 374
Muscarinic receptor blockers. *See* Anticholinergic agents
Myelodysplastic syndromes (MDS), 32, 38–39, 93, 94, 98
Myeloid growth factors. *See* Granulocyte colony-stimulating factor (G-CSF); Granulocyte macrophage colony-stimulating factor (GM-CSF)
Myeloid progenitor, 135
Myelopoiesis, 60
Myelosuppression management, supportive care in, 268–269
Myelosuppressive chemotherapy, 60, 61, 117, 136, 137, 138, 140
  toxicity of, 123
Myelotoxic chemotherapy, 115
Myofascial pain, 299

Index

Nabuphine, 309
National Cancer Institute (NCI) Common Terminology Criteria for Adverse Events (CTCAE) version 3.0 scale, 217
   for oral mucositis, 194
National Comprehensive Cancer Network (NCCN) guidelines, 4, 7, 64, 117, 129, 130, 153, 169, 173, 175, 178, 179, 182, 269, 270, 289
   cancer-related fatigue management guidelines, 13, 21, 23
   panel's guidelines, 320, 324, 329
National Institutes of Health (NIH), 7
Nausea management, supportive care in, 260, 263, 268
NCCN. *See* National Comprehensive Cancer Network (NCCN)
Neurokinin-1-receptor antagonists (NK1-RA), 169, 175
Neuroleptics, atypical, 177
Neuropathic pain, 299, 308, 311
   adjuvant agents for, 309–310
Neuropathy management, supportive care in, 270–271
Neutropenia
   causes of, 60, 63
   chemotherapy-induced. *See* Chemotherapy-induced neutropenia
   consequences of, 63
   defined, 61
   factors affecting severity of, 61
   febrile, 62, 63
      impact of primary prophylaxis with G-CSF on, 127–129
      incidence of, 123
      prevention of, 64–69
      rate of, 126, 127
      risk of, 124, 128
      treatment of, 120
   G-CSF in management of severe, 117, 118
   PIXY321 in reducing, 138
   risk models in, 369–374
   subdivided, 61
Neutropenic complications, 268, 269
Neutropenic enterocolitis, 77
Neutropenic patients, 98
   bacterial infections in, 77–78
   chemotherapy in, 97
   empiric and preemptive antifungal therapy in, 100–103
   initial management of febrile, 78–81, 82
Neutrophils
   blood, 60, 61
   developmental pathway of, 59, 60
   factors affecting levels of, 61
   as first line of host defense, 59
   glycogen supply in, 60
   granules of, 60
   production, 59, 60
   recovery of oral mucositis, 192
   transient abnormalities in function of, 60
NIH. *See* National Institutes of Health (NIH)
NMDA receptor antagonists, 311
Nociceptive pain, 298–299
Non-Hodgkin's lymphoma patients, 123, 129
Non-opioids, 260, 261
Non-small cell lung cancer (NSCLC), 43
Nonsteroidal anti-inflammatory agents (NSAID), 261, 299, 304, 305, 306, 311
Nortriptyline, 261, 310
NSCLC. *See* Non-small cell lung cancer (NSCLC)
N-telopeptide (NTX), 229, 251
NTX. *See* N-telopeptide (NTX)
Nucleus tractus solitarius (NTS), 172
Numeric rating scale (NRS), 301
Nutritional support, to patients with oral mucositis, 195–196
Nutritional therapy, for diarrhea patients, 218
Nutrition and hydration, at end-of-life, 344–345

Obesity, 286
Obsessive compulsive disorder (OCD), 324, 328
Occult blood, 217
Octreotide, 219, 312

Olanzapine, 177, 182
　transmucosal, 343
Oligospermia, 288
OMAS. *See* Oral mucositis assessment scale (OMAS)
Oncologists, role of, 280, 287. *See also* Primary care physicians (PCP)
Ondansetron, 173–174, 176
Oocyte, fertilization of, 288
OPG. *See* Osteoprotegerin (OPG)
Opiates, 195
Opioids, 212, 219, 260–261, 298, 299, 300, 304, 306, 341, 342. *See also* Morphine
Opium tincture, 219, 266, 312
Oral hygiene, maintenance of, 196
Oral microflora, 191, 192
Oral mucositis, 188
　clinical course, 192–193
　economic impacts of, 190
　incidence and severity of, 188–190
　management of, 194–201
　　nutritional support, 195–196
　　pain management, 194–195
　　therapeutic interventions, 196–201
　MASCC/ISOO clinical practice guidelines for, 196–201
　pathobiologic model of, 190–192
　in patients receiving chemotherapy before HCT, 189–190
　in patients receiving chemotherapy for solid tumors, 189
　radiation-induced. *See* Radiation-induced oral mucositis
　severity scales for, 193–194
Oral Mucositis Assessment Scale (OMAS), 193
Osmotic laxatives, 266
Osteoblastic bone metastases, 226–228
Osteoblasts
　and bone homeostasis, 224–225
　and bone metastases, 226–227
Osteoclast-mediated osteolysis, 243, 244
Osteoclasts
　and bone homeostasis, 224
　and bone metastases, 225–226
Osteolytic bone metastases, 225–226
Osteoporosis, 228, 287

Osteoprotegerin (OPG), 224
Outpatient chemotherapy, 7
Ovarian cancer
　chemotherapy-induced, 287
　secondary prevention for, 283
Ovarian stimulation, 287
Oxaliplatin, 267, 270
Oxybutynin, 311
Oxycarbazine, 310
Oxycodone, 260, 304, 307, 341
Oxymorphone, 307

Pain, 319, 320, 324, 329
　assessment, 300–301
　defined, 297–298
　diagram, 301
　dose escalation for control of, 309
　epidemiology of, 297
　etiologies of different patterns of, 298–300
　management, 303–304
　　barriers to, 312–313
　　definitions in, 313–314
　　drugs not recommended for, 308–309
　　invasive strategies for, 312
　　medication for, 304–306, 307–309, 309–312
　　nonpharmacologic strategies for, 312
　　supportive care in, 259–262
　psychosocial assessment of patients with, 301–302
　scales for measurement of, 301, 302
　treating, 302–303
Palifermin, 188, 199, 267
Palliation, defined, 297–298
Palliative and disease-focused treatments, 340
Palliative care settings, fatigue prevalence in, 14
Palliative oxygen, 342
Palonosetron, 174, 268
Pamidronate, 248–250
Pancreatic cancer, 282, 283
Panic or phobic disorder, 324
Parathyroid hormone (PTH), 224
Parathyroid hormone-related protein (PTHrP), 224, 229
　production by breast cancer cells, 226

Parentaral nutrition, 265
Parenteral iron, 36, 37
Parenteral therapy, hospital-based, 80
Paroxetine, 263
Paroxysmal sensations, 299
Parsimonious approach, 259
Pathobiologic model of oral mucositis, 190–192
Patient education for fatigue management, 21
Patient-reported HRQL outcome scores, 5
Patient-reported outcomes measurement information system (PROMIS), 7
Patient-reported outcomes (PRO)
  in chemotherapy-associated anemia treatment, 34
  instruments, 3
  issues in assessment from, 3–4
Patient-reported symptoms, 7–8. *See also* Symptom management
PDGF. *See* Platelet-derived growth factor (PDGF)
PDGF-R. *See* PDGF receptor (PDGF-R)
PDGF receptor (PDGF-R), 230
Pegfilgrastim, 117, 118, 123, 124, 131
  clinical trials of, 125–127
PEG-rHuMGDF. *See* Pegylated recombinant human MK growth and development factor (PEG-rHuMGDF)
Pegylated recombinant human MK growth and development factor (PEG-rHuMGDF), 139–140
Pegylated recombinant human thrombopoietins (rhpegTPO), 139
Pelvic floor dysfunction, 209
Penazocine, 309
Pentobarbital, 343
Peppermint as antiemetics, 178
Perianal infections in neutropenic patients, 77
Peristalsis, 216
PFS. *See* Piper fatigue scale (PFS)
PGE_2. *See* Prostaglandin E_2 (PGE_2)
Phagocytes, components of, 60
Pharmacological treatments for fatigue, 23
Phenytoin, 310
Pheohyphomycosis, 107–108

Physical therapy, 22, 286
Piperacillin-tazobactam, 80, 92
Piper fatigue scale (PFS), 18, 20
PIXY321, 137, 138
Platelet-derived growth factor (PDGF), 225, 230
Platelets. *See also* Thrombocytopenia
  causes of decreased production of, 136
  c-Mpl receptors on, 136
  development. *See* Megakaryocytopoiesis
  nadir, 138, 139, 140, 141
  transfusion, 136, 137, 139, 140, 141
Platinum-containing drugs, 270
P38 mitogen-activated protein (MAP) kinase inhibition, 232
Pneumonitis, 267
  infections in neutropenic patients, 77–78
Polyenes, 97, 103, 105, 106
Polymicrobial infections, 75, 76, 78
POMS. *See* Profile of Mood States (POMS)
Posaconazole, 98, 99, 106, 107, 108
Postmenopausal women, 152, 228, 287. *See also* Menopause
PRCA. *See* Pure red cell aplasia (PRCA)
Predictive models, 359, 369
  versus prognostic models, 364
Prednisone, 264, 268, 310
Preemptive (PE) antifungal therapy, 89, 102, 103
Pregabalin, 310
PREPIC study, 161
Primary care physicians (PCP), 280, 291, 292
PRO. *See* Patient-reported outcomes (PRO)
Procoagulants, 39–40, 150
Profile of mood states (POMS), 16, 19
Prognostic models, 359, 364
Proinflammatory cytokines, 191
PROMIS. *See* Patient-Reported Outcomes Measurement Information System (PROMIS)
Prophylactic antibiotics, meta-analysis of, 122, 124
Prophylactic anticoagulation, 42, 44

Prophylaxis, 190, 200
  in ambulatory cancer patients, 156
  antifungal, 89, 96–99
    amphotericin B. See Amphotericin B
    azoles, 92, 97, 98, 105
    factors considered before
      adopting, 96
    fluconazole, 92
    in HSCT patients, 96
    resistance rate of, 95
    in hematology patients at risk
      of IFI, 96
    itraconazole, 95, 97, 98, 99, 103, 104,
      106, 108
    ketoconazole, 97
    in leukemia patients, 99
    studies evaluating IFI, regimens,
      96–98
    voriconazole, 93, 95
  for central venous catheters (CVC),
    156–157
  in hospitalized medical cancer patients,
    154–155
  meta-analysis of, with G-CSF, 127–129
  studies of levofloxacin, 82
  suggested antiemetic, 179
  in surgery of cancer patients, 153–154
Prophylaxis in Medical Patients with
  Enoxaparin (MEDENOX)
  trial, 154, 155
Proportional hazards regression models,
  363, 364
Propoxyphene, 308
Proprionic acid, 306
Prospective Evaluation of Dalteparin
  Efficacy for Prevention of VTE
  in Immobilized Patients Trial
  (PREVENT), 154, 155
Prostaglandin analogs, 212
Prostaglandin E_2 (PGE_2), 224
Prostate cancer
  cells, 227
  osteoblastic bone metastases, 226–228
Prostate-specific antigen (PSA), 227
Proteosome inhibition, 231–232
PSA. See Prostate-specific antigen (PSA)
Pseudoaddiction in pain management, 314
Psychic pain. See Existential pain

Psychological management
  of anxiety disorders, 324, 327, 328
  of depression, 329, 330
  of distress, 320, 324
Psychopharmacologic management
  of anxiety disorders, 324, 327
  of depression, 329, 330
Psychosocial interventions in fatigue
  management, 22
Psychostimulants, 23, 346
Psychotherapy for anxiety treatment, 327,
  328, 332
Psyllium mucilloid, 266
PTH. See Parathyroid hormone (PTH)
PTHrP. See Parathyroid hormone-related
  protein (PTHrP)
PTSD, 324
Puborectalis spasm syndrome, 211
Pulmonary embolism (PE), 149
  asymptomatic, 154
  CLOT trial in, 159
  complications of recurrent, 151
Pure red cell aplasia (PRCA), 39
Pyrimidine, intravenous fluorinated, 267

QOL. See Quality of life (QOL)
Quality of life (QOL), 242, 247, 252, 298,
  300. See also Health-related
  quality of life (HRQL)
Quinolones, 64, 68, 69, 78, 79, 82

Radiation-induced fibrosis, 267
Radiation-induced oral mucositis, 197
  economic impact of, 190
  lesions in, 192–193
  ulcerations of, 189
Radiation-induced pneumonitis, 267
Radiation therapy, 267, 284, 285
  for bone metastases, 232–233
Radiopharmaceuticals, 311
RANKL. See Receptor activator of
  nuclear factor-kB ligand (RANKL)
Receiver operating characteristic (ROC)
  curve, 367, 368
Receptor activator of nuclear factor-kB
  ligand (RANKL), 224

Recombinant erythropoietin (rEPO), 31, 32–33, 34, 35
Recombinant human thrombopoietins (rhTPO), 139, 140–143
Refractory dyspnea, 340, 341, 342
Regression trees, 364
Relative dose intensity (RDI), 370
Reticulin, 144
Retinoblastoma, 288
Retrograde ejaculation, 288
Rhenium, 311
Rhoten Fatigue Scale (RFS), 19
RhpegTPO. *See* Pegylated recombinant human thrombopoietins (rhpegTPO)
Risk models. *See also* Explanatory models
  accuracy, 367
  considerations in analysis of, 366
  considerations in design of, 365
  interaction in, 362
  missing data in, 369
  model predictive performance, 365, 366–368
  neutropenia, 369–374
  uses of, 359
  validation of, 368–369
Risperidone, 343
ROC. *See* Receiver operating characteristic (ROC) curve
Rotterdam Symptom Checklist (RSCL), 16, 19
RSCL. *See* Rotterdam Symptom Checklist (RSCL)

Saforis™, 200
Salbutamol, nebulized, 311
Salicylates, 306
Salvage therapy in IA, 105
Samarium, 311
Sargramostim, 117, 118
Scedosporiosis, 107
Scedosporium species, 93, 94, 96
Scopolamine, 312, 343, 344
Screening. *See* Cancer screening
SDS. *See* Symptom Distress Scale (SDS)
Selective serotonin reuptake inhibitors (SSRI), 263, 289, 310, 324, 327, 346

Self-administered psychosocial interventions, 22
Serotonin norepinephrine reuptake inhibitors (SNRI), 310
Sertraline, 263
SIGNIFICANT trial, 122
Sildenafil citrate, 289
Skeletal morbidity, 247
Skeletal-related events (SRE), in patients with breast cancer, 242
Sleep disruptions in fatigue, 15
  treatment, 22–23
Society for Healthcare Epidemiology of America (SHEA) guidelines, 83
Sodium, docusate, 265
Solid tumors, 189, 190
  patients, causes of IFI in, 92
Somatic pain, 299
Southwest Oncology Group (SWOG) trial, 230
Spermatozoa, 288
Sperm extraction. *See* Testicular sperm extraction
Spirituality at end-of-life, 348–350
Sprycel®, 230
Squamous cell carcinoma, 193
Src, 230
SRE. *See* Skeletal-related events (SRE)
Standardized mean difference (SMD), 342
Statistical models, 363–364
Stem cell factor (SCF), 135, 136, 137, 138
Stem cell transplant (SCT), 138
Steroids, 261, 264, 268, 284
  dexamethasone, 174–175
Steyergerg procedure for model validation, 369
Subsyndromal depression, 329
Sucralfate, 201
Suicide risk, assessment of, 329
Surgery, 233, 285
  for pancreatic cancer, 282
  for patients with constipation, 216
  prophylaxis in, 153–154
Survivorship care plans, 280–281, 291
SWOG trial. *See* Southwest Oncology Group (SWOG) trial
Symptom assessment tool, 258, 262
Symptom Distress Scale (SDS), 16, 19

Symptom management, 7–9
Symptom monitoring report sample, 9

Tamoxifen, 288
   breast cancer, in treatment of, 284, 287
   endometrial cancer, in treatment of, 284
   therapy, 152
Tandutinib (MLN518), 230
Taxanes, 63, 270, 271
Tegaserod, 212
Terminal cancer, 283
Testicular sperm extraction, 288
Testosterone, 289. *See also* Steroids
TF, 150
TGF-β. *See* Transforming growth factor-β (TGF-β)
Thalidomide, 152, 156, 270
Thrombocytopenia
   chemotherapy-induced, 138, 139
   etiology of, 136, 137
   management of patients with, 137
   thrombopoietin levels in, 136
   treatment of
      AMG 531 in, 143, 144
      eltromdopag in, 144
      multifunctional cytokines in, 137–139
      PEG-rHuMGDF in, 139–140
      rhTPO in, 139, 140–143
Thromboembolism, venous. *See* Venous thromboembolism (VTE)
Thrombopoietins (TPO)
   agonist antibodies, 143
   clinical studies of, 145
   nonpeptide mimetics, 143, 144
   peptide mimetics, 143
   receptor complex, 136
   recombinant human, 139, 140–143
Thromboprophylaxis, 153, 156
Thrombosis, 44
   and cancer, 149
   venous, 39–42
Thyroid hormone, 286
Tincture of opium, 312
   for diarrhea, 219, 266
Tinzaparin, 159
Tissue factor, 39, 153

TNF. *See* Tumor necrosis factor (TNF)
Topical coating agents, 201
Topiramate, 310
Tramadol, 304, 308
Transcutaneous electrical nerve stimulation, 299
Transferrin, 37
Transforming growth factor-β (TGF-β), 225
   expression of, 226
   inhibition, 231
Traztuzumab, 270
Triazoles, 95
Trichosporon species, 93
Tricyclic, 309, 310
   antidepressants, 261, 263
Trimethoprim-sulfamethoxazole (TMP-SMZ), 64, 68, 69
Tropisetron, 174
Tumor
   burden, 14, 15
   cell hypoxia, 42
   cells, 225
   markers, 283
   progression with ESA therapy, 42–46
Tumor necrosis factor (TNF), 224
Type I cytokines, 33
Type II inflammatory cytokines, 33
Tyrosine kinase inhibition, 230

Ulcerations, of radiation therapy–induced oral mucositis, 189
Unfractionated heparin (UFH), 153, 155
   versus LMWH in initial anticoagulation, 157, 158
   use of parenteral, 157
UPA. *See* Urokinase-type plasminogen activator (uPA)
Urokinase-type plasminogen activator (uPA), 227

Vaginal dilatation, 289
Validation of risk models, 368–369
Valproic acid, 310
Vancomycin, 92
VAS. *See* Visual Analog Scale (VAS)

Index

Vasoconstriction, 196
Vena cava filters (VCF), 161
Venlafaxine, 289
Venous thromboembolism (VTE), 39–42
  anticoagulation for treatment of, 157–161
  epidemiology of, 150
  forms of. *See* Deep vein thrombosis (DVT); Pulmonary embolism (PE)
  incidence of, 150
  prevention of, 153–157
  recent trials of prophylaxis of, 154, 155
  recurrent, 157, 158, 159
    cumulative risks of, 160
  regimens for postsurgical prophylaxis for, 153, 154
  regimens for treatment of, 158
  risk factors for, 149, 150–153
  vena cava filters (VCF) for treatment of, 161
Verbal rating score (VRS), 301
Vertebroplasty, 233
Vicodan, 304
Vigor subscale of POMS, 19
Visceral pain, 299
  adjuncts for, 311–312
Visual analog scale (VAS), 17, 19, 259, 301, 341
Vitamin E, 289
Vogel study, 128–129

Voriconazole prophylaxis, 93, 95
VTE. *See* Venous thromboembolism (VTE)

Walsh's trials of empiric antifungal therapy, 101, 102
Warfarin, 156, 157
  in long-term treatment of VTE, 158, 159, 160
WHO. *See* World Health Organization (WHO)
Women's Health Initiative study, 288
World Health Organization (WHO)
  analgesic ladder, 260, 303–304, 309
  model of health, 2
  scale for oral mucositis, 194

Yoga for fatigue management, 24

Ziddani study, 129
Zingiber officinale Roscoe. *See* Ginger as antiemetics
Zoledronic acid, 247
Zometa®, 229
Zygomycetes species, 92
  infection, 96
Zygomycosis, 93, 106–107

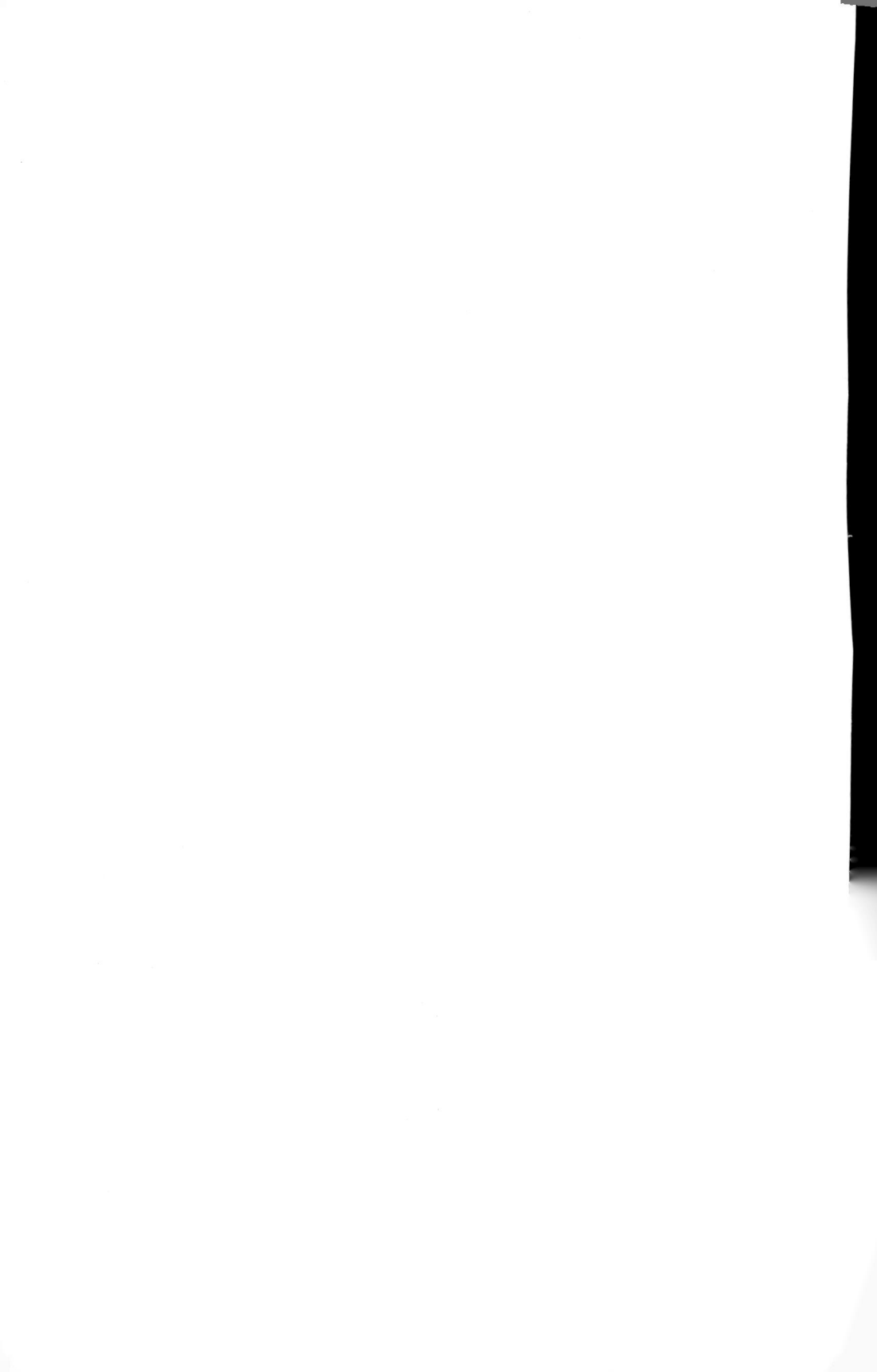